RETINAL AND CHOROIDAL MANIFESTATIONS OF SYSTEMIC DISEASE

RETINAL AND CHOROIDAL MANIFESTATIONS OF SYSTEMIC DISEASE

Edited by

LAWRENCE J. SINGERMAN, M.D.

Associate Clinical Professor
Department of Ophthalmology
Case Western Reserve University
Director, Retinal Institute
Mount Sinai Medical Center
Retina Associates of Cleveland
Cleveland, Ohio

LEE M. JAMPOL, M.D.

Louis Feinberg Professor and Chairman
Department of Ophthalmology
Northwestern University Medical School
Chicago, Illinois

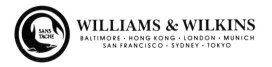

WILLIAMS & WILKINS
BALTIMORE · HONG KONG · LONDON · MUNICH
SAN FRANCISCO · SYDNEY · TOKYO

Editor: Carol-Lynn Brown
Associate Editor: Victoria M. Vaughn
Copy Editor: Clifford Malanowski
Designer: Norman W. Och
Illustration Planner: Ray Lowman
Production Coordinator: Barbara J. Felton

Copyright © 1991
Williams & Wilkins
428 East Preston Street
Baltimore, Maryland 21202, USA

Accurate indications, adverse reactions, and dosage schedules for drugs are provided in this book, but it is possible that they may change. The reader is urged to review the package information data of the manufacturers of the medications mentioned.

Printed in the United States of America

Library of Congress Cataloging-in-Publication Data

Retinal and choroidal manifestations of systemic disease / edited by
Lawrence J. Singerman, Lee M. Jampol.
    p.   cm.
    Includes bibliographical references and index.
    ISBN 0-683-07758-9
    1. Ocular manifestations of general diseases. I. Singerman,
Lawrence J. II. Jampol, Lee M.
RE65.R48   1991   90-19381
616′.047—dc20   CIP

90 91 92 93 94
1 2 3 4 5 6 7 8 9 10

To my wife, Margaret, and to my children,
Stacy and Seth

—L. J. S.

To my children, Melissa and Scott

—L. M. J.

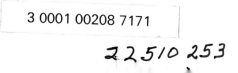

PREFACE

In October 1988 at the annual meeting of the American Academy of Ophthalmology in Las Vegas, Nevada, the Macula Society sponsored a symposium on the retinal and choroidal manifestations of systemic disease. They chose this topic to facilitate communication and cooperation between ophthalmologists and other physicians. The need to educate ophthalmologists about recent advances in other fields of medicine and to demonstrate to other physicians the value of ophthalmologic consultation and the importance of recognizing the ocular findings in their patients made this a timely topic.

The symposium served as a substrate for this book. The discussions were expanded, refined, and updated. This volume is blessed by contributions from a total of 45 authors who are all experts in their fields. The ability to stimulate these joint efforts from prominent specialists reflects the excellence of the membership and cooperative spirit that have characterized the Macula Society and its teaching activities throughout its 14-year existence. Each chapter takes a subsection of systemic disease and reviews the present core of knowledge in this area; the authors then describe the ocular manifestations of these diseases and then the treatment of both the systemic and the retinal and choroidal involvement.

We make no claim that this is a comprehensive text including all important systemic diseases. Topics were chosen because of their timeliness, especially where important new ideas and information existed. No attempt was made tō cover all the topics in an encyclopedic fashion, but pertinent systemic and ocular findings are emphasized. Extensive references are provided to aid the reader who seeks detailed information on specific topics. We specifically excluded such major topics as diabetic retinopathy and neurologic diseases because entire volumes are needed to cover these areas adequately. We feel that the mixture of internal medicine and ophthalmology in this book is almost unprecedented. We believe that those who read this text will gain practical information that will lead to better care of their patients. If this is achieved, the contributors' gratification will more than justify their prodigious efforts.

Lawrence J. Singerman, M.D.
Lee M. Jampol, M.D.

ACKNOWLEDGMENTS

We wish to thank Suzanne Hazan, James Kemp, Ellen Copeland, and Jean Kleist, all from the Retinal Institute, Mt. Sinai Medical Center of Cleveland, for their editorial assistance. Venu Kaza, a senior medical student, carefully reviewed the entire manuscript and made excellent suggestions. Kathryn Jenish and Joan Hornik of Retina Associates of Cleveland provided editorial assistance. Ms. Hornik's communication with the publisher was invaluable during the final stages of manuscript preparation. We also thank Dr. Daniel Finkelstein for co-chairing the symposium at the American Academy of Ophthalmology from which this book originated and the Program Committee for its advice. Dr. Alexander J. Brucker helped originate arrangements with the publisher. Williams & Wilkins has been very cooperative and efficient in helping develop and refine the manuscript. We particularly thank Carol-Lynn Brown, Editor; Victoria Vaughn, Associate Editor; Barbara Felton, Production Coordinator; Norman Och, Designer; and Ray Lowman, Illustration Planner, for their efforts.

CONTRIBUTORS

Gary W. Abrams, M.D., Professor and Chief, Vitreal Retinal Section, Department of Ophthalmology, Medical College of Wisconsin, Milwaukee, Wisconsin

Lloyd M. Aiello, M.D., Associate Clinical Professor of Ophthalmology, Harvard Medical School, Director of Beetham Eye Institute, Joslin Diabetes Center, Boston, Massachusetts

Gary C. Brown, M.D., Assistant Professor of Ophthalmology, Thomas Jefferson University School of Medicine, Assistant Surgeon, Retinal Service, Wills Eye Hospital, Philadelphia, Pennsylvania

Herbert L. Cantrill, M.D., Associate Clinical Professor, Department of Ophthalmology, University of Minnesota School of Medicine, Minneapolis, Minnesota

Ronald E. Carr, M.D., Professor of Ophthalmology, Department of Ophthalmology, New York University Medical Center, New York, New York

Devron H. Char, M.D., Professor, Department of Ophthalmology and Radiation Oncology, Director of Ocular Oncology Unit, Francis I. Proctor Foundation, University of California at San Francisco, San Francisco, California

Brian P. Conway, M.D., Verna Moiten Scott Professor and Chairman of the Department of Ophthalmology, University of Virginia School of Medicine, Charlottesville, Virginia

Gabriel Coscas, M.D., Clinique Ophtalmologique, Universitaire de Creteil, Université Paris-XII, Hôpital de Creteil, Paris, France

Jean-Jacques De Laey, M.D., Ph.D., Professor of Ophthalmology, Director, University Hospital Eye Clinic, University of Ghent, Ghent, Belgium

Wallace Stewart Foulds, C.B.E., Professor, Tennent Institute of Ophthalmology, University of Glasgow, Western Infirmary, Glasgow, Scotland

J. Donald M. Gass, M.D., Professor of Ophthalmology, Department of Ophthalmology, Bascom Palmer Eye Institute, University of Miami School of Medicine, Miami, Florida

Kurt A. Gitter, M.D., Chief of the Department of Ophthalmology, Touro Infirmary, Director of the Foundation for Retinal Research, New Orleans, Louisiana

Daniel H. Gold, M.D., Associate Clinical Professor, Department of Ophthalmology, University of Texas Medical Branch, Galveston, Texas

Evangelos S. Gragoudas, M.D., Associate Professor of Ophthalmology, Harvard Medical School, Director of Retina Services, Massachusetts Eye and Ear Infirmary, Boston, Massachusetts

W. Richard Green, M.D., Professor of Ophthalmology, Associate Professor of Pathology, The Johns Hopkins University School of Medicine, Baltimore, Maryland

Froncie A. Gutman, M.D., Chairman, Department of Ophthalmology, The Cleveland Clinic Foundation, Associate Professor of Ophthalmology, Case Western Reserve University, Cleveland, Ohio

Keith Henry, M.D., Director, HIV Clinics and Program, Section of Infectious Diseases, St. Paul Ramsey Medical Center, St. Paul, Minnesota, Assistant Professor of Medicine and Public Health, University of Minnesota School of Medicine, AIDS Clinical Trials Group, Minneapolis, Minnesota

Douglas A. Jabs, M.D., Associate Professor of Ophthalmology, The Wilmer Ophthalmologic Institute, The Johns Hopkins University School of Medicine, Baltimore, Maryland

Lee M. Jampol, M.D., Louis Feinberg Professor and Chairman, Department of Ophthalmology, Northwestern University Medical School, Chicago, Illinois

Robert N. Johnson, M.D., Assistant Clinical Professor of Ophthalmology, University of California at San Francisco, San Francisco, California

Mary Lou Lewis, M.D., Professor, Department of Ophthalmology, Bascom Palmer Eye Institute, University of Miami School of Medicine, Miami, Florida

H. Richard McDonald, M.D., Assistant Clinical Professor of Ophthalmology, University of California at San Francisco, San Francisco, California

Travis A. Meredith, M.D., Professor, Section of Ophthalmology, Emory University School of Medicine, Chief of Vitreoretinal Section, Emory Eye Center, Atlanta, Georgia

Robert P. Murphy, M.D., Associate Professor of Ophthalmology, The Wilmer Ophthalmologic Institute, The Johns Hopkins University School of Medicine, Baltimore, Maryland

Richard R. Ober, M.D., Associate Professor, Doheny Eye Institute, Department of Ophthalmology, School of Medicine, University of Southern California, Los Angeles, California

R. Joseph Olk, M.D., Retina Consultants, Ltd., Barnes Hospital, Associate Professor of Ophthalmology, Washington University School of Medicine, St. Louis, Missouri

David H. Orth, M.D., Associate Professor, Department of Ophthalmology, Rush-Presbyterian-St. Luke's Medical Center, Chicago, Illinois, Director, Irwin Retina Center, Ingalls Memorial Hospital, Harvey, Illinois

Stephen J. Ryan, M.D., Professor and Chairman, Department of Ophthalmology, Doheny Eye Institute, University of Southern California, Los Angeles, California

Alfredo Sadun, M.D., Ph.D., Associate Professor, Departments of Ophthalmology and Neurological Surgery, Doheny Eye Institute, University of Southern California, Los Angeles, California

Andrew P. Schachat, M.D., Associate Professor of Ophthalmology, Director of Ocular Oncology Services, The Wilmer Ophthalmologic Institute, The Johns Hopkins University School of Medicine, Baltimore, Maryland

Howard Schatz, M.D., Clinical Professor of Ophthalmology, Department of Ophthalmology, University of California, Director of Retina Research Fund, St. Mary Hospital and Medical Center, San Francisco, California

Eric P. Shakin, M.D., Instructor, Retina Services, Wills Eye Hospital, Philadelphia, Pennyslvania

Jerry A. Shields, M.D., Director of Oncology Services, Wills Eye Hospital, Philadelphia, Pennsylvania

Lawrence J. Singerman, M.D., Associate Clinical Professor, Department of Ophthalmology, Case Western Reserve University, Director, Retinal Institute, Mt Sinai Medical Center, Cleveland, Ohio

Russel S. Sobel, M.S., Clinical Research Associate, Medical Research Division, American Cyanamid Company, Pearl River, New York

Gisele Soubrane, M.D., Clinique Ophtalmologique de Creteil, Université Paris Val-de-Marne, Paris, France

Bradley R. Straatsma, M.D., Professor and Chairman, Department of Ophthalmology, UCLA School of Medicine, Director, Jules Stein Eye Institute, Los Angeles, California

Janet S. Sunness, M.D., Associate Professor, The Wilmer Ophthalmologic Institute, The Johns Hopkins University School of Medicine, Baltimore, Maryland

James S. Tiedeman, M.D., Ph.D., Assistant Professor, Department of Ophthalmology, Duke University Eye Center, Durham, North Carolina

Mark O. M. Tso, M.D., Professor of Ophthalmology, Director of the Georgiana Theobald Ophthalmic Pathology Laboratory, Director of the Macula Clinic, Medical Director of the Lions of Illinois Eye Bank, Lions of Illinois Eye Research Institute, University of Illinois College of Medicine, Chicago, Illinois

Robert C. Watzke, M.D., Professor of Ophthalmology, Department of Ophthalmology, Retina and Vitreous Division, Director of Retina and Vitreous Services, University of Oregon Health Sciences Center, Portland, Oregon

Thomas A. Weingeist, M.D., Ph.D., Professor and Head of the Department of Ophthalmology, University of Iowa College of Medicine, University of Iowa Hospitals and Clinics, Iowa City, Iowa

George A. Williams, M.D., Associate Clinical Professor, Kresge Eye Institute, Wayne State University, Detroit, Michigan, William Beaumont Hospital, Royal Oak, Michigan

Lawrence A. Yannuzzi, M.D., Surgeon Director of Ophthalmology, Director of Retinal Research, Manhattan Eye, Ear, and Throat Hospital, Associate Professor of Clinical Ophthalmology, Columbia University School of Medicine, New York, New York

CONTENTS

XV

INTRODUCTION

We are confident that *Retinal and Choroidal Manifestations of Systemic Disease*, by providing timely authoritative information important to physicians, will facilitate interactions between ophthalmology and other medical specialties. The ophthalmologist may provide valuable assistance to the internist or surgeon by diagnosing and monitoring the response to treatment of numerous systemic diseases. Unfortunately, at present, ophthalmologic skills are currently underutilized in the management of systemic diseases. The patient's interest will be most enhanced by increased involvement of ophthalmology with systemic medicine. Additionally, the ophthalmologist increases his or her skills greatly by increasing his or her knowledge of systemic medicine, as this knowledge is fundamental to the practice of ophthalmology. Also, an ophthalmologist with these skills is better able to function as a consultant to other physicians and is a better teacher or researcher. In a larger sense, the ophthalmologist who is more attuned to systemic medicine increases the cooperation and camaraderie between ophthalmology and the rest of the medical profession. This has never been more important than it is now.

The acquired diseases of connective tissue (CT) offer useful models of the interrelationship between ophthalmology and systemic medicine. These conditions often present with vague, nonspecific complaints, making diagnosis difficult. Ophthalmic manifestations are often early signs of CT diseases. For example,

in Wegener's granulomatosis, the ophthalmologist may be a front-line diagnostician, as potential early manifestations include orbital vasculitis and granuloma, leading to limited extraocular muscle movement, proptosis, and vision loss (secondary to optic nerve involvement). If a patient with Wegener's granulomatosis first presents ophthalmologically, it is critical for the ophthalmologist to suspect the diagnosis and refer the case for expeditious systemic workup and therapy, as untreated Wegener's granulomatosis can produce renal or pulmonary failure and possibly death. Giant cell arteritis (GCA) is another CT disease in which the ophthalmologist may be the initial physician involved, as the presenting complaint is often sudden visual loss or diplopia. A high suspician of GCA demands immediate institution of corticosteroids, even before the performance of the temporal artery biopsy, to prevent further visual loss. When GCA is diagnosed by the ophthalmologist, it is usually useful to consult a primary care physician regarding the management of the long-term corticosteroid therapy.

Hematologic diseases may also feature prominent retinal and choroidal manifestations. Subretinal, intraretinal, preretinal, and vitreous hemorrhage may be seen. Specific hematologic conditions cause specific ocular findings. For example, leukemia may produce "leukemic retinopathy" with retinal hemorrhages and cotton-wool spots. Venous occlusive disease, microaneurysm formation, and retinal neovascularization may be seen as a result of increased blood viscosity from very high cell counts. Furthermore, aside from the leukemia itself, therapy may produce ocular findings. As chemotherapeutic agents are often toxic to the bone marrow, producing anemia and thrombocytopenia, retinal sequelae may include hemorrhages and cotton-wool spots. Opportunistic infections may be seen. Also, systemic or local steroids may be cataractogenic, and radiation therapy may yield radiation retinopathy or radiation optic neuropathy. Hence, in managing leukemia, ophthalmologists and hematologists often need to cooperate, as leukemic ocular involvement is best controlled by treating the underlying leukemia with systemic chemotherapy and supportive measures, such as blood transfusions. Leukemic infiltrates in the retina, choroid, vitreous, or optic nerve may also necessitate ocular radiation.

Hypertension is an excellent example of an important disease in which ophthalmologists may provide a unique perspective via assessment of the vascular changes seen in the fundus. A blood pressure cuff is far more sensitive than a fundus examination in quantitating acute levels of elevated blood pressure. However, fundus findings are significant in quantitating the end-organ damage produced by systemic hypertension. Fundus evaluation may indicate the overall success of therapy in the hypertensive patient. Furthermore, retinal vascular changes may correlate with vascular changes elsewhere; for example, in the central nervous, cardiovascular, or renal systems. The authors of the chapter on hypertensive retinopathy propose a new, pathophysiologic approach to hypertensive ocular disease. As different systems of blood vessels comprise the retinal, choroidal, and optic nerve vasculature, these various vascular systems respond differently to the effects of hypertension. Based on this logic, the authors categorize hypertensive retinopathy as (a) hypertensive choroidopathy, (b) hypertensive retinopathy, and (c) hypertensive optic neuropathy. Four clinical phases of hypertensive retinopathy are discussed in

detail: (a) vasoconstrictive, (b) sclerotic, (c) exudative, and (d) complications of sclerotic phase.

The ophthalmologist may be the first physician to identify a patient with stenosis of the carotid artery from atherosclerosis, as it may first manifest as the ocular ischemic syndrome (OIS). Ninety percent of OIS patients present with good visual acuity, yet central retinal artery obstruction may follow shortly. A combination of noninvasive techniques may allow detection of high-grade carotid stenosis in 90% of cases. Particularly indicated may be referral to a vascular surgeon, who may consider carotid endarterectomy. Efficient cooperation between the ophthalmologist and vascular surgeon may even allow reversal of OIS, preventing further visual loss in the ipsilateral eye. Also, the OIS workup may identify contralateral carotid disease at a stage more amenable to effective medical or surgical intervention.

About 75% of AIDS patients will have ocular findings, most commonly AIDS retinopathy and CMV retinitis, and, appropriately, this book's AIDS chapter succinctly presents the essentials, both systemic and ophthalmic, of AIDS. Patients with AIDS may first present with ocular involvement, making the ophthalmologist a front-line AIDS physician. Early identification of CMV retinitis, which may involve one-third of AIDS cases, followed by institution of ganciclovir therapy, may preserve vision. Other opportunistic infections are also common.

The ophthalmologist plays an important role in the diagnosis of other viral diseases. Subacute sclerosing panencephalitis (SSPE) is a good example, since decreased vision from its measles maculopathy may be the presenting complaint. The viral etiologies of several chorioretinal diseases (MEWDS, APMPPE, multifocal choroiditis) are currently under investigation by the Macula Society Research Committee.

Systemic or ophthalmic drugs may damage the retina, RPE, or choroid. The ophthalmologist must be familiar with the potential ocular toxicities of these various agents. Perhaps the best known drug-induced toxic retinopathy is the bull's-eye maculopathy caused by chloroquine or hydroxychloroquine. The ophthalmologist monitoring ocular changes in conjunction with the primary care physician can help avoid visual loss from these drugs. Cancer chemotherapy may produce ocular toxicity, as when intracarotid administration is employed. Tamoxifen-treated patients may present with moderately decreased visual acuity after months of exposure. The cornea may show subepithelial whorl-like changes, and the macula may have multiple white deposits. Further, at the RPE level, yellow-white lesions may be seen, and cystoid macular edema is also possible.

Another of this book's innovative chapters is that describing optic nerve toxicity. This chapter classifies drugs and other chemicals associated with optic nerve atrophy in terms of histopathologic evidence of damage and their mechanisms of neurotoxic damage. The hierarchy proposed may allow more rational approaches to occupational and environmental medicine.

As cancer therapy improves survival, metastases, including ocular involvement, are being seen more frequently. Approximately one-third of all patients with intraocular metastases have no prior history of cancer when presenting to the ophthalmologist. Hence, the ophthalmologist may have a leading role in instigating the workup for malignancy. A suspected intraocular metastasis mandates a systemic workup, best done in conjunction with the patient's own physician. This may include a breast examination and mammogram for females, and a chest x-ray, abdominal CT, liver scan, and possibly several other studies.

Most women do not experience visual changes during pregnancy. However, preexisting retinal diseases may be affected by pregnancy, and systemic complications of pregnancy may involve the retina. Further, even a normal pregnancy may affect the retina and choroid. Pregnancy is a clinical context in which ophthalmologists may interact with obstetrics and gynecology specialists to help manage the ocular complications of pregnancy. For example, all pregnant diabetic women should have a baseline ophthalmic examination, preferably before conception or in the first trimester, with the frequency of follow-up examinations depending on the severity of the diabetic retinopathy.

The messages from this book are clear. Internists, surgeons, and other physicians should be knowledgeable about the ocular findings of their patients. Ophthalmologists, to be effective, must review current literature on the systemic diseases seen in their patients. We believe this book will facilitate these efforts.

CHAPTER 1

Ocular Complications of Acquired Diseases of Connective Tissue

Lee M. Jampol, Douglas A. Jabs, Daniel H. Gold, Stephen J. Ryan, Bradley R. Straatsma, and Alfredo Sadun

Introduction

The acquired diseases of connective tissue are a group of diseases of unknown etiology characterized by autoimmunity, vasculitis, and the presence of arthritis. They have also been called the collagen vascular diseases, connective tissue diseases, systemic rheumatic disorders, and autoimmune rheumatic disorders. The following diseases will be discussed: Wegener's granulomatosis, systemic lupus erythematosus, polymyositis-dermatomyositis, scleroderma, rheumatoid arthritis, polyarteritis, and temporal arteritis.

The ocular findings of the acquired diseases of connective tissue are not specific, although certain findings are more suggestive of one or more of the diseases than of the others. Table 1.1 provides a summary of the ocular manifestations (particularly those of the retina and choroid). A review of each disease follows, describing its pathophysiology, clinical findings, ocular findings, and treatment.

Wegener's Granulomatosis

INTRODUCTION

Wegener's granulomatosis is a distinct clinicopathological entity characterized by necrotizing granulomatous vasculitis of the upper and lower respiratory tracts, focal necrotizing glomerulonephritis, and disseminated vasculitis involving small arteries and veins of numerous organ systems (1–3).

Formulated as an entity by Wegener in 1936 (4), it is an uncommon but not rare disease. The mean age at onset is about 40 years, but it can occur in childhood or at any time thereafter. The male-to-female ratio is about 3:2, and whites are affected more frequently than blacks.

PATHOPHYSIOLOGY

The typical histopathological lesion in Wegener's granulomatosis is necrotizing vasculitis of small arteries and veins associated with granuloma formation, which may be intravascular or which may occur in the surrounding cellular infiltrates (Fig. 1.1). Respiratory tract lesions involve the nose, paranasal sinuses, nasopharynx, trachea, lung, and adjacent structures, such

1

as the orbit, eye, and ear. Renal involvement is characterized by focal glomerulitis that may evolve into rapidly progressive glomerulonephritis. The eyes, skin, and virtually any organ may be involved with vasculitis, granulomata, or both.

The etiology is unknown, but considerable evidence suggests that Wegener's granulomatosis is an immunogenic abnormality, in which both antibody and cell-mediated damage occurs. Circulating and deposited immune complexes are present in some patients; T cells may be prominent in granulomatous lesions.

CLINICAL FINDINGS

Wegener's granulomatosis usually presents with upper respiratory tract symptoms and findings such as paranasal and nasal pain, discharge, and ulceration. Nasal septum perforation may lead to saddle nose deformity. Pulmonary involvement may include asymptomatic infiltrates or may be manifest as infiltrates associated with cough, hemoptysis, pain, and dyspnea. About 95% of patients have respiratory tract disease.

Renal disease (present in 85% of patients) may smolder as a glomerulitis with proteinuria, hematuria, and red cell casts, but, unless treated, more often rapidly progresses to irreversible renal failure. Directly or indirectly, renal disease accounts for most of the mortality associated with untreated Wegener's granulomatosis.

Eye, adnexal, and orbital involvement (present in about 50% of patients) (1, 2, 5–12); skin lesions (in 45% of patients), which appear as papules, vesicles, ulcers, and nodules; nervous system disease (in 22% of patients) with cranial neuritis and focal central nervous system

Table 1.1. Ocular Manifestations of Acquired Diseases of Connective Tissue

	Wegener's granulomatosis	Systemic lupus	Polymyositis-dermatomyositis	Scleroderma	Rheumatoid arthritis	Polyarteritis	Temporal arteritis
Eyelid involvement	+ [a]	+	+	+ +		+	
Episcleritis, scleritis	+ +	+			+ +	+	
Marginal keratitis	+ +	+			+ +	+	
K. sicca	+	+		+	+ +		
Uveitis	+	?				+	+
Cranial nerve palsy ophthalmoplegia	+	+	+	+			+
CNS involvement	+	+ +				+	+
Orbital involvement	+ +	+				+	
Retinal vasculopathy or vasculitis	+	+ +	+			+	
Retinal artery occlusion		+				+	+
Cotton-wool spots, hemorrhages	+	+ +	+	+		+	+
Retinal neovascularization		+					
Retinal vein occlusion		+		+		+	
Choroidopathy (serous detachment)		+		+		+	
Optic neuropathy	+	+				+	+ +

[a]Legend: ?—possible association; +—association; + +—common association.

abnormalities; and cardiac disease (in 12% of patients) are among the manifestations of disseminated necrotizing vasculitis and granulomatosis.

While the disease is active, patients generally have symptoms and signs such as malaise, weakness, symmetric polyarticular arthralgias, fever, anorexia, and weight loss. Common laboratory findings include a sharply elevated erythrocyte sedimentation rate, mild anemia and leukocytosis, a positive test for rheumatoid factor, and mild elevation of gamma globulin, particularly of the IgA class.

The diagnosis of Wegener's granulomatosis is clinicopathological, based on clinical findings of upper and lower respiratory tract disease as well as evidence of glomerulonephritis in a patient with biopsy-proven necrotizing granulomatous vasculitis. Pulmonary tissue

offers the highest diagnostic yield, but biopsy of upper respiratory tract tissue, renal tissue, and tissue from focal lesions of the orbit and other structures may be helpful.

In its typical presentation with all of the classical features, the diagnosis of Wegener's granulomatosis is readily established. In its early stages, limited forms (11), and atypical presentations, the disease may be extremely difficult to recognize and differentiate from other vasculitides (Table 1.2) and granulomatoses. Differential conditions include allergic angiitis and granulomatosis, Goodpasture's syndrome, and infectious as well as noninfectious granulomatous diseases. For the ophthalmologist, it may be necessary to distinguish Wegener's granulomatosis from midline granuloma, which may erode through skin, soft tissue, and the bones of

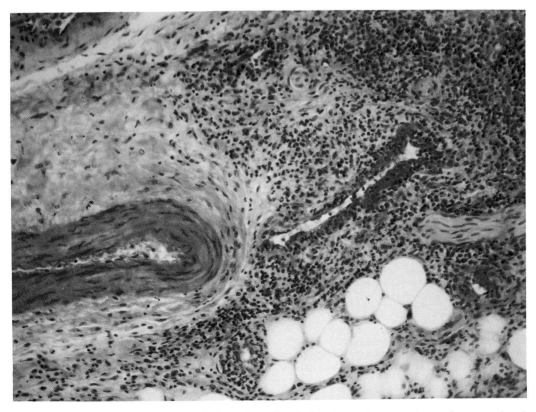

Figure 1.1. Wegener's granulomatosis. Polymorphonuclear leukocytes and mononuclear cells surround and invade small blood vessels.

the face. It should also be realized that Wegener's granulomatosis may involve an atypical lymphocytoid-plasmacytoid infiltrate of the lung, skin, central nervous system, and kidney.

Untreated Wegener's granulomatosis is usually rapidly progressive and fatal. Therefore, early diagnosis and therapy are essential to preservation of vital functions and life.

OCULAR MANIFESTATIONS

Ophthalmic findings resulting from Wegener's granulomatosis may contribute to prompt diagnosis and are present in about 50% of patients, with a range in

frequency from 28% (7) to 58% (1) in published reports. Virtually any vascularized part of the eye, adnexae, orbit, and visual pathways of the central nervous system may be involved (1, 5–10, 12–18, Table 1.3).

Orbital disease is the most common ophthalmic manifestation of Wegener's granulomatosis. It is usually secondary to nasal or paranasal sinus disease. Orbital vasculitis and granuloma may commence with a presentation resembling idiopathic pseudotumor or cellulitis with pain, tenderness, erythema, limited extraocular movement, and proptosis. Necrosis accompanied by tissue loss and skin ulceration, as well as optic nerve compression causing loss of vision, are other indications of orbital disease. Prompt medical management or surgical decompression sometimes restores vision even after the optic nerve compression has caused no light perception for 1 to 2 days.

Eye manifestations may be unilateral or bilateral and may include a distinctive corneal marginal infiltration often associated with ulceration (Fig. 1.2), episcle-

Table 1.2.   Clinical Classification of Vasculitis Syndromes[a]

Polyarteritis nodosa group
    Classic polyarteritis nodosa
    Allergic angiitis and granulomatosis of Churg-
        Strauss
    Polyarteritis overlap syndrome

Hypersensitivity vasculitis
    Exogenous stimuli
        Henoch-Schönlein purpura
        Serum sickness and similar reactions
        Other drug-induced vasculitides
    Endogenous stimuli
        Vasculitis associated with neoplasms
        Vasculitis associated with connective tissue
            disease
        Vasculitis associated with other diseases
        Vasculitis associated with congenital
            deficiencies in complement system

Wegener's granulomatosis

Giant cell arteritis
    Temporal or cranial arteritis
    Takayasu's arteritis

Other vasculitic syndromes
    Lymphomatoid granulomatosis
    Mucocutaneous lymph node syndrome
        (Kawasaki's disease)
    Behcet's disease
    Isolated central nervous system vasculitis
    Thromboangiitis obliterans (Buerger's disease)
    Miscellaneous vasculitides

[a]Adapted from Braunwald E, Isselbacher KJ, Petersdorf RG, et al., eds. Harrison's principles of internal medicine, 11th Ed. New York: McGraw-Hill, 1987; and Wyngaarden JB, Smith LH Jr, eds. Cecil textbook of medicine, 18th ed. Philadelphia: WB Saunders, 1988.

Table 1.3.   Ophthalmic Manifestations of Wegener's Granulomatosis

Orbit
    Orbital vasculitis-granulomatosis with
        pseudotumor-like or cellulitis presentation
    Orbital vasculitis-granulomatosis with ulceration
    Orbital vasculitis-granulomatosis with optic nerve
        compression

Eye
    Keratitis, marginal infiltrates with ulceration
    Scleritis and episcleritis
    Conjunctivitis
    Uveitis
    Retinal vasculitis
    Optic nerve vasculitis and compression

Ocular adnexae
    Lacrimal gland disease
    Dacryocystitis
    Nasolacrimal duct obstruction
    Eyelid erythema and granulomata

Central nervous system
    Cranial nerve palsies
    Cortical blindness

ritis, conjunctivitis, and scleritis, which may be nodular or necrotizing. Uveitis may involve the ciliary body and/or the choroid and may be associated with intravitreal "snowballs," cystoid macular edema, or chorioretinal scars. Retinal vasculitis is associated with arterial and venous abnormalities, hemorrhages, edema, and cotton-wool spots.

Optic nerve vasculitis may present as disc edema, hemorrhages, or ischemia. Optic nerve ischemia may also be compressive and secondary to orbital vasculitis and granulomata. Vision may be lost in one or both eyes as a consequence of optic nerve disease and compression (5, 7).

Adnexal disease is apt to involve the lacrimal system, potentially yielding lacrimal gland inflammation and keratoconjunctivitis sicca, dacryocystitis, and naso-lacrimal duct obstruction. Surgical dacryocystorhinostomy may be associated with wound necrosis (15). Eyelid edema and discrete eyelid granulomata are also reported.

Central nervous system disease affecting the visual system is uncommon but may consist of cranial nerve palsies or cortical blindness (16).

TREATMENT

Cyclophosphamide and corticosteroid therapy have dramatically improved the prognosis for arrest of the disease and maintenance of life. Cyclophosphamide in dosages of 2 mg/kg/day orally is the treatment of choice. Leukopenia may occur. Other potential complications of cyclophosphamide therapy include hemor-

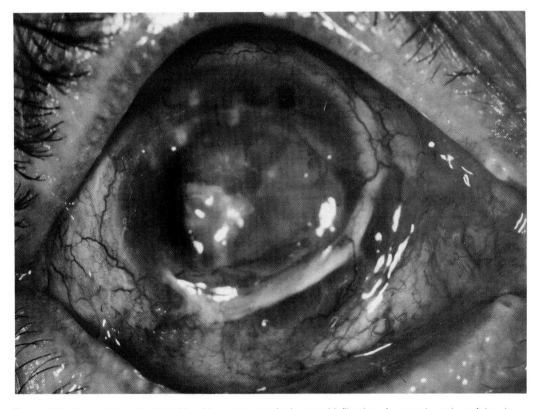

Figure 1.2. Necrotizing sclerokeratitis with severe marginal corneal infiltration. A corneal patch graft has been sewn in place but is now melting.

rhagic cystitis, cytomegalovirus retinitis, and azoospermia or ovarian dysfunction. 1 year following complete remission of the disease, gradually tapered, and discontinued thereafter (1).

Corticosteroids should be administered at the initiation of cytotoxic treatment. They can be given as prednisone, 1 mg/kg/day initially, gradually converted to alternate-day schedule, and discontinued after approximately 6 months of use (1). Corticosteroids given systemically are apt to be particularly effective in limiting ocular tissue damage and in promptly reducing optic nerve compression associated with orbital inflammation.

With this treatment regimen, long-term remission and control of ophthalmic manifestations are achieved in 90% of patients. Even patients who have developed irreversible renal failure may undergo successful renal transplantation, and, when indicated, appropriate ophthalmic plastic and reconstructive surgery may be performed.

References

1. Fauci AS, Haynes BF, Katz P, Wolff SM. Wegener's granulomatosis: prospective clinical and therapeutic experience with 85 patients for 21 years. Ann Intern Med 1983;98:76–85.
2. Braunwald E, Isselbacher KJ, Petersdorf RG, et al., eds. Harrison's principles of internal medicine, 11th ed. New York: McGraw-Hill, 1987.
3. Wyngaarden JB, Smith LH Jr, eds. Cecil textbook of medicine, 18th ed. Philadelphia: WB Saunders, 1988.
4. Wegener F. On generalized septic vessel diseases. (Transl.) Verhandl Deutsch Pathol Gesellsch 1937;29:202–210.
5. Straatsma BR. Ocular manifestations of Wegener's granulomatosis. Am J Ophthalmol 1957;44:789–799.
6. Haynes BF, Fishman ML, Fauci AS, Wolff SM. The ocular manifestations of Wegener's granulomatosis: fifteen years experience and review of the literature. Am J Med 1977;63:131–141.
7. Bullen CL, Liesegang TJ, McDonald TJ, DeRemee RA. Ocular complications of Wegener's granulomatosis. Ophthalmology 1983;90:279–290.
8. Robin JB, Schanzlin DJ, Meisler DM, deLuise VP, Clough JD. Ocular involvement in the respiratory vasculitides. Surv Ophthalmol 1985;30:127–140.
9. Rao NA, Marak GE, Hidayat AA. Necrotizing scleritis: a clinico-pathologic study of 41 cases. Ophthalmology 1985;92:1542–1549.
10. Littlejohn GO, Ryan SJ, Holdsworth SR. Wegener's granulomatosis: clinical features and outcome in seventeen patients. Aust NZ J Med 1985;15:241–245.
11. Carrington CB, Liebow AA. Limited forms of angiitis and granulomatosis of Wegener's type. Am J Med 1966;41:497–527.
12. Spalton DJ, Graham EM, Page NGR, Sanders MD. Ocular changes in limited forms of Wegener's granulomatosis. Br J Ophthalmol 1981;65:553–563.
13. Koyama T, Matsuo N, Watanabe Y, Ojima M, Koyama T. Wegener's granulomatosis with destructive ocular manifestations. Am J Ophthalmol 1984;98:736–740.
14. Parelhoff ES, Chavis RM, Friendly DS. Wegener's granulomatosis presenting as orbital pseudotumor in children. J Pediatr Ophthalmol Strabismus 1985;22:100–104.
15. Jordan DR, Miller D, Anderson RL. Wound necrosis following dacryocystorhinostomy in patients with Wegener's granulomatosis. Ophthalmic Surg 1987;18:800–803.
16. Payton CD, Jones JM. Cortical blindness complicating Wegener's granulomatosis. Br Med J (Clin Res) 1985;290:676.
17. Noritake DT, Weiner SR, Bassett LW, Paulus HE, Weisbart R. Rheumatic manifestations of Wegener's granulomatosis. J Rheumatol 1987;14:949–951.
18. Hodges EJ, Turner S, Doud RB. Refractory scleritis due to Wegener's granulomatosis. West J Med 1987;146:361–363.

Systemic Lupus Erythematosus

INTRODUCTION

Systemic lupus erythematosus (SLE), an idiopathic, multisystem inflammatory disorder, is characterized by hyperactivity of the immune system and prominent autoantibody production. Acute exacerbations of disease activity are followed by periods of remission, and its course and spectrum of clinical manifestations are variable.

About 80% to 90% of SLE patients are women (1, 2). Although increased frequency and severity of the disease have been reported in blacks, these data may be an artifact of referral bias and socioeconomic factors (1, 2). The average age of onset is about 30 years, with a range from infancy to old age.

PATHOPHYSIOLOGY

Genetic Considerations

A definite genetic predisposition to SLE exists, though the precise nature of these genetic factors and their role in the pathophysiology of the disease remains unknown. The earliest evidence for this genetic basis was the widely recognized increased incidence of SLE, related "connective tissue disorders," or serologic abnormalities in family members of lupus patients. In addition, identical twins are concordant for lupus in 35% to 65% of cases (3, 5). But the fact that there is not a 100% concordance indicates that postnatal, environmental factors play a critical role in inducing the disease in genetically predisposed individuals.

More sophisticated evidence for a genetic role in SLE comes from HLA typing. The major histocompatibility complex (MHC) is a closely linked set of genes located on the short arm of chromosome six. This genetic complex includes three loci, A, B, and C, which are responsible for the production of glycoprotein antigens found on every nucleated cell in the body. Still another region, HLA-D, encodes antigens found on various cells in the immune system, including B cells, activated T cells, and macrophages (4, 6). The HLA antigen system is an important part of the body's immunoregulation system, and, although reports have been inconsistent, a significantly higher incidence of HLA-DR2 and HLA-DR3 seems to exist in lupus patients. Significant HLA associations also seem to exist with various SLE subsets (see clinical findings below) and with specific autoantibodies. Since some of these autoantibodies are associated with specific clinical manifestations of SLE, the HLA region

clearly exerts some effect on the clinical presentation of this disease (4, 6).

Immunological Abnormalities

Autoimmune phenomena are the hallmark of SLE. Autoantibodies to a number of nuclear and cytoplasmic constituents may be present and may be the result of a generalized polyclonal B cell hyperactivity (3, 7, 8). Antinuclear antibodies include anti–ds DNA (anti–native double-stranded DNA, very specific for SLE), anti–ss DNA (single-stranded DNA, common but nonspecific), and anti-Ro/SSA and anti-La/SSB antibodies. The latter, Ro/SSA and La/SSB, are ribonucleoprotein (RNP) antigens detectable in both the nucleus and cytoplasm, and antibodies against them are highly associated with certain subsets of lupus, including ANA-negative lupus, subacute cutaneous lupus erythematosus (SCLE), neonatal lupus, and lupus associated with inherited disorders of complement (4, 6–10).

Autoantibodies to cytoplasmic antigens include a group reactive against phospholipids. These antibodies, including "lupus anticoagulant" (LA) and anticardiolipin (ACA), are a heterogeneous group of immunoglobulins, apparently of major clinical significance. They are thrombogenic on the basis of complex interactions with the coagulation cascade, and they may react directly with phospholipid antigens in platelets and the cell membranes of endothelial cells. LA and ACA have been associated with recurrent arterial and venous thromboses, recurrent abortions, thrombocytopenia, and most of the neurological complications of lupus (11–13). The antiphospholipid antibodies are reactive with the cardiolipin used in standard screening tests for syphilis, which explains the "biologic false positive" test for syphilis long associated with lupus and related disorders. These antibodies appear to have clinical significance far beyond their importance in producing many of the clinical manifestations of lupus; they are found in nonlupus patients as well (11, 12).

Still another important group of lupus autoantibodies is the group reactive against brain constituents. These antineuronal antibodies are associated with active CNS lupus, especially diffuse disease (e.g., psychosis, organic brain syndrome), as opposed to focal CNS disease (14).

Antibodies play a dual role in the pathophysiology of lupus. Some may be reactive against cell constituents and may have direct toxic effects on their target cells (e.g., antineuronal antibodies, anti-RBC or anti-platelet antibodies). Others may form antigen-antibody immune complexes, which form in the circulation or in situ in tissues and provide an alternative pathway for disease production. These immune complexes, bound with complement, may induce a destructive inflammatory response, most typically an immune-complex vasculitis (8, 14).

Still another immunological abnormality in systemic lupus is that of T cell function. Although its precise pathophysiological role is unknown, T cell dysfunction and its relationship to the critical issues of immune regulation and the recognition of "self" may prove an important contributor to the overall disease process (5).

Drug-Induced Lupus

A systemic inflammatory disorder that usually fulfills the traditional criteria for SLE may be induced by a number of drugs. Those generally accepted as producing drug-induced lupus include chlorpromazine, hydralazine, methyldopa, isoniazid, and procainamide (15). The pathophysiological mechanism by which this induction occurs remains unknown, and the associated systemic complications are typically mild.

CLINICAL FINDINGS

Classic SLE

The most common clinical manifestations of SLE involve the skin and the musculoskeletal system (1, 16–19). Muco-

cutaneous complications include the classic, butterfly malar rash, photosensitivity eruptions, mucosal ulcers, and discoid skin lesions. The term "discoid" refers to a specific type of skin lesion, not to a subtype of lupus. Discoid lesions are chronic lesions exhibiting a characteristic histopathology. They resolve with both scarring and atrophy. Although usually found in patients with limited or no systemic involvement, they may be seen in all forms of lupus, including classic SLE. Those lupus patients with widespread discoid disease are more likely to develop systemic complications than are those with localized discoid lupus (18).

Musculoskeletal changes may be due to the disease process itself or secondary to the drugs used to treat it. Inflammatory arthralgias and arthritis are frequent findings. Aseptic bone necrosis is caused both by lupus and corticosteroids, while lupus myopathy may also be due to steroids and/or antimalarial drugs (19).

Lupus serositis includes pleurisy, pericarditis, and peritonitis. Renal disease accounts for a significant portion of the mortality from lupus. Circulating immune complexes localize in the kidney, resulting in lupus nephritis, the nephrotic syndrome, and renal failure (17, 20).

Neurological involvement is also responsible for much morbidity and mortality in SLE. Diffuse CNS manifestations include organic brain syndrome, generalized seizures, and psychosis/neurosis. Focal seizures, strokes, movement disorders, and cranial and peripheral neuropathies are also seen. Headaches, including classic migraines with scotomata, are a frequent finding. These neurological complications occur on the basis of small vessel occlusive disease as well as direct autoantibody damage to neuronal tissue (14, 21). A very significant association exists between CNS involvement in lupus and the presence of thrombogenic antiphospholipid antibodies (lupus anticoagulant and/or anticardiolipin antibodies) (11, 12, 14).

Lupus vasculitis, Raynaud's phenomenon, myocarditis, endocarditis (Libman-

Sacks), pneumonitis, and diffuse interstitial fibrosis are other major complications of SLE (22).

No single specific test exists that is diagnostic of SLE. The American Rheumatism Association (ARA) has identified a series of eleven clinical and laboratory criteria, any four or more of which must be present to establish a diagnosis of SLE (2, 16, 23).

SLE Subsets

Advances in genetic and immunological studies have aided in the identification of more homogeneous subsets within the broad clinical spectrum of SLE. These subsets include subacute cutaneous lupus erythematosus (SCLE), neonatal lupus, ANA-negative lupus, lupus associated with complement deficiency disorders, and late-onset lupus. These lupus subsets are characterized by primarily cutaneous involvement, minimal systemic complications, and a high incidence of circulating anti-Ro (SSA) antibodies. SCLE patients often have a high incidence of HLA-DR3 antigen, as do the mothers of infants with neonatal lupus (1, 4, 6, 9, 10, 16, 24).

OCULAR MANIFESTATIONS

SLE can affect many ocular and adnexal structures; "lupus retinopathy" is a classic feature of the disorder. Ocular complications tend to occur in acutely ill patients with active system disease (25–27), which explains the discrepancy between an incidence of eye findings of 10% to 28% in the earliest series and an incidence of 3.3% found by Gold et al. (25). The latter series consisted of treated lupus patients, with inactive disease, seen in an outpatient setting. Earlier reports described mostly inpatients seen during episodes of acute disease activity.

The retina is the most frequently involved site in the eye (25). Cotton-wool spots and retinal hemorrhages are the most frequently reported findings (Fig. 1.3), but retinal edema, hard exudates, microaneu-rysms, arterial narrowing, venous engorgement, and vascular tortuosity have also been noted (25–27). Although many of these changes are part of the clinical picture of hypertensive retinopathy and hypertension is often present secondary to lupus renal disease, lupus retinopathy can occur as an independent manifestation of the underlying disease process in the absence of hypertension (25–27).

Retinal vascular occlusive disease is a potentially visually devastating complication of SLE (28–30). Arterial occlusion may involve the central retinal artery or a single branch retinal artery, but it most often occurs as a multifocal occlusion of multiple retinal arteries that is accompanied by extensive nonperfusion of the retinal capillary bed (Fig. 1.4). The involved arteries are sheathed or reduced to thin, white, nonperfused cords, and patches of gray-white, infarcted retina may be present. Retinal hemorrhages may be seen, but they are usually not prominent. As is true in many other disorders in which retinal nonperfusion and hypoxia are present, lupus arterial occlusive disease can lead to disc and retinal neovascularization, vitreous hemorrhage, and traction retinal detachment. Optic atrophy may develop, depending on the extent and severity of the occlusive process.

Fluorescein angiography demonstrates the arterial and capillary nonperfusion, leakage from neovascular fronds, and occasional staining of the walls of the involved vessels. Vascular incompetence and fluorescein leakage have been found on angiography even in eyes that appear normal clinically (26).

Central retinal vein occlusion has also been reported in SLE, but this occurrence appears to be less common than the arterial occlusive disease described above (25, 26, 31, 32).

Although the retinal vascular complications of lupus are usually bilateral, unilateral or asymmetric disease can be noted (30–33).

Lupus choroidopathy results in multifocal serous detachments of the retina and underlying retinal pigment epithelium (RPE), sometimes progressing to large, exudative retinal detachments (34–36) (Fig. 1.5A). Fluorescein angiography demonstrates multiple sites of leakage from the choroid into the sub-RPE and subretinal spaces (Fig. 1.5B). Visual loss is variable, depending upon the extent of macular involvement, and the detachments may regress with improved control of the systemic disease (34).

The precise pathophysiology underlying the vasculopathy of lupus in the eye is uncertain, but evidence points to a critical role for autoimmune mechanisms. Histopathological studies have documented occlusion of retinal and choroidal vessels, including the choriocapillaris (37–40). Although a true, active vasculitis is occasionally noted, most occluded vessels have either a mild perivasculitis or no evidence of active inflammation. This situation closely resembles that seen in histopathological studies of the CNS in lupus, in which widely scattered microinfarcts are associated with a generally noninflammatory vasculopathy (14, 41).

Immunofluorescent techniques reveal immune reactants (immunoglobulins and complement) deposited in blood vessel walls within the retina, choroid, ciliary body, sclera, and bulbar conjunctiva, as well as Schlemm's canal, the basement membranes of the bulbar conjunctiva, ciliary body, and corneal epithelium, and along nerve fibers in the ciliary body and bulbar conjunctiva (36, 37). In one patient, extensive immune reactants were found in retinal vessels in areas of focal nerve fiber layer infarcts where cotton-wool spots had been observed clinically. Vessels containing immune deposits showed a variety of changes including thrombosis, endothelial swelling, and focal perivasculitis. A

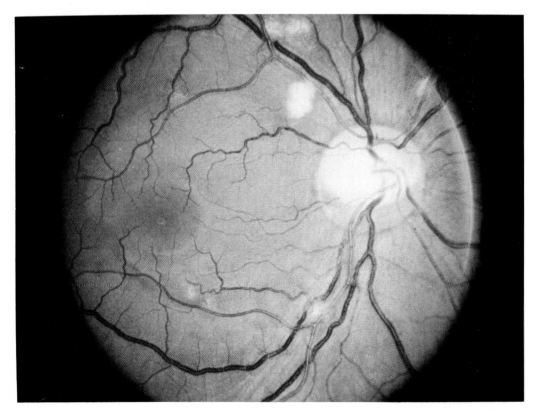

Figure 1.3. Lupus retinopathy with cotton-wool spots in the absence of hypertension.

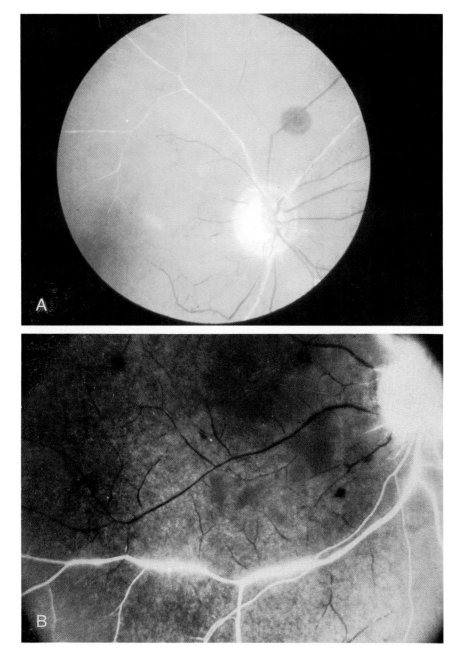

Figure 1.4. A. Lupus erythematosus. Arteries are severely narrowed and sheathed with extensive capillary closure. **B.** Fluorescein angiogram of a patient with lupus shows severe capillary closure. (Reprinted with permission from Arch Ophthalmol 1986;104:560, American Medical Association. Copyright 1986.)

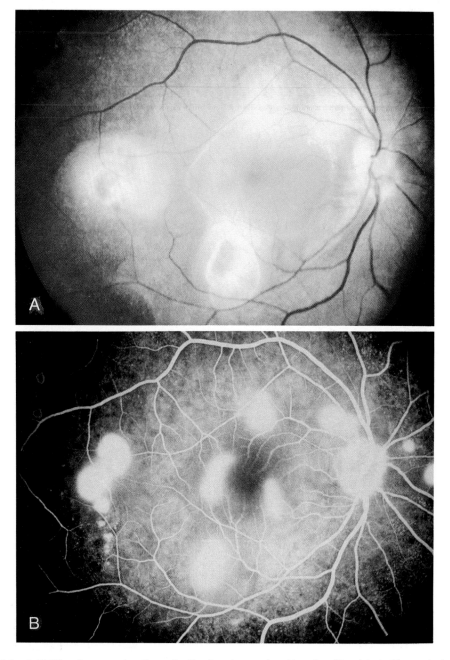

Figure 1.5. A. Multifocal serous elevations of retina from lupus choroidopathy. (Reprinted with permission from Arch Ophthalmol 1988;106:231, American Medical Association. Copyright 1988.) **B.** Fluorescein angiogram shows filling of neurosensory retinal detachments.

nongranulomatous uveitis was sometimes seen associated with immune reactants in uveal blood vessels. Focal RPE destruction and subretinal hemorrhage were found in an area of choroidal infarction and fibrin occlusion of the choriocapillaris. Ocular immune deposits were much more extensive in patients in whom the clinical and immunological evidence of active systemic disease was the most pronounced. Despite well-documented evidence that immune-complex mediated inflammatory vasculitis produces systemic complications of lupus, immune reactants in the eye and elsewhere in the body are fairly widespread, while histological evidence of active inflammation tends to be much less common and more localized (37).

Since histopathological evidence indicates that autoimmune mechanisms are involved in producing the ocular vascular lesions of lupus and that a true inflammatory vasculitis is very uncommon, one or more additional pathways are thought to be involved. Lupus anticoagulant, anticardiolipin antibodies, and other antiphospholipid antibodies are the likely candidates playing a major role in this process. These autoantibodies are thrombogenic (see immunological abnormalities discussed above) and are associated with both CNS (11, 12) and ocular vaso-occlusive phenomena (11, 13, 29). A clinical association also appears to exist between severe retinal vascular occlusion and the presence of CNS lupus (28, 30). The so-called "bland vasculopathy" seen histopathologically in CNS lupus (14, 41) may, in fact, be directly visualized clinically in lupus patients with multifocal retinal artery occlusions.

Embolic disease (e.g., from a coexisting endocarditis) or in situ thrombosis induced by other, as yet unknown, mechanisms is also a potential factor in the production of retinal vascular occlusions.

Regardless of the underlying mechanism, vessel wall damage may result in vascular occlusion and also in loss of vascular integrity, manifesting itself clinically as hemorrhage or edema. Choroidal vascular damage and/or occlusion produces multifocal serous retinal and RPE detachments. An associated hypertension can contribute to vessel wall damage as well as provide greater hydrostatic pressure, forcing fluid and blood cells out of the intravascular compartment and into the surrounding tissues.

CNS lupus can also produce a host of neuro-ophthalmological signs and symptoms (21, 42–45). Cranial nerve palsies may result in ophthalmoplegias accompanied by diplopia, ptosis, and/or pupillary abnormalities. Homonymous visual field defects, cortical blindness, internuclear ophthalmoplegia, nystagmus, visual hallucinations, pseudotumor cerebri with papilledema, and migraine-like headaches with fortification or other scotomata have also been reported. Direct involvement of the optic nerve can occur as acute retrobulbar neuritis, acute anterior optic neuritis (papillitis with a swollen disc), anterior ischemic optic neuropathy, or slowly progressive visual loss (43, 46, 47). Both optic neuropathy and retinal arterial occlusive disease can result in optic atrophy. Immune complex vasculitis, lupus anticoagulant and related antiphospholipid antibodies, and possibly antineuronal autoantibodies may play a role in the pathogenesis of these neuro-ophthalmologic complications (11, 12, 14, 21, 47).

Secondary Sjögren's syndrome is a frequent finding in SLE. It may produce clinical ocular manifestations such as keratoconjunctivitis sicca and is strongly associated with the presence of HLA-DRW52 antigen and anti-Ro (SSA) and anti-La (SSB) antibodies (1, 4, 6).

Orbital inflammation in SLE may result in episodes of acute proptosis, lid edema, conjunctival chemosis and hyperemia, and limited ocular motility. Elevated intraocular pressure and myositis with enlargement of the extraocular muscles on CT scanning have also been reported (48, 49).

The eyelid may be involved in the cutaneous facial changes of lupus. Discoid lesions of the eyelids can mimic chronic blepharitis (50).

Other, less common ocular complications of lupus include conjunctivitis, episcleritis, scleritis, keratitis, corneal staining, uveitis, and anterior segment neovascularization (25, 28).

In addition to lupus-induced eye problems, the drugs used to treat the systemic disease have potential ocular side effects. Corticosteroids may induce cataracts and glaucoma, and antimalarials can cause retinal toxicity. The retinopathy of chloroquine or hydroxychloroquine may cause subtle, asymptomatic, reversible macular pigment mottling in its "premaculopathy" early phase and profound irreversible visual loss with a bulls-eye pattern, pigmentary maculopathy in its later phases. Although the risk of developing maculopathy has been thought to depend on the total cumulative dose of the drugs, the size of the daily dose rather than the total dosage or duration of treatment may be the most important factor. Dosages of 400 mg/day or 6.5 mg/kg body weight/day of hydroxychloroquine, whichever is less, may permit very high total drug intake without inducing clinical retinal toxicity (51).

TREATMENT

The three major classes of drugs used in treating SLE are nonsteroidal anti-inflammatory agents, corticosteroids, and immunosuppressives (52–54). Nonsteroidals (including aspirin) and antimalarials (usually hydroxychloroquine) are useful for nonspecific manifestations such as fever and arthralgias, as well as for arthritis and serositis. Systemic corticosteroids are used orally and intravenously for major organ involvement and for the hematological complications such as hemolytic anemia and thrombocytopenia. Immunosuppressive drugs, especially azathioprine, are used when life-threatening complications of lupus do not respond to steroids. Cyclophosphamide, chlorambucil, nitrogen mustard, methotrexate, and cyclosporine A have also been employed in the treatment of SLE. Plasmapheresis can reduce levels of circulating immune complexes and antibodies (53, 54). Hemodialysis and renal transplantation are used in lupus patients with renal failure. Thrombotic events associated with antiphospholipid antibodies (lupus anticoagulant and anticardiolipin antibodies) are often treated with oral anticoagulants, though no treatment exists that is consistently effective for this class of major lupus-associated complications (11, 12). Anticoagulation may prevent recurrent thrombosis, and there is a recognized tendency for rebound thrombosis if anticoagulation therapy is stopped. Cutaneous lesions may respond to topical or intralesional steroids, antimalarials, systemic steroids, immunosuppressives, topical or systemic steroids, topical or systemic retinoids, or oral gold (18). Sunscreens are useful in preventing photosensitivity skin eruptions.

Appropriate therapy for specific complications of SLE is also important and may include antihypertensive agents for lupus-induced hypertension and antibiotics for infections in these immune-compromised patients. Varying combinations of drugs and other modes of therapeutic intervention have dramatically improved the prognosis for SLE patients. Survival rates have increased from less than 50% after 4 years of disease, as reported in 1954, to over 90% 20 years later (55).

Since the ocular complications of SLE are generally associated with active disease elsewhere in the body, control of the systemic disease may resolve its ocular manifestations (23, 24). Systemic steroids, with or without immunosuppressive agents, have been used in the treatment of lupus optic neuropathy (46, 47), choroidopathy (34, 36), orbital inflammation (48), and pseudotumor cerebri (42). Simultaneous control of any associated systemic hypertension is also important.

Treatment of the sequelae of retinal vascular occlusive disease has generally been limited to local ocular measures. Retinal neovascularization responds to scatter laser photocoagulation in a manner similar to that observed in diabetic retinopathy, retinal vein occlusion, and other retinal neovascular disorders (29, 30, 56). Anterior segment ischemia has been observed as a complication following laser treatment in a patient with SLE (56). Vitrectomy and scleral buckling may be required for cases involving vitreous hemorrhage or retinal detachment.

These modalities involve therapy of the complications of retinal vascular occlusion but not of the vaso-occlusive process itself. The possible thrombogenic role of antiphospholipid antibodies in the pathophysiology of retinal vaso-occlusion has not been systematically addressed. Meaningful information on the subject might best be collected by pooling the collective experiences of investigators working at different centers. Perhaps anticoagulation, in combination with other types of systemic therapy, should be considered in treating this problem. Of course, prior laser photocoagulation of any neovascularization would be necessary to reduce the risk of intraocular hemorrhage. A similar, multicenter approach might yield important information about the role of antiphospholipid antibodies in the pathogenesis of lupus choroidopathy or optic neuropathy and about the possible role of antineuronal antibodies in producing lupus optic neuropathy.

SUMMARY

The significance of the ocular manifestations of lupus are not limited to the eye. Their presence should alert the clinician to the likely presence of disease activity elsewhere (25, 28, 30, 34, 56). Severe retinal arterial occlusive disease (28, 30, 56) and lupus optic neuropathy (46, 47) have been particularly associated with CNS lupus; lupus choroidopathy (34) (or other ocular complications) may coexist with widespread, systemic vascular disease. All patients with ocular lupus should be carefully evaluated from a systemic perspective for potentially treatable and preventable complications of the disease.

References

1. Hochberg MC, Boyd RE, Ahearn JM, et al. Systemic lupus erythematosus: a review of clinico-laboratory features and immunogenetic markers in 150 patients with emphasis on demographic subsets. Medicine 1985;64:285–295.
2. Wallace DJ, Dubois EL. Definition, classification and epidemiology of systemic lupus erythematosus. In: Wallace DJ, Dubois EL, eds. Dubois' lupus erythematosus. 3rd ed. Philadelphia: Lea & Febiger, 1987:15–32.
3. Steinberg AD, Klinman DM. Pathogenesis of systemic lupus erythematosus. Rheum Dis Clin North Am 1988;14:25–41.
4. Arnett FC. Familial SLE, the HLA system, and the genetics of lupus erythematosus. In: Wallace DJ, Dubois EL, eds. Dubois' lupus erythematosus. 3rd ed. Philadelphia: Lea & Febiger, 1987:161–184.
5. Shen HH, Winchester RJ. Susceptibility genetics of systemic lupus erythematosus. Springer Semin Immunopathol 1986;9:143–159.
6. Arnett FC. HLA and genetic predisposition to lupus erythematosus and other dermatologic disorders. J Am Acad Dermatol 1985;13:472–481.
7. Mackay IR. Autoimmunity in relation to lupus erythematosus. In: Wallace DJ, Dubois EL, eds. Dubois' lupus erythematosus. 3rd ed. Philadelphia: Lea & Febiger, 1987:44–52.
8. Harley JB, Gaither KK. Autoantibodies. Rheum Dis Clin North Am 1988;14:43–56.
9. Tsokos GC, Pillemer SR, Klippel JH. Rheumatic disease syndromes associated with antibodies to the Ro (SS-A) ribonuclear protein. Semin Arthritis Rheum 1987;16:237–244.
10. Reichlin M. Significance of the Ro antigen system. J Clin Immunol 1986;6:339–348.
11. Levine SR, Welch KMA. The spectrum of neurologic disease associated with antiphospholipid antibodies. Lupus anticoagulants and anticardiolipin antibodies. Arch Neurol 1987;44:876–883.
12. Hughes GRV, Harris NN, Gharavi AE. The anticardiolipin syndrome. J Rheumatol 1986;13:486–489.
13. Glueck HI, Kant KS, Weiss MA, et al. Thrombosis in systemic lupus erythematosus. Relation to the presence of circulating anticoagulants. Arch Intern Med 1985;145:1389–1395.
14. Bluestein HG, Pischel KD, Woods VL Jr. Immunopathogenesis of the neuropsychiatric manifestations of systemic lupus erythematosus. Springer Semin Immunopathol 1986;9:237–249.
15. Solinger AM. Drug-related lupus. Clinical and etiologic considerations. Rheum Dis Clin North Am 1988;14:187–202.
16. Stevens MB. Systemic lupus erythematosus clinical issues. Springer Semin Immunopathol 1986;9:251–270.
17. Dubois EL, Wallace DJ. Clinical and laboratory manifestations of systemic lupus erythematosus. In: Wallace DJ, Dubois EL, eds. Dubois' lupus erythematosus. 3rd ed. Philadelphia: Lea & Febiger, 1987:317–449.
18. Callen JP. Mucocutaneous changes in patients with lupus erythematosus. The relationship of

these lesions to systemic disease. Rheum Dis Clin North Am 1988;14:79–97.

19. Cronin ME. Musculoskeletal manifestations of systemic lupus erythematosus. Rheum Dis Clin North Am 1988;14:99–116.

20. Balow JE, Austin HA III. Renal disease in systemic lupus erythematosus. Rheum Dis Clin North Am 1988;14:117–133.

21. McCune WJ, Golbus J. Neuropsychiatric lupus. Rheum Dis Clin North Am 1988;14:149–167.

22. Carette S. Cardiopulmonary manifestations of systemic lupus erythematosus. Rheum Dis Clin North Am 1988;14:135–147.

23. Tan EM, Cohen AS, Fries JF, et al. The 1982 revised criteria for the classification of systemic lupus erythematosus. Arthritis Rheum 1982;25:1271–1277.

24. Agnello V. Lupus diseases associated with hereditary and acquired deficiencies of complement. Springer Semin Immunopathol 1986;9:161–178.

25. Gold DH, Morris DA, Henkind P. Ocular findings in systemic lupus erythematosus. Br J Ophthalmol 1972;56:800–804.

26. Lanham JG, Barrie T, Kohner EM, Hughes GRV. SLE retinopathy: evaluation by fluorescein angiography. Ann Rheum Dis 1982;41:473–478.

27. Klinkhoff AV, Beattie CW, Chalmers A. Retinopathy in systemic lupus erythematosus: relationship to disease activity. Arthritis Rheum 1986;29:1152–1156.

28. Gold D, Feiner L, Henkind P. Retinal arterial occlusive disease in systemic lupus erythematosus. Arch Ophthalmol 1977;95:1580–1585.

29. Hall S, Buettner H, Luthra HS. Occlusive retinal vascular disease in systemic lupus erythematosus. J Rheumatol 1984;11:846–850.

30. Jabs DA, Fine SL, Hochberg MC, et al. Severe retinal vaso-occlusive disease in systemic lupus erythematosus. Arch Ophthalmol 1986;104:558-563.

31. Kremer I, Gilad E, Cohen S, Ben Sira I. Combined arterial and venous retinal occlusion as a presenting sign of systemic lupus erythematosus. Ophthalmologica 1985;191:114–118.

32. Laroche L, Saraux H. Unilateral central retinal vein occlusion in systemic lupus erythematosus. Ophthalmologica 1984;189:128–129.

33. Terhorst DR, Campo RV, Abrams GW. Unilateral systemic lupus erythematosus retinopathy. Am J Ophthalmol 1983;95:840–841.

34. Jabs DA, Hanneken AM, Schachat AP, Fine SL. Choroidopathy in systemic lupus erythematosus. Arch Ophthalmol 1988;106:230–234.

35. Matsuo T, Nakayama T, Koyama T, Matsuo N. Multifocal pigment epithelial damages with serous retinal detachment in systemic lupus erythematosus. Ophthalmologica 1987;195:97–102.

36. Aronson AJ, Ordonez NG, Diddie KR, Ernest JT. Immune-complex deposition in the eye in systemic lupus erythematosus. Arch Intern Med 1979;139:1312–1313.

37. Karpik AG, Schwartz MM, Dickey LE, et al. Ocu-lar immune reactants in patients dying with systemic lupus erythematosus. Clin Immunol Immunopathol 1985;35:295–312.

38. Graham EM, Spalton DJ, Barnard RO, et al. Cerebral and retinal vascular changes in systemic lupus erythematosus. Ophthalmology 1985;92:444–448.

39. Cordes FC, Aiken SD. Ocular changes in acute disseminated lupus erythematosus; report of a case with microscopic findings. Am J Ophthalmol 1947;30:1541–1555.

40. Goldstein I, Wexler D. Retinal vascular disease in a case of acute lupus erythematosus disseminatus. Arch Ophthalmol 1932;8:852–857.

41. Johnson RT, Richardson EP. The neurological manifestations of systemic lupus erythematosus; a clinical-pathological study of 24 cases and review of the literature. Medicine 1968;47:337–369.

42. Delgiudice GC, Scher CA, Athreya BH, Diamond GR. Pseudotumor cerebri and childhood systemic lupus erythematosus. J Rheumatol 1986;13:748–752.

43. Lessell S. The neuro-ophthalmology of systemic lupus erythematosus. Doc Ophthalmol 1979;47:13–42.

44. Brandt KD, Lessell S, Cohen AS. Cerebral disorders of vision in systemic lupus erythematosus. Ann Intern Med 1975;83:163–169.

45. Brandt KD, Lessell S. Migrainous phenomena in systemic lupus erythematosus. Arthritis Rheum 1978;21:7–16.

46. Jabs DA, Miller NR, Newman SA, et al. Optic neuropathy in systemic lupus erythematosus. Arch Ophthalmol 1986;104:564–568.

47. Oppenheimer S, Hoffbrand BI. Optic neuritis and myelopathy in systemic lupus erythematosus. Can J Neurol Sci 1986;13:129–132.

48. Fossaluzza V, Dal Mas P. Proptosis and systemic lupus erythematosus. Clin Exp Rheumatol 1987;5:192–193.

49. Grimson BS, Simons KB. Orbital inflammation, myositis, and systemic lupus erythematosus. Arch Ophthalmol 1983;101:736–738.

50. Huey C, Jakobiec FA, Iwamoto T, et al. Discoid lupus erythematosus of the eyelids. Ophthalmology 183;90:1389–1398.

51. Johnson MW, Vine AK. Hydroxychloroquine therapy in massive total doses without retinal toxicity. Am J Ophthalmol 1987;104:139–144.

52. Kimberly RP. Treatment. Corticosteroids and anti-inflammatory drugs. Rheum Dis Clin North Am 1988;14:203–221.

53. Lieberman JD, Schatten S. Treatment. Disease-modifying therapies. Rheum Dis Clin North Am 1988;14:223–243.

54. Miescher PA. Treatment of systemic lupus erythematosus. Springer Semin Immunopathol 1986;9:271–282.

55. Ginzler EM, Schorn K. Outcome and prognosis in systemic lupus erythematosus. Rheum Dis Clin North Am 1988;14:67–78.

56. Jost BF, Olk RJ, Patz A, et al. Anterior segment ischaemia following laser photocoagulation in a

patient with systemic lupus erythematosus. Br J Ophthalmol 1988;72:11–16.

Polymyositis and Dermatomyositis

INTRODUCTION

Polymyositis and dermatomyositis are inflammatory diseases of skeletal muscle and are characterized by pain and weakness in the involved muscle groups. In the typical case, weakness begins insidiously and involves the proximal muscle groups, particularly those of the shoulders and hips. Dermatomyositis is distinguished from polymyositis by the presence of cutaneous lesions. The skin lesions of dermatomyositis are an erythematous to violaceous rash that variably affects the eyelids (heliotrope rash), cheeks, nose, chest, and extensor surfaces. The knuckles of the fingers may develop plaques known as Gottron's papules (1–3).

The estimated incidence of myositis in the United States is 5 new cases/1,000,000 population/year (4). Females exceed males in adult myositis.

Bohan and Peter (5, 6) have classified polymyositis and dermatomyositis into five groups as outlined in Table 1.4. They include (a) primary idiopathic polymyositis, (b) primary idiopathic dermatomyositis, (c) dermatomyositis or polymyositis associated with neoplasia, (d) childhood dermatomyositis or polymyositis often associated with vasculitis, and (e) polymyositis or dermatomyositis associated with other acquired disease of connective tissue (overlap syndrome).

Malignancy occurs in perhaps 13% of adults with dermatomyositis. These patients are likely to be age 45 years and above and will more often have dermatomyositis than polymyositis. The tumors occur at typical cancer sites and are usually diagnosed either concurrently with the diagnosis of myositis or within one year of it. Extensive laboratory screening examinations other than the standard history, physical, and basic laboratory examination do not appear to be effective in finding occult malignancies (7–9). Vasculitis is common in patients with childhood dermatomyositis. Inflammatory myositis with a defined acquired disease of connective tissue is seen most often in association with systemic lupus erythematosus or with scleroderma.

PATHOPHYSIOLOGY

The etiology of myositis is unknown. The pathogenesis appears to be an inflammatory attack mounted against the muscle fibers, although the exact mechanisms remain to be elucidated. Muscle biopsy specimens often show vascular deposits of immunoglobulin and complement, particularly in childhood dermatomyositis, although this finding has not been seen in all cases (10, 11). These vascular deposits possibly represent immune complexes producing vascular damage. This finding in patients with childhood dermatomyositis is consistent with the high frequency of vasculitis in this subgroup. A noninflammatory vasculopathy has also been seen in childhood dermatomyositis (11). More recently, microvascular deposition of the complement-membrane attack complex has been demonstrated in dermatomyositis, suggesting that a vasculopathy may contribute to this disease process (12). The presence of a vasculopathy in patients

Table 1.4. Classification of Polymyositis and Dermatomyositis

Group	Name
1	Primary idiopathic polymyositis
2	Primary idiopathic dermatomyositis
3	Dermatomyositis or polymyositis associated with neoplasia
4	Childhood dermatomyositis or polymyositis associated with vasculitis
5	Polymyositis or dermatomyositis associated with other acquired disease of connective tissue (overlap syndrome)

without frank vasculitis may help explain the occasional occurrence of a retinopathy in patients with dermatomyositis.

Cellular immune mechanisms have also been suggested. Some investigators have found lymphocyte proliferation in response to skeletal muscle antigens (13, 14).

Immunogenetic studies have suggested that HLA-DR3 is associated with primary idiopathic polymyositis but not with dermatomyositis (15). This HLA type has also been associated with juvenile dermatomyositis but not with adult dermatomyositis (16). These studies have been interpreted as suggesting a genetic predisposition and potential immune mechanism.

Although autoantibodies are generally not present in patients with myositis, antibodies to a saline extractable nuclear antigen Jo-1 have been found in approximately 25% of patients with myositis. Some investigators have suggested that anti-Jo-1 antibodies are found only in those patients with myositis who develop an associated interstitial pulmonary fibrosis (17, 18).

CLINICAL FINDINGS

The typical case of muscle weakness begins insidiously either in the lower or the upper limbs. The patient slowly becomes aware of difficulty in running, climbing stairs, and getting out of a chair. Ultimately, the gait may become clumsy, and the patient will have difficulty arising without assistance. Systemic symptoms, including malaise and weight loss, are common.

On examination, proximal upper and lower limb weakness is found to some extent in almost every patient. The distribution of weakness is usually symmetrical. By definition, cutaneous lesions are found in patients with dermatomyositis but not in those with polymyositis.

Laboratory abnormalities include an elevated erythrocyte sedimentation rate and elevated skeletal muscle enzymes, the latter being released into the serum as a consequence of skeletal muscle dam-

age. Serum autoantibodies, such as the antinuclear antibody (ANA) and rheumatoid factor (RF), are found much less frequently. The potentially abnormal muscle enzymes include creatine phosphokinase (CPK), aldolase, serum glutamic oxaloacetic transaminase (SGOT), serum glutamic pyruvic transaminase (SGPT), and lactic dehydrogenase (LDH). Of these, the CPK is most frequently abnormal, although the pattern of abnormal enzymes will vary from individual to individual. Electromyographical abnormalities are present in over 90% of patients with myositis. The characteristic changes consist of an increase in insertional activity of the muscle, numerous fibrillation potentials, and positive sharp waves at rest. Motor unit action potentials show myopathic changes with decreased amplitude and duration and an increase in the proportion of polyphasic potentials. Bizarre, high frequency, repetitive discharges are also common features.

Muscle biopsy reveals degeneration of muscle fibers; regeneration is seen less commonly. Interstitial muscle necrosis is present in approximately 60%, and interstitial fibrosis is found in another 20%. Inflammatory infiltrates in muscle are the hallmark of myositis but are present in only 75% of muscle biopsies. The inflammatory infiltrate consists primarily of lymphocytes, with lesser numbers of plasma cells. Vasculitis is sometimes seen, particularly in childhood dermatomyositis.

OCULAR MANIFESTATIONS

Although a heliotrope rash of the lids is common with dermatomyositis, ocular involvement due to inflammatory myositis is relatively uncommon. Occasionally, ophthalmoplegia due to involvement of the extraocular muscles by myositis may occur (19, 20).

Cotton-wool spots have occasionally been reported in association with polymyositis and dermatomyositis (21–29). The vast majority of these cases are children with dermatomyositis, although adults with dermatomyositis have been reported as well. Even more rarely, intraretinal hemorrhages in association with cotton-wool spots have been reported. Cotton-wool spots reported in children with dermatomyositis may represent the vasculitis commonly seen in these patients. However, clinicians have reported an occasional patient with dermatomyositis with retinal vasculopathy without demonstrable systemic vasculitis (30). The finding of inflammatory mediators in the microvasculature of patients with myositis may help to account for the occasional associated retinal vascular lesion.

TREATMENT

Corticosteroids remain the mainstay of treatment for myositis. Steroids are usually started at a dosage of 1 mg/kg/day (60–80 mg daily) and continued until the muscle enzymes have normalized. At that time, tapering of the steroids can be initiated, with continued monitoring of the skeletal muscle enzymes. No randomized, double-masked controlled studies have been performed to demonstrate the efficacy of steroids in the treatment of myositis, but most authors agree that they are significantly beneficial.

When steroids fail or when steroid complications become unacceptable, immunosuppressive agents such as methotrexate or azathioprine have been used to treat the myositis (31, 32). These agents appear to have a steroid-sparing effect.

References

1. Bradley WG. Inflammatory diseases of muscle. In: Kelley WN, Harris ED Jr, Ruddy S, Sledge CB, eds. Textbook of rheumatology. 2nd ed. Philadelphia: WB Saunders, 1985:1225–1245.
2. Bohan A, Peter JB, Bowman RL, Pearson CM. Computer-assisted analysis of 153 patients with polymyositis and dermatomyositis. Medicine 1977;56:255–286.
3. Benbassat J, Gefel D, Larholt K, et al. Prognostic factors in polymyositis/dermatomyositis: a computer-assisted analysis of 92 cases. Arthritis Rheum 1985;28:249–255.
4. Medsger TA Jr, Dawson WN Jr, Masi AT. The epidemiology of polymyositis. Am J Med 1970;48:715–723.
5. Bohan A, Peter JB. Polymyositis and dermatomyositis (first of two parts). N Engl J Med 1975;292:344–347.
6. Bohan A, Peter JB. Polymyositis and dermatomyositis (second of two parts). N Engl J Med 1975;292:403–407.
7. Barnes BE. Dermatomyositis and malignancy; a review of the literature. Ann Intern Med 1976;84:68–76.
8. Callen JP, Hyla JF, Bole GG Jr, Kay DR. The relationship of dermatomyositis and polymyositis to internal malignancy. Arch Dermatol 1980;116:295–298.
9. Hochberg MC. Polymyositis/dermatomyositis and malignancy. In: Brooks PM, York JR, eds. Rheumatology-85; Proceedings of the XVIth International Congress of Rheumatology, Sydney, 1985. Amsterdam: Excerpta Medica, 1985:279–282.
10. Whitaker JN, Engle WK. Vascular deposits of immunoglobulin and complement in idiopathic inflammatory myopathy. N Engl J Med 1972;286:333–338.
11. Crowe WE, Bove KE, Levinson JE, Hilton PK. Clinical and pathogenic implications of histopathology in childhood polydermatomyositis. Arthritis Rheum 1982;25:126–139.
12. Kissel JT, Mendell JR, Rammohan KW. Microvascular deposition of complement membrane attack complex in dermatomyositis. N Engl J Med 1986;314:329–334.
13. Currie S, Saunders M, Knowles M, Brown AE. Immunological aspects of polymyositis: the in vitro activity of lymphocytes on incubation with muscle antigen and with muscle cultures. Q J Med 1971;40:63–84.
14. Esiri MM, MacLennan ICM, Hazleman BL. Lymphocyte sensitivity to skeletal muscle in patients with polymyositis and other disorders. Clin Exp Immunol 1973;14:25–35.
15. Hirsch TJ, Enlow RW, Bias WB, Arnett FC. HLA-D related (DR) antigens in various kinds of myositis. Human Immunol 1981;3:181–186.
16. Friedman JM, Pachman LM, Maryjowski ML, et al. Immunogenetic studies of juvenile dermatomyositis: HLA-DR antigen frequencies. Arthritis Rheum 1983;26:214–216.
17. Arnett FC, Hirsch TJ, Bias WB, et al. The Jo-1 antibody system in myositis: relationships to clinical features and HLA. J Rheumatol 1981;8:925–930.
18. Yoshida S, Akizuki M, Mimori T, et al. The precipitating antibody to an acidic nuclear protein antigen, the Jo-1, in connective tissue diseases; a marker for a subset of polymyositis with interstitial pulmonary fibrosis. Arthritis Rheum 1983;26:604–611.
19. Susac JO, Garcia-Mullin R, Glaser JS. Ophthalmoplegia in dermatomyositis. Neurology 1973;23:305–310.
20. Arnett FC, Michels RG. Inflammatory ocular my-

opathy in systemic sclerosis (scleroderma); a case report and review of the literature. Arch Intern Med 1973;132:740–743.

21. Bruce GM. Retinitis in dermatomyositis. Trans Am Ophthalmol Soc 1938;36:282–297.

22. Lisman JV. Dermatomyositis with retinopathy; report of a case. Arch Ophthalmol 1947;37:155–159.

23. London RD. Dermatomyositis. J Pediatr 1950; 36:817–820.

24. De Vries S. Retinopathy in dermatomyositis. Arch Ophthalmol 1951;46:432–435.

25. Munro S. Fundus appearances in a case of acute dermatomyositis. Br J Ophthalmol 1959;43:548–558.

26. Klien BA. Comments on the cotton-wool lesion of the retina. Am J Ophthalmol 1965;59:17–23.

27. Liebman S, Cook C, Donaldson DD. Retinopathy with dermatomyositis. Arch Ophthalmol 1965;74:704–705.

28. Henkind P, Gold DH. Ocular manifestations of rheumatic disorders. Natural and iatrogenic. Rheumatology 1973;4:13–59.

29. Fruman LS, Ragsdale CG, Sullivan DB, Petty RE. Retinopathy in juvenile dermatomyositis. J Pediatr 1976;88:267–269.

30. Zamora J, Pariser K, Hedges T, Nicholas O. Retinal vasculitis in polymyositis-dermatomyositis. Abstract. Arthritis Rheum 1987;30(suppl 4):S106.

31. Metzger AL, Bohan A, Goldberg LS, Bluestone R. Polymyositis and dermatomyositis: combined methotrexate and corticosteroid therapy. Ann Intern Med 1974;81:182–189.

32. Bunch TW, Worthington JW, Combs JJ, et al. Azathioprine with prednisone for polymyositis; a controlled, clinical trial. Ann Intern Med 1980;92:365–369.

Scleroderma

INTRODUCTION

Scleroderma is an idiopathic, systemic connective tissue disease characterized by fibrous and degenerative changes in the skin and viscera. In addition to the thickening and fibrous replacement of the dermis of the skin, vascular insufficiency and vasospasm occur. The hallmark of scleroderma is the skin change, which consists of thickening, tightening, induration, and subsequent contracture and loss of mobility (1–3). Localized forms of scleroderma, such as linear scleroderma and morphea, exist (4); however, in this section, we will consider only the systemic variant, sometimes also known as systemic sclerosis. The disease characteristically affects middle-aged women and has a peak age of onset of 30 to 50 years. The incidence has been calculated at 2.7/million population/year (5).

PATHOPHYSIOLOGY

The etiology of scleroderma is unknown. Its most characteristic feature is the increased collagen content in the skin and visceral organs (6). In vitro studies of fibroblasts from patients with scleroderma have demonstrated increased collagen production (7, 8), although this phenomenon has not been found by all investigators (9). A second feature of scleroderma is the vascular disease, including Raynaud's phenomenon and the diffuse microvasculopathy. Several theories of pathogenesis have been proposed, including a primary vascular disorder, a primary abnormality of fibroblast function, and a primary immunological disorder. To date, none has been proven.

Vascular theories suggest that the primary lesion is a vascular disorder, which subsequently triggers a fibroblastic response, resulting in the abnormal collagen deposition. These theories suggest that the fibroblastic response further aggravates the problem by the intimal proliferation seen in blood vessels and the increase in dermal collagen seen in the skin (1, 20). In support of the primary vascular theories, several investigators have found that sera from patients with scleroderma is cytotoxic for endothelial cells (10, 11), but this phenomenon has not been found by all investigators (12). Abnormalities of platelet aggregation and platelet activation have also been detected in patients with scleroderma (13). However, it is not known whether these changes represent primary problems or are secondary to platelet activation as the platelets pass through damaged blood vessels.

Because a mononuclear inflammatory cell infiltrate is present in the dermis of patients with scleroderma (14), and because lymphocyte function is abnormal (15), a primary immunological pathogenesis has been proposed. The lymphocytes in the skin of patients with scleroderma consist largely of T lymphocytes with a predominance of T helper cells (CD-4) (16). In vitro studies have demonstrated that lymphocytes can produce lymphokines, which can augment collagen production by fibroblasts (17). Furthermore, dermal antigens have been shown to stimulate lymphocytes from patients with scleroderma. The patients also show polyclonal hypergammaglobulinemia, and the majority will have autoantibodies, such as antinuclear antibodies (ANA). Studies of peripheral blood have shown a decrease in the number of CD8+ suppressor/cytotoxic T lymphocytes (18), further suggesting an immunological pathogenesis.

CLINICAL FINDINGS

Scleroderma is defined by skin changes that include thickening, tightening, induration, and hidebound changes, which result in contracture and loss of mobility. The disease most characteristically begins peripherally and involves the fingers and hands, with a subsequent centripetal spread up the arms to involve the face and body. Early in the disease, an edematous phase of the skin changes may exist, but late stage disease consists of contractured, shiny, taut, hidebound skin. Telangiectasia and calcinosis are common (1–3).

Skin biopsy results depend upon the stage of cutaneous involvement. Early on, subcutaneous edema, perivascular round cell infiltrates, and interstitial cellular collections are present. With progression, subcutaneous cellular infiltration is replaced by subcutaneous fibrosis, which is the diagnostic histological finding. Late stages of disease demonstrate thinning and loss of the epidermis and absence of epidermal appendages (1).

Vascular disease is common in patients with scleroderma. Over 95% of patients with scleroderma will have Raynaud's phenomenon, which consists of pallor, cyanosis, suffusion, and tingling that occur in an abrupt and phasic manner after a known exposure. Most often, this exposure is to cold, but other precipitating factors include emotion and exposure to vibration tools. Raynaud's disease and Raynaud's syndrome often refer to Raynaud's phenomenon in the absence of any associated systemic disease. Raynaud's phenomenon is due to an exaggerated vasospasm and subsequent vasodilatation in response to the stimulus. Isolated Raynaud's phenomenon is a benign condition. If it is present for more than 2 to 3 years, there is little likelihood that scleroderma or another acquired disease of connective tissue will emerge.

These microvascular abnormalities in systemic sclerosis are widespread, and capillary abnormalities can be detected in the nailfold beds of patients with scleroderma (1). Raynaud's phenomenon may be more systemic in nature, and some studies have suggested that similar events can be detected in the cardiac and renal vasculature upon cold exposure. Histologically, the blood vessels often show intimal proliferation, which sometimes may be associated with fibrinoid necrosis in those patients with severe vascular disease. As a consequence of Raynaud's phenomenon and vascular insufficiency, digital ulcers may develop in patients with scleroderma.

Gastrointestinal involvement is also common and may occur in over 75% of patients with scleroderma. The esophagus is most frequently involved and may show dysmotility, gastroesophageal reflux, and stricture formation. Small bowel involvement is considerably less common and presents with decreased motility, bacterial overgrowth, and malabsorption. Large bowel involvement produces widemouth diverticula.

Pulmonary disease is present in 75% to 90% of patients at autopsy (1) but is less frequently detected clinically. Characteristically, the patients develop pulmonary fibrosis and may have exertional dyspnea, decreased lung capacity, and a restrictive lung disease. As a consequence of this lung disease, they may develop pulmonary hypertension and, in some cases, right heart failure (19, 20). Cardiac disease, which can be detected in approximately one-third of patients, can also develop from fibrotic involvement of the cardiac conducting system, resulting in conduction abnormalities and arrhythmias (21).

Renal disease is a major cause of mortality and is often associated with the onset of malignant hypertension and a rapid progression to renal failure (22, 23). This process, sometimes known as "scleroderma renal crisis" or "scleroderma kidney," was almost uniformly fatal until the late 1970s, but aggressive antihypertensive therapy can reverse the scleroderma renal crisis (24–28).

Musculoskeletal lesions may also occur and are most commonly polyarthralgias or tendon friction rubs (4). Polyarticular arthritis is unusual. Myositis occasionally may occur as an overlap syndrome, sometimes known as sclerodermatomyositis (1–3).

The central nervous system is not usually involved in scleroderma. Peripheral neuropathy can occur and is usually an entrapment neuropathy, apparently caused by fibrosis impinging upon the nerve. Trigeminal neuralgia is the most common example of this neuropathy (29). These lesions generally occur after scleroderma has been present for many years.

The spectrum of disease for systemic sclerosis ranges from the more mild CREST syndrome to the more severe, diffuse scleroderma variant. The CREST syndrome was so named for its features of Calcinosis, Raynaud's phenomenon, Esophageal disease, Sclerodactyly, and Telangiectasia. This syndrome appears to be relatively benign and more slowly progressive. In these patients, visceral involvement is less common than with diffuse scleroderma, although it may occur. However, late stage, CREST syndrome patients may appear similar in nature to early stage, diffuse scleroderma patients. The CREST syndrome is often associated with anticentromere antibodies, which appear to be a marker for this variant (30–33).

Patients with diffuse scleroderma, sometimes known as progressive systemic sclerosis, have a more rapidly progressive skin disease and a more severe and rapidly progressive visceral involvement. These patients have a poorer prognosis than do patients with the CREST variant.

Overlap syndromes occur between scleroderma and other diseases. The best known overlap syndrome is Mixed Connective Tissue Disease (MCTD), which has features of systemic lupus erythematosus, systemic sclerosis, and myositis (34). It is characterized by antibodies to RNP (ribonuclear protein) and a steroid responsiveness of some of the clinical features. Long-term follow-up studies have suggested that MCTD generally evolves into systemic sclerosis (35), and some experts no longer consider MCTD a separate entity.

OCULAR MANIFESTATIONS

Several studies have demonstrated the common involvement of the eye in patients with scleroderma (36, 37). Most often, this involvement consists of scleroderma of the eyelids, resulting in tightness of the lids and blepharophimosis. Lid involvement occurs in 30% to 65% of patients. Despite the frequent involvement of the eyelids, corneal exposure is uncommon. Conjunctival vascular anomalies, including telangiectasia and vascular sludging, can occur, with prevalence estimates as high as 71%. These changes in the conjunctival vasculature may be analogous to those seen in the nailfold capillary bed. Keratoconjunctivitis sicca with a Sjögren's-like picture has been described (36–39). Minor salivary gland biopsy studies have suggested that two different pathogenetic mechanisms may be present (38). Some patients have inflammation of the glands, similar to Sjögren's syndrome, and this mechanism seems to be associated more often with the CREST syndrome. The other pathogenetic mechanism appears to be glandular fibrosis, which has been seen more often in patients with diffuse systemic sclerosis. Whereas earlier studies suggested good correlation with these two variants (28), later studies have suggested that the issue is not as clearcut (39).

Other lesions have included periorbital edema occurring as part of the early edematous phase of scleroderma (40), cranial nerve pareses (41), and extraocular muscle myositis occurring in a patient with sclerodermatomyositis (42). All of these have been described as case reports but are not common.

In patients without scleroderma renal disease, retinal vascular lesions are relatively uncommon, occurring in less than 5% of patients. Findings described include retinal hemorrhage, branch retinal vein occlusion, and central retinal vein occlusion in a patient with secondary polycythemia from scleroderma lung disease (36, 37, 43). Rarely, retinal nonperfusion and neovascularization can be seen.

By far, the most commonly described retinal lesion in patients with scleroderma has been the retinopathy of malignant hypertension (44–49), including cotton-wool spots, intraretinal hemorrhage, and optic disc edema. Both clinical and histological studies have demonstrated that the picture is identical to that of idiopathic malignant hypertension. These patients have malignant hypertension due to scleroderma renal crisis. Pathological studies have shown early hyalinization of the ciliary arteries, microinfarcts of the nerve fiber layer exhibiting multiple cytoid bodies, neuroretinal edema, subretinal exudates, optic disc edema, and fibrinoid changes consisting of fibrin plugs in the choroidal arterioles and the choriocapillaris.

In contrast to the infrequent findings of retinopathy in patients with scleroderma, fluorescein angiographic studies have suggested more frequent abnormalities of the choroid (50–53). Grenan and Foster (50) have reported patchy and irregular perfusion of the choroid in patients with systemic sclerosis. Fluorescein angiography was performed in 10 patients with systemic sclerosis, all of whom had normal ophthalmoscopy. Five patients had patchy choroidal nonperfusion, which was not related to hypertension. In only one case was the patient found to have abnormal retinal vessels and microaneurysms. Clinically, these lesions were silent. In their histological study, Farkas et al. (51) reported extensive choroidal disease with sclerosis of the choroidal precapillary arterioles, PAS-positive material in the vessel walls, decreased lumina of the choroidal vessels, endothelial hypertrophy, and areas of obliteration of the choriocapillaris. The patient had microinfarcts of the nerve fiber layer and a serous detachment in the fovea. On electron microscopy, the basement membrane of the choriocapillaris was thickened up to 6 to 10 times normal, with endothelial cell swelling and islets of totally degenerated choriocapillaris. Larger vessels contained swollen endothelial cells. These changes were similar to the vascular abnormalities found elsewhere in the body and were probably due in part to the patient's associated hypertension. More recently, Serup et al. (52) have demonstrated abnormalities of choroidal fluorescence in one-third of 21 patients studied with fluorescein angiography. Again, the lesions were clinically silent and ophthalmoscopy was normal. Angiographic abnormalities consisted of variable hyperfluorescence of the pigment epithelial layer and, in two cases, of minute hyperfluorescence of the retinal layer. These angiographic abnormalities were interpreted as damage to the retinal pigment epithelium caused by vascular lesions in the choroid. The authors concluded that abnormalities of the choroidal vasculature could be detected by fluorescein angiography in one-third of patients with generalized scleroderma.

In general, retinal complications are uncommon in patients with scleroderma unless hypertension is present. Occasionally, retinal vascular disease can herald the onset of malignant hypertension and a medical emergency for the scleroderma patient. Choroidal vascular changes may be more common but are generally clinically silent.

TREATMENT

No specific treatment has been definitely determined to be efficacious in altering the progression of scleroderma and, traditionally, treatment has been directed toward management of the complications and symptomatic relief. More recently, D-penicillamine therapy has attracted considerable attention as a potential agent for treating the sclerodermatous process (53). Steroids have not proven to be of benefit in the treatment of scleroderma but may occasionally be used for treatment of an associated myositis in patients with an overlap syndrome. In this situation, the steroids are used for the myositic component rather than for the sclerodermatous component. Immunosuppressive agents have not shown any consistent value in the treatment of scleroderma.

Scleroderma renal crisis, which was previously a fatal complication, can often be controlled by aggressive treatment of the hypertension and dialysis for renal failure. Control of the hypertension generally involves the use of multiple antihypertensive agents including angiotensin-converting enzyme inhibitors. Long-term successful outcomes have been accomplished using this medication (25–28).

Raynaud's phenomenon is most often treated with calcium channel antagonists, particularly nifedipine (54, 55). Studies have generally shown that this agent is effective for symptomatic relief and reduction of the number of attacks in patients with Raynaud's phenomenon. The studies generally show that calcium channel antagonists are more effective in patients with idiopathic Raynaud's phenomenon than in those with scleroderma. This finding may reflect the fixed, vascular changes caused by the luminal narrowing in patients with scleroderma. Serotonin antagonists have also been tried in the treatment of Raynaud's phenomenon (56).

D-penicillamine has been used to treat systemic sclerosis. It inhibits the cross-linking of collagen and may be of benefit in reducing the cutaneous fibrosis, which is the hallmark of the disease. Retrospective analysis (53) of D-penicillamine therapy has suggested that the extent of the skin thickening, rate of new visceral organ involvement, and survival are improved in patients treated with this agent. To date, no randomized, placebo-controlled, prospective study has documented the efficacy of D-penicillamine in the treatment of scleroderma.

References

1. LeRoy EC. Scleroderma (systemic sclerosis). In: Kelley WN, Harris ED Jr, Ruddy S, Sledge CB, eds. Textbook of rheumatology. 2nd ed. Philadelphia: WB Saunders, 1985:1183–1205.
2. Tuffanelli DL, Winkelmann RK. Systemic scleroderma; a clinical study of 727 cases. Arch Dermatol 1961;84:359–371.
3. Rodnan GP. The natural history of progressive systemic sclerosis (diffuse scleroderma). Bull Rheum Dis 1963;13:301–304.
4. Falanga V, Medsger TA Jr, Reichlin M, Rodnan GP. Linear scleroderma; clinical spectrum, prognosis, and laboratory abnormalities. Ann Intern Med 1986;104:849–857.
5. Medsger TA Jr, Masi AT. Epidemiology of systemic sclerosis (scleroderma). Ann Intern Med 1971;74:714–721.
6. Rodnan GP, Lipinski E, Luksick J. Skin thickness and collagen content in progressive systemic sclerosis and localized scleroderma. Arthritis Rheum 1979;22:130–140.
7. LeRoy EC. Increased collagen synthesis by scleroderma skin fibroblasts in vitro: a possible defect in the regulation or activation of the scleroderma fibroblast. J Clin Invest 1974;54:880–889.
8. Buckingham RB, Prince RK, Rodnan GP, Taylor F. Increased collagen accumulation in dermal fibroblast cultures from patients with progressive systemic sclerosis (scleroderma). J Lab Clin Med 1978;92:5–21.
9. Perlish JS, Bashey RI, Stephens RE, Fleischmajer R. Connective tissue synthesis by cultured scleroderma fibroblasts. I. In vitro collagen synthesis by normal and scleroderma dermal fibroblasts. Arthritis Rheum 1976;19:891–901.
10. Kahaleh MB, Sherer GK, LeRoy EC. Endothelial cell injury in scleroderma. J Exp Med 1979;149:1326–1335.
11. Cohen S, Johnson AR, Hurd E. Cytotoxicity of sera from patients with scleroderma; effects on human endothelial cells and fibroblasts in culture. Arthritis Rheum 1983;26:170–178.
12. Shanahan WR Jr, Korn JH. Cytotoxic activity of sera from scleroderma and other connective tissue diseases; lack of cellular and disease specificity. Arthritis Rheum 1982;25:1391–1395.
13. Kahaleh MB, Osborn I, LeRoy EC. Elevated levels of circulating platelet aggregates and beta-thromboglobulin in scleroderma. Ann Intern Med 1982;96:610–613.
14. Haynes DC, Gershwin ME. The immunopathology of progressive systemic sclerosis (PSS). Semin Arthritis Rheum 1982;11:331–351.
15. Kondo H, Rabin BS, Rodnan GP. Cutaneous an-

tigen-stimulating lymphokine production by lymphocytes of patients with progressive systemic sclerosis (scleroderma). J Clin Invest 1976;58:1388–1394.

16. Roumm AD, Whiteside TL, Medsger TA Jr, Rodnan GP. Lymphocytes in the skin of patients with progressive systemic sclerosis; quantification, subtyping, and clinical correlations. Arthritis Rheum 1984;27:645–653.

17. Johnson RL, Ziff M. Lymphokine stimulation of collagen accumulation. J Clin Invest 1976;58:240–252.

18. Whiteside TL, Kumagai Y, Roumm AD, et al. Suppressor cell function and T lymphocyte subpopulations in peripheral blood of patients with progressive systemic sclerosis. Arthritis Rheum 1983;26:841–847.

19. Steen VD, Owens GR, Fino GJ, et al. Pulmonary involvement in systemic sclerosis (scleroderma). Arthritis Rheum 1985;28:759–767.

20. Ungerer RG, Tashkin DP, Furst D, et al. Prevalence and clinical correlates of pulmonary arterial hypertension in progressive systemic sclerosis. Am J Med 1983;75:65–74.

21. Roberts NK, Cabeen WR Jr, Moss J, et al. The prevalence of conduction defects and cardiac arrhythmias in progressive systemic sclerosis. Ann Intern Med 1981;94:38–40.

22. Cannon PJ, Hassar M, Case DB, et al. The relationship of hypertension and renal failure in scleroderma (progressive systemic sclerosis) to structural and functional abnormalities of the renal cortical circulation. Medicine 1974;53:1–46.

23. Kovalchik MT, Guggenheim SJ, Silverman MH, et al. The kidney in progressive systemic sclerosis: a prospective study. Ann Intern Med 1978;89:881–887.

24. Mitnick PD, Feig PU. Control of hypertension and reversal of renal failure in scleroderma. N Engl J Med 1978;299:871–872.

25. Wasner C, Cooke CR, Fries JF. Successful medical treatment of scleroderma renal crisis. N Engl J Med 1978;299:873–875.

26. Lopez-Ovejero JA, Saal SD, D'Angelo WA, et al. Reversal of vascular and renal crises of scleroderma by oral angiotensin-converting-enzyme blockade. N Engl J Med 1979;300:1417–1419.

27. Sorensen LB, Paunicka K, Harris M. Reversal of scleroderma renal crisis for more than two years in a patient treated with captopril. Arthritis Rheum 1983;26:797–800.

28. Thurm RH, Alexander JC. Captopril in the treatment of scleroderma renal crisis. Arch Intern Med 1984;144:733–735.

29. Teasdall RD, Frayha RA, Shulman LE. Cranial nerve involvement in systemic sclerosis (scleroderma): a report of 10 cases. Medicine 1980;59:149–159.

30. Fritzler MJ, Kinsella TD, Garbutt E. The CREST syndrome: a distinct serologic entity with anticentromere antibodies. Am J Med 1980;69:520–526.

31. Tan EM, Rodnan GP, Garcia I, et al. Diversity of antinuclear antibodies in progressive systemic sclerosis. Anticentromere antibody and its relationship to CREST syndrome. Arthritis Rheum 1980;23:617–625.

32. McCarty GA, Rice JR, Bembe ML, Barada FA Jr. Anticentromere antibody; clinical correlations and association with favorable prognosis in patients with scleroderma variants. Arthritis Rheum 1983;26:1–7.

33. Powell FC, Winkelmann RK, Venecie-Lemarchand F, et al. The anticentromere antibody: disease specificity and clinical significance. Mayo Clin Proc 1984;59:700–706.

34. Sharp GC, Irvin WS, Tan EM, et al. Mixed connective tissue disease—an apparently distinct rheumatic disease syndrome associated with a specific antibody to an extractable nuclear antigen (ENA). Am J Med 1972;52:148–159.

35. Nimelstein SH, Brody S, McShane D, Holman HR. Mixed connective tissue disease: a subsequent evaluation of the original 25 patients. Medicine 1980;59:239–248.

36. Horan EC. Ophthalmic manifestations of progressive systemic sclerosis. Br J Ophthalmol 1969;53:388–392.

37. West RH, Barnett AJ. Ocular involvement in scleroderma. Br J Ophthalmol 1979;63:845–847.

38. Cipoletti JF, Buckingham RB, Barnes EL, et al. Sjogren's syndrome in progressive systemic sclerosis. Ann Intern Med 1977;87:535–541.

39. Osial TA Jr, Whiteside TL, Buckingham RB, et al. Clinical and serologic study of Sjogren's syndrome in patients with progressive systemic sclerosis. Arthritis Rheum 1983;26:500–508.

40. Dorwart BB. Periorbital edema in progressive systemic sclerosis. Ann Intern Med 1974;80:273.

41. Rush JA. Isolated superior oblique paralysis in progressive systemic sclerosis. Ann Ophthalmol 1981;13:217–220.

42. Arnett FC, Michels RG. Inflammatory ocular myopathy in systemic sclerosis (scleroderma); a case report and review of the literature. Arch Intern Med 1973;132:740–743.

43. Saari KM, Rudenberg HA, Laitinen O. Bilateral central retinal vein occlusion in a patient with scleroderma. Ophthalmologica 1981;182:7–12.

44. Pollack IP, Becker B. Cytoid bodies of the retina in a patient with scleroderma. Am J Ophthalmol 1962;54:655–660.

45. Manschot WA. Generalized scleroderma with ocular symptoms. Ophthalmologica 1965;149:131–137.

46. Klien BA. Comments on the cotton-wool lesion of the retina. Am J Ophthalmol 1965;59:17–23.

47. Ashton N, Coomes EN, Garner A, Oliver DO. Retinopathy due to progressive systemic sclerosis. J Pathol Bacteriol 1968;96:259–268.

48. Maclean H, Guthrie W. Retinopathy in scleroderma. Trans Ophthalmol Soc UK 1969;89:209–220.

49. Henkind P, Gold DH. Ocular manifestations of rheumatic disorders; natural and iatrogenic. Rheumatology 1973;4:13–59.

50. Grennan DM, Forrester J. Involvement of the eye in SLE and scleroderma; a study using fluorescein angiography in addition to clinical ophthalmic assessment. Ann Rheum Dis 1977;36:152–156.

51. Farkas TG, Sylvester V, Archer D. The choroidopathy of progressive systemic sclerosis (scleroderma). Am J Ophthalmol 1972;74:875–886.

52. Serup L, Serup J, Hagdrup H. Fundus fluorescein angiography in generalized scleroderma. Ophthalmic Res 1987;19:303–308.

53. Steen VD, Medsger TA Jr, Rodnan GP. D-penicillamine therapy in progressive systemic sclerosis (scleroderma); a retrospective analysis. Ann Intern Med 1982;97:652–659.

54. Rodeheffer RJ, Rommer JA, Wigley F, Smith CR. Controlled double-blind trial of nifedipine in the treatment of Raynaud's phenomenon. N Engl J Med 1983;308:880–883.

55. White CJ, Phillips WA, Abrahams LA, et al. Objective benefit of nifedipine in the treatment of Raynaud's phenomenon; double-blind controlled study. Am J Med 1986;80:623–625.

56. Seibold JR, Jaganeau AHM. Treatment of Raynaud's phenomenon with ketanserin, a selective antagonist of the serotonin$_2$ (5-HT$_2$) receptor. Arthritis Rheum 1984;27:139–146.

Rheumatoid Arthritis

INTRODUCTION

Rheumatoid arthritis is the most common inflammatory rheumatic disorder, with an estimated prevalence of 0.3% to 2.1% in the general population (1). Rheumatoid arthritis is a clinical diagnosis, characterized by an additive, symmetrical, deforming polyarthritis (2). Eighty percent of the patients demonstrate a positive rheumatoid factor, which is an autoantibody directed against IgG. It cannot be overemphasized, however, that rheumatoid factor does not define rheumatoid arthritis and that rheumatoid arthritis is a clinical diagnosis. Therefore, the American Rheumatism Association has devised criteria for the diagnosis of rheumatoid arthritis. These criteria have recently been revised (3) and are outlined in Table 1.5.

PATHOPHYSIOLOGY

The etiology of rheumatoid arthritis is unknown. However, a genetic predisposition to the disease appears to be evident, as there is a statistical association of rheumatoid arthritis and the HLA type DR4 (4).

Current theories of the pathogenesis of rheumatoid arthritis postulate an inciting immunologic event, either one involving immune complexes or one of a cellular nature, producing inflammation within the joint, subsequently leading to synovial proliferation and joint destruction (4–6). Immunohistological studies of the joint space have shown an early accumulation of T lymphocytes, sometimes surrounding germinal centers of B cells (7). Plasma cells are also present. Subsequently, proliferation of synovial fibroblasts occurs, with synovial hypertrophy and pannus formation. Class II antigen expression can be detected in all phases of the disease. In addition, in established rheumatoid arthritis, an accumulation of polymorphonuclear leukocytes (PMNs) occurs in the synovial fluid, suggesting recruitment of PMNs to this compartment. Possibly this is due to immune complexes and complement activation.

Studies of peripheral blood mononuclear cells in rheumatoid arthritis have generally revealed no consistent abnormalities, with variable CD-4:CD-8 ratios reported. More recent studies have suggested that there may be a deficiency of that subset of helper/inducer T lymphocytes that induces suppressor T cells (CD 4, 2H-4) in patients with rheumatoid arthritis (8). The contribution of rheumatoid factors to the pathogenesis of the disease remains unclear, although they are a useful marker for the disease itself (except in children). Circulating immune complexes can be detected in patients with rheumatoid arthritis, although it is uncertain whether they are pathogenic for the arthritis. Most likely, they contribute to the rheumatoid vasculitis seen in a small percentage of patients with rheumatoid arthritis (9).

CLINICAL FINDINGS

The onset of rheumatoid arthritis is generally insidious. However, in 10% to 20% of patients with rheumatoid arthritis, an explosive onset may occur. The arthritis, classically an additive, symmetrical, deforming polyarthritis, is described as peripheral, affecting the small joints of the hands and feet, though all joints can be involved. The disease is characterized by a gel phenomenon, the most common manifestation of which is morning stiffness. X-rays of the affected joints show erosions of the bone at the joint margin, with subsequent joint destruction in longstanding disease. Because of the damage to the surrounding structures, joint laxity may develop, one manifestation of which is characteristic ulnar deviation of the fingers (2). Extra-articular features are common (2, 4).

The most common extra-articular lesion in patients with rheumatoid arthritis is rheumatoid nodules. These nodules occur in approximately 25% of patients, and are classically located on the extensor surfaces. They have a characteristic histological picture of central fibrinoid necrosis exhibiting a palisade of elongated, histiocyte-like cells around the necrotic zone. This core is enveloped by an outer zone of the mononuclear inflammatory cells, primarily lymphocytes and plasma cells (4). Immunohistochemical analysis has demonstrated that class II antigen expression is present throughout the lesion and that the cells within the palisading layer stain for monocyte markers. The peripheral lymphocytes are predominantly T cells (10).

Possible pulmonary lesions include pleurisy, plumonary effusions, and pleural nodules. Pulmonary nodules may occasionally be seen, and interstitial fibrosis may be present. Caplan's syndrome consists of a severe pneumoconiosis in association with rheumatoid arthritis. In Caplan's syndrome, the two processes are synergistic, and a violent, fibroblastic reaction is seen in the lungs,

Table 1.5. The 1987 Revised Criteria for the Classification of Rheumatoid Arthritis[a, b]

Criterion	Definition[c]
1. Morning stiffness	Morning stiffness in and around the joints, lasting at least 1 hour before maximal improvement.
2. Arthritis of 3 or more joint areas	At least 3 joint areas simultaneously have had soft tissue swelling or fluid (not bony outgrowth alone) observed by a physician. The 14 possible areas are right or left PIP, MCP, wrist, elbow, knee, ankle, and MTP joint.
3. Arthritis of hand joints	At least 1 area swollen (as defined above) in a wrist, MCP, or PIP joint.
4. Symmetrical arthritis	Simultaneous involvement of the same joint areas (as defined in 2) on both sides of the body (bilateral involvement of PIPs, MCPs, or MTPs is acceptable without absolute symmetry).
5. Rheumatoid nodules	Subcutaneous nodules, over bony prominences, or extensor surfaces, or in juxtaarticular regions, observed by a physician.
6. Serum rheumatoid factor	Demonstration of abnormal amounts of serum rheumatoid factor by any method for which the result has been positive in <5% of normal control subjects.
7. Radiographical changes	Radiographical changes typical of rheumatoid arthritis on posteroanterior hand and wrist radiographs, which must include erosions or unequivocal bony decalcification localized in, or most marked adjacent to, the involved joints (osteoarthritis changes alone do not qualify).

[a]Arnett FC, Edworthy SM, Bloch DA, et al. The American Rheumatism Association 1987 revised criteria for the classification of rheumatoid arthritis. Arthritis Rheum 1988;31:315–324.
[b]For classification purposes, a patient shall be said to have rheumatoid arthritis if he has satisfied at least 4 of these 7 criteria.
[c]Abbreviations: PIP—proximal interphalangeal joints; MCP—metacarpal-phalangeal joint; MTP—metatarsal-phalangeal joint.

accompanied by an ultimately obliterative granulomatous fibrosis. This disease, characteristically seen in miners, has become less severe as the respiratory environment in mines has improved (2).

Cardiac involvement includes pericarditis, detected in up to 50% of patients at autopsy but much less frequently at clinical evaluation. Cardiac conduction defects can occur as a consequence of rheumatoid nodules present in the conducting system, and rheumatoid nodules have been detected on the heart valves (2).

Rheumatoid vasculitis, also known as rheumatoid arteritis, is seen in less than 1% of patients with rheumatoid arthritis. It often will present with a polyneuropathy or skin ulceration and infection. Digital gangrene and visceral ischemia may also be seen. Nonhealing peripheral leg ulcers are common findings (11–13).

Felty's syndrome consists of rheumatoid arthritis, splenomegaly, and leukopenia. The etiology of the leukopenia is unknown. Other characteristic features include hyperpigmentation of the skin, chronic leg ulcers, and recurrent infections (14).

OCULAR MANIFESTATIONS

The eye is frequently involved in patients with rheumatoid arthritis, and the most common ocular problems are keratoconjunctivitis sicca (Sjögren's syndrome) and scleritis (15).

Sjögren's syndrome was originally defined as dry eyes, dry mouth, and rheumatoid arthritis. It has subsequently become evident that Sjögren's syndrome can exist as secondary Sjögren's syndrome, in which the sicca complex is associated with acquired disease of connective tissue, or as primary Sjögren's syndrome, in which the sicca complex has no definable associated connective tissue disease. In Sjögren's syndrome, there is a lymphocytic infiltration in the lacrimal and salivary glands, resulting in glandular destruction and dysfunction. As a consequence of this process, the characteristic loss of tear and saliva production occurs. Approximately 11% to 13% of patients with rheumatoid arthritis will have secondary Sjögren's syndrome (16).

Scleral inflammation is the second most common problem in patients with rheumatoid arthritis. Watson (15) has classified scleral disease as episcleritis and scleritis. Scleritis is characterized by more severe ocular discomfort (often pain), deeper inflammation, more frequent ocular complications, and greater association with systemic disease than is episcleritis. Scleritis may be classified as anterior, posterior, or necrotizing. Anterior scleritis may be further classified as either diffuse or nodular (Fig. 1.6). In addition to the characteristic necrotizing scleritis (Fig. 1.6) with an active inflammatory process, scleromalacia perforans, in which there is a more insidious but equally destructive scleral process, may be seen in patients with rheumatoid arthritis. Most often, anterior scleritis is present in rheumatoid arthritis patients, although any type may be seen. Necrotizing scleritis (Fig. 1.7) may be seen in association with rheumatoid vasculitis.

Approximately 1% of patients with rheumatoid arthritis will have scleral disease (16), although estimates have run as high as 6% (17). Of patients with scleritis, 10% to 33% will have rheumatoid arthritis (15, 16), which is the most commonly seen acquired disease of connective tissue in patients with scleritis. Several retrospective studies have suggested that scleritis is associated with more severe systemic disease, in particular, a greater frequency of extraarticular manifestations (11, 13, 16). Necrotizing scleritis appears to be associated with a poor prognosis, possibly due to its relationship with rheumatoid vasculitis.

Another less common ocular lesion in rheumatoid arthritis is the marginal furrow (19, 20), which may be benign or noninflammatory and can be treated with local measures (21), or which may be necrotizing in nature and require aggressive medical therapy (18). Brown's syndrome has been described in a few patients and appears to be secondary to a stenosing tenosynovitis of the superior oblique tendon (22, 23). Ocular chrysiasis consists of deposition of gold crystals in the cornea of patients treated with gold compounds but generally does not affect vision (24).

Posterior segment lesions due to rheumatoid arthritis are uncommon (25, 26). Meyer et al. (27) reported a 67-year-old woman with rheumatoid arthritis, pericarditis, and cotton-wool spots responsive to oral corticosteroids. Posterior scleritis (Fig. 1.7) has also been infrequently described in patients with rheumatoid arthritis (28).

Probably the most common reason for performing an ophthalmic evaluation of the posterior segment in a patient with rheumatoid arthritis is to monitor the patient for antimalarial drug toxicity (29–33). The antimalarial drugs chloroquine and hydroxychloroquine have an anti-inflammatory effect, and because of their relative lack of toxicity, they are commonly used as first-line remittive agents in treating rheumatoid arthritis. Hydroxychloroquine is now used almost exclusively because it is apparently less toxic

than chloroquine (31). Both drugs are accumulated in pigmented tissues, such as the retinal pigment epithelium, and may cause a "bull's-eye" pigmentary retinopathy. The retinopathy of antimalarial drugs is said to be reversible if discovered early, but it may be irreversible, even progressive, despite discontinuation of the drug, if not detected early. Because of this toxicity, patients receiving antimalarial drugs are often given screening ophthalmic examinations so that the earliest signs of antimalarial toxicity can be detected. These examinations are generally conducted every 6 months while the patient is on hydroxychloroquine. Studies (32) have suggested that the frequency of retinopathy is less than 5% when dosages less than 6.5 mg/kg/day of hydroxychloroquine are used (generally less than 400 mg/day), and that patients can be treated with large total doses without evidence of toxicity when these daily doses are used (33).

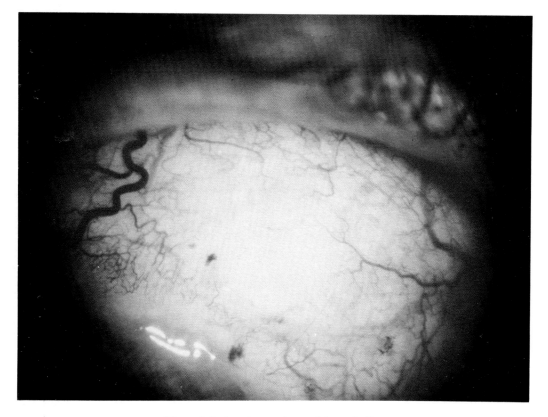

Figure 1.6. Local area of necrotizing scleritis.

TREATMENT

Treatment of rheumatoid arthritis is instituted in a stepwise, additive fashion, with the initial therapy being a nonsteroidal antiinflammatory drug (NSAID) (2). All of the different NSAIDs (e.g., aspirin, indomethacin, naproxen, sulindac, piroxicam, etc.) appear to be approximately equally efficacious, although the response of the individual patient may vary from drug to drug. The second step in treatment is to add a remittive agent, sometimes also known as a slow-acting antirheumatic drug (SAARD) (34). Remittive agents include hydroxychloroquine, gold, and penicillamine. They often take several months to have an effect, but they can induce a remission of the active rheumatoid arthritis. Hydroxychloroquine is used first by some rheumatologists because of its relative lack of toxicity. Gold has been demonstrated to be effective in randomized controlled studies (35) and is given as a first choice by some as an intramuscular injection. More recently, an oral form of gold has become available and has demonstrated efficacy in the treatment of rheumatoid arthritis (36). D-Penicillamine is almost as effective as gold, although an individual patient may respond better to one drug than to the other. Because of their toxicity, the immunosuppressive drugs (e.g., azathioprine and cyclophosphamide) are reserved for severe cases only (37). They are often used to treat rheumatoid vasculitis (12). Low-dose prednisone (e.g., 5 to 10 mg/day or every other day) is sometimes added to the treatment regimen to increase the patient's mobility and functional capacity. If a patient fails treatment with an NSAID only, most rheumatologists will then add a remittive agent with or without low-dose corticosteroids.

Newer forms of therapy include intrave-

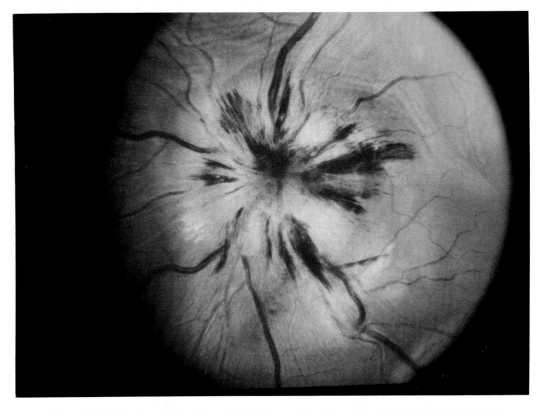

Figure 1.7. Posterior scleritis with a choked disc, papillary hemorrhages, and venous dilatation.

nous pulse methylprednisolone (38), methotrexate therapy (39–41), combined drug therapy (42), and total lymphoid irradiation (43–46). Intravenous pulse methylprednisolone, given as an infusion of 1 gm of methylprednisolone, often has a dramatic benefit in rheumatoid arthritis. However, this benefit is often short-lived. The drug is useful as an initial adjunct to therapy while waiting for a remittive agent to take effect. Some investigators have used regular monthly "pulses" with success (38).

Several studies have demonstrated that methotrexate is also an effective agent for managing refractory rheumatoid arthritis (39–41). The improvement generally is lost when the drug is discontinued. Methotrexate may cause cirrhosis, but the methotrexate is felt to be considerably less toxic than azathioprine or cyclophosphamide. Thus, it has found a role in treating rheumatoid arthritis, usually after failure of a drug like gold or hydroxychloroquine.

In very severe or refractory rheumatoid arthritis, some authors have tried combination chemotherapy with cyclophosphamide, azathioprine, and hydroxychloroquine (42), or total lymphoid irradiation (43–46). These regimens are currently considered investigational, and their long-term utility remains to be determined.

Keratoconjunctivitis sicca in patients with Sjögren's symdrome should be treated with the frequent instillation of tear substitutes. Bland corneal melts can be treated with lubrication, local measures to promote reepithelialization, and tissue adhesive, if necessary (21). Necrotizing marginal keratitis requires systemic antiinflammatory medications (18) or conjunctival recession or resection. Grafting may be necessary in severe cases to maintain or restore the integrity of the globe. Anterior scleritis can be treated with indomethacin, which seems to be more effective than many other NSAIDs (15). Posterior scleritis and necrotizing scleritis often require treatment with systemic corticosteroids, generally at an initial dosage of prednisone of 1 mg/kg/day; necrotizing scleritis (like necrotizing keratitis) may sometimes require treatment with immunosuppressive drugs in addition to systemic corticosteroids (15, 18).

References

1a. Wolfe AM. The epidemiology of rheumatoid arthritis: a review. I. Surveys. Bull Rheum Dis 1968;19:518–523.

1b. Wolfe AM, Kellgren JH, Masi AT. The epidemiology of rheumatoid arthritis: a review. II. Incidence and diagnostic criteria. Bull Rheum Dis 1968:19:524–529.

2. Harris ED Jr. Rheumatoid arthritis: the clinical spectrum. In: Kelley WN, Harris ED Jr, Ruddy S, Sledge CB, eds. Textbook of rheumatology. 2nd ed. Philadelphia: WB Saunders, 1985:915–950.

3. Arnett FC, Edworthy SM, Bloch DA, et al. The American Rheumatism Association 1987 revised criteria for the classification of rheumatoid arthritis. Arthritis Rheum 1988;31:315–324.

4. Stastny P. Immmunogenetic factors in rheumatoid arthritis. Clin Rheum Dis 1977;3:315–332.

5. Zvaifler NJ. The immunopathology of joint inflammation in rheumatoid arthritis. Adv Immunol 1973;16:265–336.

6. Decker JL, Malone DG, Haraoui B, et al. Rheumatoid arthritis: evolving concepts of pathogenesis and treatment. Ann Intern Med 1984;101:810–824.

7. Young CL, Adamson TC III, Vaughan JH, Fox RI. Immunohistologic characterization of synovial membrane lymphocytes in rheumatoid arthritis. Arthritis Rheum 1984;27:32–39.

8. Emery P, Gentry KC, Mackay IR, et al. Deficiency of the suppressor inducer subset of T lymphocytes in rheumatoid arthritis. Arthritis Rheum 1987;30:849–856.

9. Hurd ER. Extraarticular manifestations of rheumatoid arthritis. Semin Arthritis Rheum 1979;8:151–176.

10. Hedfors E, Klareskog L, Lindblad S, et al. Phenotypic characterization of cells within subcutaneous rheumatoid nodules. Arthritis Rheum 1983;26:1333–1339.

11. Schmid FR, Cooper NS, Ziff M, McEwen C. Arteritis in rheumatoid arthritis. Am J Med 1961;30:56–83.

12. Abel T, Andrews BS, Cunningham PH, et al. Rheumatoid vasculitis: effect of cyclophosphamide on the clinical course and levels of circulating immune complexes. Ann Intern Med 1980;93:407–413.

13. Scott DGI, Bacon PA, Tribe CR. Systemic rheumatoid vasculitis: a clinical and laboratory study of 50 cases. Medicine 1981;60:288–297.

14. Goldberg J, Pinals RS. Felty syndrome. Semin Arthritis Rheum 1980;10:52–65.

15. Watson PG, Hazleman BL. The sclera and systemic disorders. Philadelphia: WB Saunders, 1976.

16. Williamson J. Incidence of eye disease in cases of connective tissue disease. Trans Ophthalmol Soc UK 1974;94:742–752.

17. Jayson MIV, Jones DEP. Scleritis and rheumatoid arthritis. Ann Rheum Dis 1971;30:343–347.

18. Foster CS, Forstot SL, Wilson LA. Mortality rate in rheumatoid arthritis patients developing necrotizing scleritis or peripheral ulcerative keratitis; effects of systemic immunosuppression. Ophthalmology 1984;91:1253–1263.

19. Brown SI, Grayson M. Marginal furrows; a characteristic corneal lesion of rheumatoid arthritis. Arch Ophthalmol 1968;79:563–567.

20. Lyne AJ. "Contact lens" cornea in rheumatoid arthritis. Br J Ophthalmol 1970;54:410–415.

21. Weiss JL, Williams P, Lindstrom RL, Doughman DJ. The use of tissue adhesive in corneal perforations. Ophthalmology 1983;90:610–615.

22. Sandford-Smith JH. Intermittent superior oblique tendon sheath syndrome; a case report. Br J Ophthalmol 1969;53:412–417.

23. Killian PJ, McClain B, Lawless OJ. Brown's syndrome; an unusual manifestation of rheumatoid arthritis. Arthritis Rheum 1977;20:1080–1084.

24. McCormick SA, DiBartolomeo AG, Raju VK, Schwab IR. Ocular chrysiasis. Ophthalmology 1985;92:1432–1435.

25. Henkind P, Gold DH. Ocular manifestations of rheumatic disorders. Rheumatology 1973;4:13–59.

26. Scherbel AL, Mackenzie AH, Nousek JE, Atdjian M. Ocular lesions in rheumatoid arthritis and related disorders with particular reference to retinopathy. A study of 741 patients treated with and without chloroquine drugs. N Engl J Med 1965;273:360–366.

27. Meyer E, Scharf J, Miller B, et al. Fundus lesions in rheumatoid arthritis. Ann Ophthalmol 1978;10:1583–1584.

28. Hurd ER, Snyder WB, Ziff M. Choroidal nodules and retinal detachments in rheumatoid arthritis. Improvement with fall in immunoglobulin levels following prednisolone and cyclophosphamide therapy. Am J Med 1970;48:273–278.

29. Hobbs HE, Sorsby A, Freedman A. Retinopathy following chloroquine therapy. Lancet 1959;2:478–480.

30. Shearer RV, Dubois EL. Ocular changes induced by long-term hydroxychloroquine (Plaquenil) therapy. Am J Ophthalmol 1967;64:245–252.

31. Finbloom DS, Silver K, Newsome DA, Gunkel R. Comparison of hydroxychloroquine and chloroquine use and the development of retinal toxicity. J Rheumatol 1985;12:692–694.

32. Tobin DR, Krohel GB, Rynes RI. Hydroxychloroquine; seven year experience. Arch Ophthalmol 1982;100:81–83.

33. Johnson MW, Vine AK. Hydroxychloroquine therapy in massive total doses without retinal toxicity. Am J Ophthalmol 1987;104:139–144.

34. Bunch TW, O'Duffy JD. Disease-modifying drugs for progressive rheumatoid arthritis. Mayo Clin Proc 1980;55:161–179.

35. Research Subcommittee of the Empire Rheumatism Council. Gold therapy in rheumatoid arthritis: final report of a multicentre controlled trial. Ann Rheum Dis 1961;20:315–334.

36. Ward JR, Williams HJ, Egger MJ, et al. Comparison of auranofin, gold sodium thiomalate, and placebo in the treatment of rheumatoid arthritis; a controlled clinical trial. Arthritis Rheum 1983;26:1303–1315.

37. Townes AS, Sowa JM, Shulman LE. Controlled trial of cyclophosphamide in rheumatoid arthritis. Arthritis Rheum 1976;19:563–573.

38. Liebling MR, Leib E, McLaughlin K, et al. Pulse methylprednisolone in rheumatoid arthritis: a double-blind cross-over trial. Ann Intern Med 1981;94:21–26.

39. Williams HJ, Willkens RF, Samuelson CO Jr, et al. Comparison of low-dose oral pulse methotrexate and placebo in the treatment of rheumatoid arthritis; a controlled clinical trial. Arthritis Rheum 1985;28:721–730.

40. Andersen PA, West SG, O'Dell JR, et al. Weekly pulse methotrexate in rheumatoid arthritis; clinical and immunologic effects in a randomized, double-blind study. Ann Intern Med 1985;103:489–496.

41. Kremer JM, Lee JK. The safety and efficacy of the use of methotrexate in long-term therapy for rheumatoid arthritis. Arthritis Rheum 1986;29:822–831.

42. Csuka ME, Carrera GF, McCarty DJ. Treatment of intractable rheumatoid arthritis with combined cyclophosphamide, azathioprine, and hydroxychloroquine: a follow-up study. JAMA 1986;255:2315–2319.

43. Kotzin BL, Strober S, Engleman EG, et al. Treatment of intractable rheumatoid arthritis with total lymphoid irradiation. N Engl J Med 1981;305:969–976.

44. Trentham DE, Belli JA, Anderson RJ, et al. Clinical and immunologic effects of fractionated total lymphoid irradiation in refractory rheumatoid arthritis. N Engl J Med 1981;305:976–982.

45. Field EH, Strober S, Hoppe RT, et al. Sustained improvement of intractable rheumatoid arthritis after total lymphoid irradiation. Arthritis Rheum 1983;26:937–946.

46. Strober S, Tanay A, Field E, et al. Efficacy of total lymphoid irradiation in intractable rheumatoid arthritis; a double-blind, randomized trial. Ann Intern Med 1985;102:441–449.

Polyarteritis Nodosa

INTRODUCTION

Polyarteritis nodosa (PAN) is an uncommon, although not rare, multisystem disorder. It is characterized by necrotizing vasculitis of small- and medium-sized arteries throughout the body, with a particular predilection for renal and visceral arteries. PAN also affects various ocular structures. Approximately 30% of cases of PAN are associated with circulating or localized deposits of immune complexes in the affected vessels. These complexes may contain hepatitis B antigen. In the classic form, as described initially by Kussmaul and Maier, PAN spares the pulmonary arteries. In addition to the classic form of PAN, there are cases showing typical features of PAN but with additional lesions characteristic of other vasculitides, such as allergic angiitis and granulomatosis of Churg-Strauss with significant eosinophilia. The exact incidence of PAN is not known, due to the lack of specific diagnostic serological testing and to the focal distribution of the lesions, which makes blind biopsy relatively insensitive. Males are 2.5 times more commonly affected than are females. The disease can occur at any age, but the mean age at onset is 45 years (1).

PATHOPHYSIOLOGY

PAN is an inflammatory disease affecting small- and medium-sized arteries, especially at sites of bifurcation and branching. The inflammation involves all layers of the arteries, so the term polyarteritis is more appropriate than the previous name periarteritis. In advanced stages, adjacent vessels and connective tissues are also involved. In the acute stage, the inflammation is characterized by a predominantly polymorphonuclear leukocytic infiltration throughout all layers of the artery, with occasional mononuclear cells and eosinophils. In the chronic stage, the infiltration consists of mononuclear cells. Edema, exudation, and fibrinoid necrosis can occur. The arterial wall, weakened from the inflammation and under sustained intra-arterial pressure, develops an aneurysm that infrequently ruptures possibly causing hemorrhagic necrosis of the involved tissue. The aneurysmal dilatation accounts for the name, polyarteritis *nodosa*. Other complications, such as thrombosis, infarction, and hemorrhage, can also occur from occlusion of vessels. Ultimately, the necrotic area is replaced by fibrovascular scar. The most commonly affected sites are the kidneys, heart, liver, gastrointestinal tract, musculoskeletal system, pancreas, testes, peripheral nerves, the central nervous system, and the skin.

It is commonly believed that the basic pathological changes are due to deposition of immune complexes in the arterial wall. These complexes, often composed of hepatitis B antigen and immunoglobulin, were noted in 30% of cases in one series (2). Some of these patients also have circulating hepatitis B antigen. Occasionally, lesions identical to those of PAN are seen in patients with systemic lupus erythematosus (SLE), particularly those who have levels of circulating immune complexes (3). Similarly, circulating or tissue deposits of tumor-related antigens have been demonstrated in some patients with PAN. All of these associated disorders suggest that the necrotizing vasculitis observed in PAN is mediated by deposition of immune complexes (4), even though the precise mechanisms for such deposition in the vessel walls are unknown. However, once immune complexes are deposited within the arterial walls, the tissue damage is initiated by activation of complement components, particularly C5a, which is strongly chemotactic for polymorphonuclear leukocytes. The polymorphonuclear leukocytes phagocytose the immune complexes and release various chemical mediators, including proteolytic lysosomal enzymes and oxygen free radicals. The proteolytic enzymes and the free radicals are known to cause damage to the vessel wall.

CLINICAL FINDINGS

Clinical findings secondary to arterial necrosis are widespread and involve multiple organ systems. Patients commonly present with nonspecific symptoms including fever, weight loss, malaise, headaches, abdominal pain, migratory arthralgia, and myalgia. However, patients can also present with complaints related specifically to the organs involved, such as renal failure, heart failure, pain in the umbilical region, arthritis, peripheral neuropathy, or skin nodules. Differential diagnosis includes allergic angiitis, Churg-Strauss granulomatosis, Wegener's granulomatosis, giant cell arteritis, and rheumatoid arthritis, as well as a host of infectious and lymphomatous diseases.

No serological test is available for the definitive diagnosis of this disease. Polymorphonuclear leukocytosis is seen in over 75% of cases, and an elevated erythrocyte sedimentation rate is almost invariably present. Eosinophilia is not usually present. Hypergammaglobulinemia and hepatitis B surface antigen may be present in some cases. Hypocomplementemia is infrequently present, except in a form of vasculitis associated with urticaria and leukocytoclastic angiitis.

Arteriograms rarely show the aneurysmal dilatation that is usually present in the smaller-sized arteries of the kidneys and abdominal viscera. Larger aneurysms may be demonstrated. The laboratory findings are nonspecific; therefore, diagnosis depends upon demonstrating the characteristic histopathological findings in biopsy specimens of the involved organ. Because the arterial involvement is segmental and often patchy, it is advisable to obtain the biopsy from a suspected site of involvement and then perform multiple cuts of the vessel. Where biopsy material is not available, angiographic demonstration of aneurysmal involvement of arteries of the renal, hepatic, and gastrointestinal systems suggests the disease. The demonstration of circulating hepatitis B antigen, if found, supports the clinical diagnosis.

OCULAR MANIFESTATIONS

Although ocular involvement due to polyarteritis nodosa is uncommon, ocular manifestations may be the initial sign. Since 10% of patients show some ocular findings (5, 6), ophthalmologists should be aware of the varied manifestations of this disorder. An unknown number of cases of eye involvement remain undetected due to minimal symptoms. Ocular lesions can involve any part of the eye, although choroidal vasculitis is most common. In the anterior segment, chemosis, subconjunctival hemorrhages, and raised yellow plaques due to inflammation of conjunctival vessels have been reported (7, 8). Vessels supplying the extraocular muscles, sclera, and cornea may also be affected, leading to necrotizing scleritis, episcleritis, and marginal keratitis (9–11). Scleritis may cause exudative retinal detachment (11). Scleral necrosis may lead to perforation (12). Iritis and iridocyclitis are quite uncommon and, when present, are secondary to ciliary and iris vessel involvement (8, 13). Orbital vascular involvement may lead to exophthalmos and pseudotumor formation, which may be the earliest manifestation of this disease (14–18). Thrombophlebitis of the orbital veins may lead to chemosis of the conjunctivae and varicosities of the eyelids. Inflammation of adjacent paranasal sinuses can also affect the orbit (16, 19).

Posterior segment involvement in PAN can occur due to localized vasculitis or may be secondary to systemic hypertension (20). Posterior ciliary artery and choroidal vessels are commonly affected, and vasculitis of these vessels can lead to choroidal infarction, secondary retinal detachment (21), and transient ischemic attacks (22). Retinal vascular involvement can cause retinal edema, retinal vasculitis (23), cotton-wool spots (22), retinal or subhyaloid hemorrhages, and retinal exudates (20). Inconsistency of the caliber of retinal vessels, with or without aneurysm formation, has been observed (24, 25). Retinal vascular occlusions, especially of the central retinal artery and vein, can be seen (12, 26–29). Optic nerve involvement can precipitate ischemic optic neuropathy, disc edema, and hemorrhages (26, 30).

TREATMENT

Polyarteritis nodosa can be a fatal disease if not treated. Systemic steroids, often

40 to 60 mg of prednisone, can produce symptomatic relief and, to a limited extent, increase survival. Combination therapy using corticosteroids and immunosuppressive agents has significantly improved the prognosis. This combination therapy consists of prednisone 1 mg/kg/day and cyclophosphamide 2 mg/kg/day. Cyclophosphamide has been found to be the most effective cytotoxic drug. Cyclophosphamide may be given as a large, intravenous loading dose, administered in divided doses within a span of 2 to 5 days. If the response is favorable, the patient may be kept on a maintenance dose of 2 to 3 mg/kg/day orally. Treatment at lower doses may be necessary for more than a year.

The major side effect of this treatment is marked leukopenia, but white blood cell counts return to normal within 7 to 10 days after discontinuation of therapy. There has been marked improvement in the survival rate since the introduction of this immunosuppressive regimen (31). When a high dose, systemic steroid alone was given, the 5-year survival rate was 50%; combination therapy with systemic steroids and immunosuppressive agents has increased the survival rate to 80% (32). Death results usually from renal failure, myocardial infarction, congestive heart failure, hepatic failure, bowel perforation, or cerebral infarction and hemorrhage.

References

1. Cupps TR, Fauci AS. The vasculitides. Philadelphia: WB Saunders, 1981.
2. Michalak T. Immune complexes of hepatitis B surface antigen in the pathogenesis of periarteritis nodosa; a study of seven necropsy cases. Am J Pathol 1978;90:619–632.
3. Paronetto F, Deppisch L, Tuchman LR. Lupus erythematosus with fatal hemorrhage into the liver and lesions resembling those of periarteritis nodosa and malignant hypertension; immunocytochemical observations. Am J Med 1964;36:948–955.
4. Elkon KB, Hughes GRV, Catovsky D, et al. Hairy-cell leukaemia with polyarteritis nodosa. Lancet 1979;2:280–282.
5. Wise GN. Ocular periarteritis nodosa; report of two cases. Arch Ophthalmol 1952;48:1–11.
6. Stillerman ML. Ocular manifestations of diffuse collagen disease. Arch Ophthalmol 1951;45:239–250.
7. Duke-Elder S, ed. System of ophthalmology. Vol 15: Summary of systemic ophthalmology. St. Louis: CV Mosby, 1976.
8. Purcell JJ Jr, Birkenkamp R, Tsai CC. Conjunctival lesions in periarteritis nodosa; a clinical and immunopathologic study. Arch Ophthalmol 1984;102:736–738.
9. Cogan DG. Corneoscleral lesions in periarteritis nodosa and Wegener's granulomatosis. Trans Am Ophthalmol Soc 1955;53:321–344.
10. Moore JG, Sevel D. Corneo-scleral ulceration in periarteritis nodosa. Br J Ophthalmol 1966;50:651–655.
11. Kielar RA. Exudative retinal detachment and scleritis in polyarteritis. Am J Ophthalmol 1976;82:694–698.
12. Herbert F, McPherson SD Jr. Scleral necrosis associated with periarteritis nodosa: report of a case. Arch Ophthalmol 1947;37:688–693.
13. Gold DH. Ocular manifestations of connective tissue (collagen) diseases. In: Duane TD, ed. Clinical ophthalmology. Philadelphia: Harper & Row, 1984: Vol 5, Chap 26.
14. Hope-Robertson WJ. Pseudo-tumour of the orbit as a presenting sign in periarteritis nodosa. Trans Ophthalmol Soc NZ 1955;8:56–66.
15. Walton EW. Pseudo tumour of the orbit and polyarteritis nodosa. J Clin Pathol 1959;12:419–426.
16. Aström KE, Lidholm SO. Extensive intracranial lesions in a case of orbital non-specific granuloma combined with polyarteritis nodosa. J Clin Pathol 1963;16:137–143.
17. Van Wien S. Merz EH. Exophthalmos secondary to periarteritis nodosa. Am J Ophthalmol 1963;56:204–208.
18. Harcourt RB. Orbital granulomata associated with widespread angiitis. Br J Ophthalmol 1964;48:673–677.
19. Castleman B, ed. Case records of the Massachusetts General Hospital; case 23–1974. N Engl J Med 1974;290:1365–1372.
20. Sheehan B, Harriman DGF, Bradshaw JPP. Polyarteritis nodosa with ophthalmic and neurological complications. Arch Ophthalmol 1958;60:537–547.
21. Jakobiec FA, Jones IS. Orbital inflammations. In: Duane TD, ed. Clinical ophthalmology. Philadelphia: Harper & Row, 1984: Vol 2, Chap 35.
22. Brown GC, Brown MM, Hiller T, Fischer D, Benson WE, Magargal LE. Cotton-wool spots. Retina 1985;5:206–214.
23. Morgan CM, Foster CS, D'Amico DJ, Gragoudas ES. Retinal vasculitis in polyarteritis nodosa. Retina 1986;6:205–209.
24. Kincaid J, Schatz H. Bilateral retinal arteritis with multiple aneurysmal dilatations. Retina 1983;3:171–178.
25. Goldsmith J. Periarteritis nodosa with involvement of the choroidal and retinal arteries. Am J Ophthalmol 1946;2:435–446.
26. Ford RG, Siekert RG. Central nervous system manifestations of periarteritis nodosa. Neurology 1965;15:114–122.

27. Boeck J. Ocular changes in periarteritis nodosa. Am J Ophthalmol 1956;42:567–577.

28. Wise GN, Dollery CT, Henkind P. The retinal circulation. New York: Harper & Row, 1971:290–294.

29. Leung AC, McLay A, Boulton-Jones JM. Polyarteritis presenting with thrombocytosis and central retinal vein thrombosis. Scott Med J 1987;32:24–26.

30. Kimbrell OC Jr, Wheliss JA. Polyarteritis nodosa complicated by bilateral optic neuropathy. JAMA 1967;201:61–62.

31. Foster CS, Regan CDJ. Retinal vascular diseases: management. Int Ophthalmol Clin 1986;26(2):55–71.

32. Leib ES, Restivo C, Paulus HE. Immunosuppressive and corticosteroid therapy of polyarteritis nodosa. Am J Med 1979;67:941–947.

Giant Cell Arteritis (GCA)

INTRODUCTION

In 1890, Hutchinson described a patient having scalp tenderness that was attributed to thrombosis of his temporal artery (1). Further description of this syndrome followed (2–4). In 1957, Barber described polymyalgia rheumatica as a presentation of giant cell arteritis (GCA) (5).

Three recent reports have added a great deal to our understanding of GCA. Keltner (6) has written an excellent review of giant cell arteritis particularly in regards to general symptomatology and demographics. More recently the reviews of McDonnell et al. (6a) and Raskin (6b) have elucidated the difficulties of diagnosis and definition. Recognition of the histopathologic features of active or healed GCA can increase the sensitivity of a temporal artery biopsy (6a).

GCA is predominantly a disease of the elderly. Several cases have been reported describing its appearance in patients as young as 50, but it is seldom seen in people under the age of 60 years. Its incidence continues to increase after age 70 and beyond. In the 60s, there is a specific prevalence of GCA of 33/100,000; over age 80, the prevalence has increased more than 20-fold (7). The preponderance of women may simply reflect their greater number in these older age groups. The disease occurs in blacks but appears to be rarer in this group than in Caucasians of European ancestry. GCA is probably markedly underdiagnosed. Random autopsies in patients over 60 years of age have revealed a prevalence of occult cases of approximately 2.5% (8). Interestingly, the prevalence of GCA increases with each decade (6, 9), suggesting either recent better recognition of this disorder or a change in its actual incidence.

PATHOPHYSIOLOGY

The histological changes of GCA include arteritis accompanied by cellular infiltration, the presence of multinucleated giant cells, and the breakdown of the internal elastic lamina (Fig. 1.8). A granulomatous reaction is usually seen around the fragmented elastica. At a minimum, the demonstration of epithelioid cells and a ruptured elastica are needed for the diagnosis. Ultrastructural changes in the muscular media take place. Degeneration of smooth muscle cells is noted, with adjacent collections of macrophages. In early stages of the vasculitis, there is intimal proliferation that may consist of an inner, thicker zone composed of loosely packed cellular fibrous tissue and an outer, thinner zone of granulomatous tissue. Neutrophils, lymphocytes, and other mononuclear cells may be seen in varying numbers in the outer granulomatous zone. Eosinophils are rarely found. Often multinucleated giant cells (usually Langhans', less often foreign body type) are found near the disrupted internal elastica. Less often, the giant cells are in the adjacent intima and, rarely, in the adventitia. Less commonly, foci of fibrinoid necrosis are seen.

Following steroid administration, the number of inflammatory cells decreases. Generally, giant cells or epithelioid cells remain for 3 weeks after initiation of steroids. However, the elastica remains fragmented long after the initiation of steroid treatment. Occluded vessels may recanalize. While resumption of blood flow will lead to the reversal of some signs and symptoms (e.g., ophthalmoplegia), ischemic damage to the optic nerve usually is irreversible.

The origin of the vasculitis remains uncertain. A predisposition to temporal arteritis has been reported in patients with certain HLA types, but these findings have not been confirmed by other studies. Other theories as to the origin of the vasculitis include infectious causes (e.g., the herpes virus) or immune complex deposition. Takayasu's disease resembles GCA histopathologically, but it is seen predominantly in young females.

CLINICAL FINDINGS

Polymyalgia rheumatica is a disease characterized by an aching and stiffness of the neck, shoulder, hips, and other joints accompanied by an elevated erythrocyte sedimentation rate. It is seen in 50% of patients with GCA and may precede other symptoms. In classical GCA, the patient presents with a history of headaches with swelling, tenderness, and pain over the temporal scalp. Jaw claudication, arthralgias, myalgias, malaise, anorexia, and weight loss are common. Low-grade fever and vertigo may also be described. Laboratory testing usually shows a markedly elevated erythrocyte sedimentation rate (ESR) and mild anemia (6, 9). Less frequently, other systemic signs and symptoms may be present, such as intermittent leg claudication or peripheral neuropathy (10).

"Occult" GCA is often misdiagnosed. The systemic signs and symptoms described above are not evident, and the symptom-

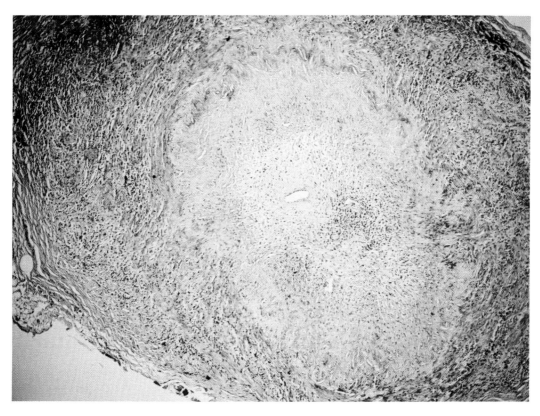

Figure 1.8. Temporal artery biopsy. Almost total closure of vessel demonstrated with cellular infiltration and destruction of the internal elastic lamina.

atology may be vague. However, the physician must still consider the diagnosis of GCA and obtain an ESR, which is usually very high; a positive temporal artery biopsy confirms the diagnosis. Any elderly patient presenting with ischemic optic neuropathy, central retinal artery occlusion, or unexplained ophthalmoplegia should have an ESR obtained immediately. If this is elevated, or temporal arteritis is strongly suspected, an arterial biopsy should be considered.

Temporal Artery Biopsy

Biopsy of the superficial temporal artery provides the most reliable evidence for the diagnosis of GCA. Although some authors feel that a negative biopsy does not exclude GCA because of the possibility of skip lesions (11), most authors feel that careful pathological assessment of longitudinal as well as multiple cross-sectional views of the temporal artery will usually confirm the diagnosis of GCA.

The superficial temporal artery and the extradural vertebral arteries are involved in almost 100% of cases of GCA. The ophthalmic artery and the posterior ciliary arteries are involved about 75% of the time.

Laboratory Findings

Internists, rheumatologists, and ophthalmologists rely on the ESR as a nonspecific indicator of GCA. A raised ESR is characteristic of GCA, even in the absence of other clinical symptoms, but it may be seen in association with inflammatory types of arthritis, infection, and other common systemic inflammations. ESRs can be measured by the Westergren or Wintrobe methods; the former is more reliable (6, 12). No absolute value of the ESR can be considered pathognomonic for the disease. Many authors have suggested that the upper normal limit for Westergren ESR is 40 mm; however, usually patients with GCA have ESRs above 80 mm. It is rare for patients with GCA to have ESRs (Westergren) below 40 (10). It should be kept in mind that anti-inflammatory agents, including

aspirin, can lower the ESR. In fact, patients with arthritis or individuals who are on chronic doses of aspirin often present with an occult GCA that is difficult to diagnose because the ESR is only moderately elevated.

Most patients with GCA have at least a mild degree of normochromic normocytic anemia (hematocrits of 28 to 35%). Other laboratory abnormalities include impairment in liver function, elevated haptoglobin, and elevated fibrinogen (10).

Jacobson and Slamovits reviewed 24 patients with biopsy-proven GCA. Of these, four had ESRs less than 40 mm, eight had ESRs between 41 mm and 80 mm, and twelve had ESRs greater than 81 mm. Jacobson and Slamovits also found a linear and inverse relationship between ESR and the patient's hematocrit. ESRs of about 140 mm were seen with hematocrits of about 26%; ESRs of about 50 mm were generally seen with hematocrits of 38% (13).

Untreated GCA may lead to bilateral blindness and even death. Despite the fact that some authors have not found a significantly reduced survivorship (7), GCA can lead to occlusion of the vertebral arteries and subsequent stroke or occlusion of the coronary arteries with subsequent myocardial infarction.

OCULAR MANIFESTATIONS

GCA may manifest itself ophthalmologically through either sudden loss of vision or diplopia. Severe visual loss occurs in one-third to one-half of untreated cases of GCA (9, 14). Sudden visual loss is most often attributed to involvement of the posterior ciliary vessel supply to the optic nerve, which leads to an anterior ischemic optic neuropathy. Alternatively, occlusion of the central retinal artery may occur. Less frequently, there is posterior ischemic optic neuropathy. Thus, the ophthalmoscopic picture can vary from that of a classical central retinal artery occlusion (white retina, cherry-red spot, arteriolar constriction), to anterior ischemic optic neuropathy (disc edema accompanied by peripapillary hemorrhages and cotton-wool spots), to an almost normal-appearing fundus.

Occasionally, transient obscurations of vision may precede the sudden visual failure. More often, the first ophthalmological manifestation is profound, irreversible visual loss.

Diplopia may be the first ocular symptom in GCA and is due to an ophthalmoplegia (6). Approximately 10% of patients with GCA show this manifestation. Histopathological studies suggest that the ophthalmoplegia is due to ischemia within the orbit (15). Some authors have suggested that there is ischemia of the extraocular muscle itself, yet many cases present with a pattern of a third, fourth, or sixth cranial nerve involvement.

Rarely, GCA may present as an ischemic uveitis due to anterior segment ischemia (16). Rubeosis iridis, cataract, hypotony, or secondary glaucoma may be seen. Abnormalities of the choroidal circulation have also been noted (17).

TREATMENT

As soon as the patient is suspected of having temporal arteritis, administration of prednisone or another corticosteroid should be started immediately. A dose of 60 to 100 mg prednisone orally has usually been used. Pulsed, high dose intravenous steroids are also used by some (18). A biopsy should be scheduled within the next few days. Several studies have demonstrated that the temporal artery biopsy will be positive in cases of GCA for at least 3 weeks after appropriate corticosteroid treatment (19). Some authors suggest that a temporal artery biopsy is unnecessary because, in many cases, the classic presentation of GCA together with a very high ESR is sufficient to make the diagnosis. However, the patient may experience severe side effects from long-term corticosteroid therapy, at which time a temporal artery biopsy may no longer be reliably used to confirm the diagnosis of GCA. However, if the patient is suffering from

life-threatening manifestations of chronic corticosteroid use (e.g., bleeding, peptic ulcers) or even the severely debilitating manifestations of Cushing's syndrome (e.g., myopathies), then there may be considerable pressure from both the patient and his or her internist or rheumatologist to discontinue the corticosteroids. The ophthalmologist would be best prepared to discuss the relative risks and benefits of the discontinuation of therapy if he were to have already obtained a baseline temporal artery biopsy.

The temporal artery biopsy should be obtained from the side that appears to have the most tenderness or nodularity to palpation. Some authors suggests that it should be taken from the side ipsilateral to the involved eye in unilateral cases. We recommend that the superficial temporal artery be palpated beside the hairline near the ear. The artery should then be marked prior to shaving the adjacent hair, prepping the skin, and administering local anesthetic (2% lidocaine with epinephrine). A straight incision can then be made through the scalp along the previously marked temporal artery for a length of approximately 4 cm. The incision should be brought through the skin to the underlying fascia. Blunt tip scissors can then be used to further the dissection until the temporal artery is visualized for a length of at least 3 cm. 4–0 or 5–0 silk can be used to tie off the proximal and distal ends of the temporal artery. A double tie can be used on the proximal artery. Care should be taken that any small branches from the temporal artery are also ligated. The isolated segment of the temporal artery is excised, placed in formalin, and sent for pathological examination. Subcutaneous vicryl and running silk skin sutures can be used to close the wound.

Occasionally, cases have been reported describing significant recovery of vision after profound visual loss from GCA (20). However, the most important reason for placing the patient on corticosteroid treatment is to prevent any further vascular occlusions. Once a patient is receiving an adequate amount of corticosteroids, the ESR is found to drop dramatically, and the patient is almost free of the risk of further ischemic episodes. Evidence in the rheumatological literature suggests that alternate day administration of corticosteroids is inadequate because the patient may show manifestations of polymyalgia rheumatica on the days that he or she is not treated.

No firm studies have established the exact required steroid dosage, although the patient's weight and the presence of other systemic diseases are issues that need to be kept in mind. We recommend that an internist or rheumatologist monitor the patient. The patient should be kept on daily doses of corticosteroids, with the ESR as one means of establishing the dose. We try to keep the ESR below 30 mm with an allowance for systemic diseases that may be influencing the ESR (e.g., arthritis). Usually, the prednisone dose can be tapered down to 20 mg/day within 6 to 8 weeks after the onset of therapy. The patient may need to be given corticosteroids at a low dose (10 mg to 15 mg/day) for a prolonged period. Therapy is further decreased or discontinued when the ESR does not rise above 30 mm after a decrease in dosage. If the patient redevelops symptoms of polymyalgia rheumatica, or if the ESR dramatically rises, then the patient should again be given significantly higher dosages of corticosteroids.

References

1. Hutchinson J. On a peculiar form of thrombotic arteritis of the aged which is sometimes productive of gangrene. Arch Surg (London) 1890;1:323–329.
2. Horton BT, Magath TB, Brown GE. An undescribed form of arteritis of the temporal vessels. Mayo Clin Proc 1932;7:700–701.
3. Jennings GH. Arteritis of the temporal vessels. Lancet 1938;1:424–428.
4. Cooke WT, Cloake PCP, Govan ADT, Colbeck JC. Temporal arteritis: a generalized vascular disease. Quart J Med 1946;15:47–75.
5. Barber HS. Myalgic syndrome with constitutional effects; polymyalgia rheumatica. Ann Rheum Dis 1957;16:230–237.
6. Keltner JL. Giant-cell arteritis; signs and symptoms. Ophthalmology 1982;89:1101–1110.
6a. McDonnell PJ, Moore GW, Miller NR, Hutchins GM, Green R. Temporal arteritis, a clinicopathologic study. Ophthalmology 1986;93:518–530.
6b. Raskin NH. Headache. 2nd ed. New York: Churchill Livingstone, 1988:317–332.
7. Hauser WA, Ferguson RH, Holley KE, Kurland LT. Temporal arteritis in Rochester, Minnesota, 1951 to 1957. Mayo Clin Proc. 1971;46:597–602.
8. Ainsworth RW, Gresham GA, Balmforth GV. Pathological changes in temporal arteries removed from unselected cadavers. J Clin Pathol 1961;14:115–119.
9. Cullen JF, Coleiro JA. Ophthalmic complications of giant cell arteritis. Surv Ophthalmol 1976;20:247–260.
10. Healey LA, Wilske KR. The systemic manifestations of temporal arteritis. New York: Grune & Stratton, 1978.
11. Cohen DN, Smith TR. Skip areas in temporal arteritis: myth versus fact. Trans Am Acad Ophthalmol Otolaryngol 1974;78:OP772–OP783.
12. Schrader WH. Erythrocyte sedimentation rate. Postgrad Med 1963;34(5):A42–52.
13. Jacobson DM, Slamovits TL. Erythrocyte sedimentation rate and its relationship to hematocrit in giant cell arteritis. Arch Ophthalmol 1987;105:965–967.
14. Coomes EN, Ellis RM, Kay AG. A prospective study of 102 patients with polymyalgia rheumatica syndrome. Rheumatol Rehabil 1976;15:270–279.
15. Barricks ME, Traviesa DB, Glaser JS, Levy IS. Ophthalmoplegia in cranial arteritis. Brain 1977;100:209–221.
16. Winter BJ, Cryer TH, Hameroff SB. Anterior segment ischemia in temporal arteritis. South Med J 1977;70:1479–1481.
17. Fastenberg DM, Feldon SE. Reversible choroidal vascular insufficiency without infarction in temporal arteritis. Graefes Arch Clin Exp Ophthalmol 1982;218:327–330.
18. Rosenfeld SI, Kosmorsky GS, Klingele TG, Burde RM, Cohen EM. Treatment of temporal arteritis with ocular involvement. Am J Med 1986;80:143–145.
19. Fulton AB, Lee RV, Jampol LM, et al. Active giant cell arteritis with cerebral involvement. Findings following four years of corticosteroid therapy. Arch Ophthalmol 1976;94:2068–2071.
20. Schneider HA, Weber AA, Ballen PH. The visual prognosis in temporal arteritis. Ann Ophthalmol 1971;3:1215–1230.

CHAPTER 2

Retinal and Choroidal Manifestations of Hematological Diseases

W. Richard Green, George A. Williams, Andrew P. Schachat, R. Joseph Olk, and Robert P. Murphy

PLATELET DISORDERS

Platelets play a primary role in normal hemostasis. They form hemostatic plugs at sites of vascular disruption and are also important in the activation of the coagulation system. Platelet disorders may result in a broad spectrum of ocular manifestations, ranging from hyphema to serous retinal detachments. The majority of clinically significant platelet disorders are secondary to either thrombocytopenia or platelet dysfunction syndromes.

Platelet Destruction

A common cause of thrombocytopenia is accelerated platelet destruction due to either immunological or nonimmunological mechanisms (1). Immune-mediated mechanisms result in the production of antiplatelet antibodies. This antibody production occurs in *idiopathic thrombocytopenic purpura* (ITP) or following drug exposure.

ITP is an autoimmune disease that may occur acutely as a self-limited condition following a viral infection in children or, more typically, as a chronic disorder of young and middle-aged women. ITP is associated with antibodies against unknown platelet antigens. Systemic manifestations range from petechiae to intracranial hemorrhage. Ocular manifestations of ITP include retinal hemorrhages (2) and an interesting association with Graves' disease (3). The development of thrombocytopenia in Graves' disease probably involves either autoimmunity or secondary effects of thyrotoxicosis (3). This association should be considered in patients with Graves' disease and unexplained ocular bleeding and particularly in Graves' patients undergoing ocular or orbital surgery.

A second type of immune-mediated thrombocytopenia occurs after drug exposure. Certain drugs act as haptens. When a drug acts as a hapten, the ensuing drug-antibody complex then binds to the platelet, resulting in platelet destruction (1). Quinine and quinidine are the best-studied drugs related to platelet destruction, but many others, including the sulfonamides, heparin, phenytoin, diazepam, and acetaminophen, have been implicated. A thorough drug history is necessary to determine drug exposure.

Drug-induced thrombocytopenia may cause a variety of ocular bleeding events. Vitreous hemorrhage, subconjunctival hemorrhage, and postsurgical bleeding following lid surgery have all been attributed to drug-induced thrombocytopenia (4, 5). Bilateral serous retinal detachments

(6) and disc edema have also been described.

The prototype of nonimmunological accelerated destruction of platelets is *thrombotic thrombocytopenic purpura* (TTP). The hallmark of this enigmatic entity is diffuse platelet activation and aggregation resulting in five major clinical manifestations: (*a*) microangiopathic hemolytic anemia, (*b*) thrombocytopenia, (*c*) fever, (*d*) central nervous system dysfunction, and (*e*) renal disease (1). In the past, TTP has been confused with disseminated intravascular coagulation (DIC) (7). Although both entities involve thrombocytopenia, only DIC results in widespread activation of coagulation and fibrinolysis. Coagulation tests, which are categorically abnormal in DIC, are unaffected in TTP (1). TTP and DIC are now regarded as separate diseases.

The most common ocular manifestations of TTP include papilledema, extraocular muscle palsies, and visual field defects, all of which are usually secondary to concomitant central nervous system involvement (8–10). Retinal findings consist of hemorrhages and serous detachments (Fig. 2.1) (8–11). The etiology of the serous detachments appears to be focal occlusion of the choriocapillaris, resulting in retinal pigment epithelial damage and disruption of the blood-retinal barrier (9, 11). The picture depicted by fluorescein angiography is characterized by focal areas of nonperfusion of the choriocapillaris associated with late leakage into the subretinal space (Fig. 2.2) (9). This picture is consistent with histopathological studies, which demonstrate occlusion of the choriocapillaris (Fig. 2.3) and the large choroidal vessels (Fig. 2.4) by fibrin, with overlying necrosis of the pigment epithelium (8, 9).

Clinically, the development of serous retinal detachments is usually associated with exacerbations of TTP and the development of acute hypertension. Although serous retinal detachments have been described as a preterminal event, a recent report (11) demonstrated resolution of the detachments accompanied by subsequent pigment epithelial changes when the underlying hypertension and thrombocytopenia were controlled.

Thrombocytopenia may also occur due

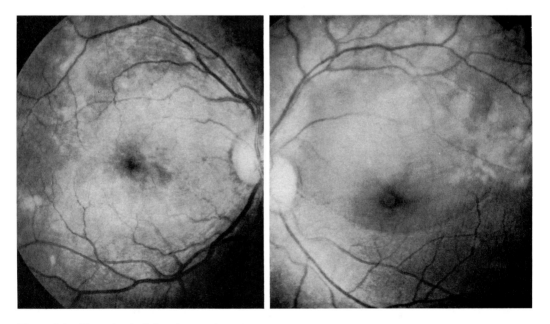

Figure 2.1. Bilateral retinal detachments in a 28-year-old woman with thrombotic thrombocytopenic purpura. (From: Wyszynski RE, Frank KE, Grossniklaus HE. Graefes Arch Clin Exp Ophthalmol 1988;226:501–504.)

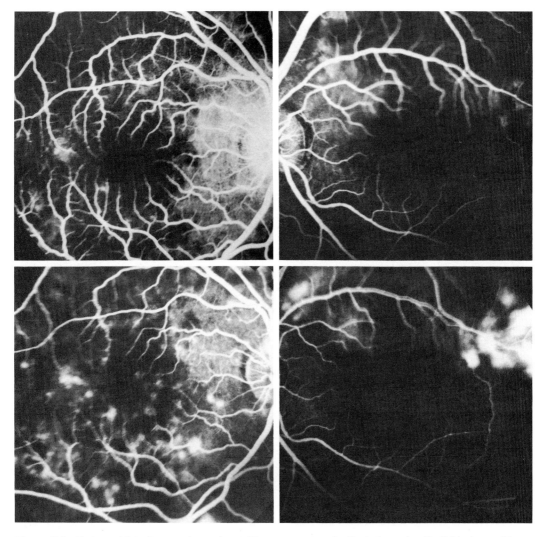

Figure 2.2. Early and late fluorescein angiographic appearance of retinal pigment epithelial leakage. (From: Wyszynski RE, Frank KE, Grossniklaus HE. Graefes Arch Clin Exp Ophthalmol 1988;226:501–504.)

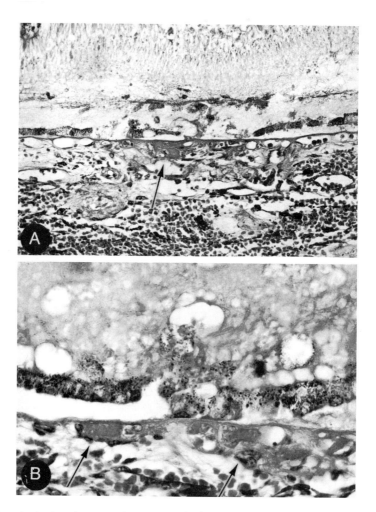

Figure 2.3. Thrombotic thrombocytopenic purpura with focal fibrin occlusion of the choriocapillaris (*arrows*), disruption of the retinal pigment epithelium, and serous detachment of the retina (hematoxylin and eosin: **A**, ×230; **B**, ×450).

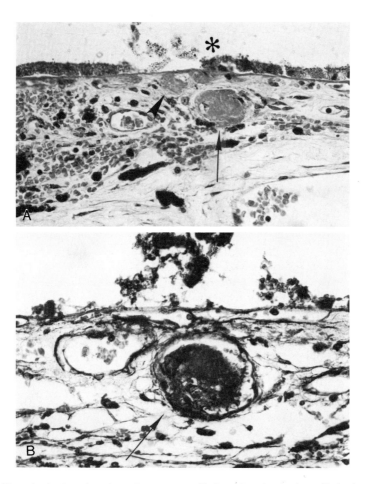

Figure 2.4. **A**. Thrombotic thrombocytopenic purpura with thrombus in choriocapillaris (*arrowhead*) and in choroidal vein (*arrow*), and focal necrosis of the retinal pigment epithelium (*asterisk*) (hematoxylin and eosin: ×380). **B**. Fibrin-containing thrombus in large choroidal vein (*arrow*) and extensive degeneration of the retinal pigment epithelium (phosphotungstic acid hematoxylin: ×380).

to bone marrow suppression or infiltration, which is the case in diseases such as aplastic anemia, leukemia, or lymphoma. Retinal hemorrhage and/or vitreous hemorrhage are more likely to occur when thrombocytopenia is accompanied by anemia (2).

Platelet Dysfunction Syndromes

These syndromes may occur as congenital or acquired defects of platelet metabolism. These abnormalities can involve platelet adhesion, aggregation, or release. A variety of ocular findings and diseases have been associated with these disorders.

Thrombasthenia

Thrombasthenia is an autosomal recessive disorder characterized by failure of platelets to aggregate in response to adenosine diphosphate. These platelets have abnormal binding sites for fibrinogen and fibronectin, resulting in poor platelet aggregation and clot retraction (1). Spontaneous preretinal and vitreous hemorrhages may result (12).

Familial Exudative Vitreoretinopathy

Familial exudative vitreoretinopathy (FEVR) is a retinal vascular disorder possibly associated with congenital platelet aggregation defects. Two families with FEVR have been described in whom abnormal platelet aggregation was seen in response to arachidonic acid (13). Whether this thrombocytopathy plays a role in the pathogenesis of FEVR is unknown.

Retinitis Pigmentosa

Abnormalities of platelet amino acid metabolism and protein content have been associated with some types of retinitis pigmentosa (14). It is not known if these disorders of platelet function play any role in the pathogenesis of retinitis pigmentosa.

Acquired Platelet Disorders

Acquired platelet dysfunction may occur with diabetes, liver disease, uremia, or macroglobulinemia but most commonly occurs after ingestion of aspirin or other nonsteroidal anti-inflammatory agents. These drugs affect platelet prostaglandin metabolism by inhibiting platelet cyclo-oxygenase, which is important in platelet aggregation and granule release. Unlike other nonsteroidal anti-inflammatory agents, aspirin irreversibly acetylates cyclo-oxygenase at doses as low as 20 mg. This irreversible inhibition of platelet function will prolong the bleeding time for about 7 days (15).

Despite the marked in vitro effects of aspirin or salicylates on platelet function, the incidence of retinal or choroidal bleeding associated with these drugs appears low (16). Massive subretinal and vitreous hemorrhage occurring in age-related macular degeneration has been associated with the use of aspirin (17). The aspirin is thought to predispose choroidal neovascularization to bleeding. Other ocular sequelae of these drugs involve rebleeding with hyphema and postsurgical bleeding (18, 19).

Acquired abnormalities of platelet function have been implicated in the pathogenesis of diabetic retinopathy. However, a review of the literature (20) produces a confusing picture of the importance of platelet dysfunction in diabetic retinopathy. Multiple parameters of platelet function, including aggregation, platelet survival, and release of platelet factor 4 and beta thromboglobulin, have been correlated with diabetic retinopathy (21). It remains uncertain, however, whether these changes represent a primary event in the pathogenesis of diabetic retinopathy or simply epiphenomena. Because platelet dysfunction is assumed to be involved in diabetic retinal microangiopathy, the Early Treatment Diabetic Retinopathy Study is examining the effect of aspirin on the course of diabetic retinopathy in almost 4000 patients (22). The results of this study, presented at the 1989 meeting of the American Academy of Ophthalmology, showed virtually no effect of aspirin on the development or complications of diabetic retinopathy.

Acquired platelet abnormalities have also been described in retinal arterial occlusive disease (23) and acute retinal necrosis (24). Antiplatelet therapy has been recommended for both of these diseases.

ABNORMALITIES OF WHITE BLOOD CELLS

Fundus changes seen in patients with white blood cell disease are protean. White cell abnormalities can be classified into diseases characterized by overproduction of white cells, underproduction of white cells, or production of abnormally functioning white cells, although there may be overlap between these categories. For example, the leukemias generally are characterized by overproduction of white cells, but in some of the leukemias there may be a phase of underproduction of white cells.

Leukemia

In most cases, the leukemias can be classified according to their cell of origin (25). Chronic lymphocytic leukemia may be of T cell or B cell origin. Most cases of acute lymphocytic leukemia are of B cell origin, and the various monocytic leukemias are primarily derived from histiocytic cell lines. Acute lymphocytic leukemia is the predominant leukemia type in children, and acute myelogenous leukemia is the predominant leukemia type in adult patients.

Accurate data are scant regarding the incidence and prevalence of various fundus findings in patients with leukemia. Autopsy series will presumably show the highest prevalence rates and will most likely overstate the frequency with which clinical disease can be detected. Allen and Straatsma (26) found that 50% of patients had ocular involvement; Nelson and coworkers (27) found a 28% prevalence rate; and Kincaid and Green (28) found that 75% of patients with chronic leukemias and 82% of patients with acute leukemias had intraocular involvement at the time of death.

Clinical series show variable prevalence rates. Ridgway (29) noted ocular involvement in 52 (9%) of 657 patients. Duke-Elder (30) estimated that up to 90% of patients will have abnormal eye findings at some point during the course of their disease.

Leukemic infiltrates may be seen in the retina, choroid (Figs. 2.5, 2.6), or vitreous. In general, they are thought to be an ominous prognostic sign associated with high blood counts, fulminant disease, and early demise (29). Multifocal retinal pigment epithelial defects (Fig. 2.7) and serous detachments of the retinal pigment epithelium (31) and retina (Fig. 2.8) (32, 33) may occur in areas overlying choroidal infiltration (34, 35). Prominent pigment epithelial changes may be seen following resolution of retinal and/or choroidal infiltrates (35–37). Vitreous infiltrates have been diagnosed following vitreous aspirates in a few cases (28, 38, 39).

The term "leukemic retinopathy" is most often used to describe the fundus manifestations of anemia, thrombocytopenia, and increased blood viscosity (Fig. 2.9) (40). Retinal hemorrhages are seen most often at the posterior pole. They may involve all layers of the retina and may be accompanied by bleeding into the vitreous cavity. The hemorrhages are described as dot- or blotch-shaped or as flame-shaped; they may have associated white centers. The white area associated with such hemorrhages is most likely due to the accumulation of platelets and fibrin (41, 42) but rarely may be due to accumulation of leukemic cells (Fig. 2.10) (42) or septic emboli. Cotton-wool spots are common and may be the abnormality that precipitates the systemic evaluation leading to the diagnosis of leukemia (43).

Patients with chronic leukemia may exhibit peripheral retinal microaneurysms (44, 45), capillary nonperfusion, and, occasionally, localized retinal neovascularization (46, 47). Elevated white blood cell counts may lead to whole blood hyperviscosity, which, in turn, can cause venous occlusive disease, microaneurysm formation, retinal hemorrhages, and retinal neovascularization (48).

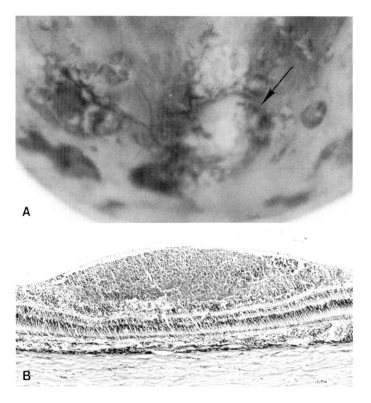

Figure 2.5. A. Gross appearance of retinal hemorrhages and tumor infiltrates (*arrow*) in a 39-year-old woman who died from chronic myelogenous leukemia. **B**. Subinternal limiting membrane leukemic infiltrate and hemorrhage (hematoxylin and eosin: **B**, ×60). (From: Kincaid MC, Green WR. Ocular and orbital involvement in leukemia. Surv Ophthalmol 1983;27:211–232.)

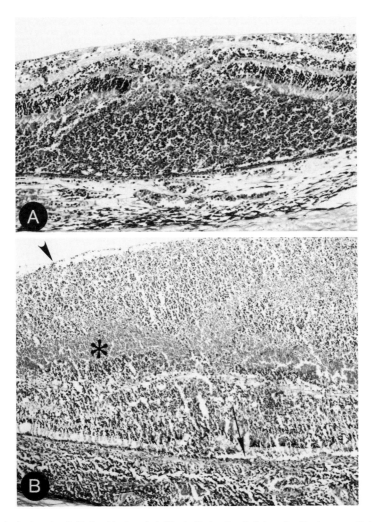

Figure 2.6. Acute leukemia. **A**. Retinal leukemic infiltrate that extends into subretinal space. Subadjacent retinal pigment epithelium is intact, and stroma of choroid is free of tumor. Choroidal vessels contain leukemia cells (hematoxylin and eosin: × 130). **B**. Section through retinal nodule shows a large tumor infiltrate under the internal limiting membrane (*arrowhead*), hemorrhage (*asterisk*), and tumor infiltrate of the remainder of the retina and choroid. Retinal pigment epithelium is discontinuous (*arrow*) (hematoxylin and eosin: × 100). (From: Kincaid MC, Green WR. Ocular and orbital involvement in leukemia. Surv Ophthalmol 1983;27:211–232.)

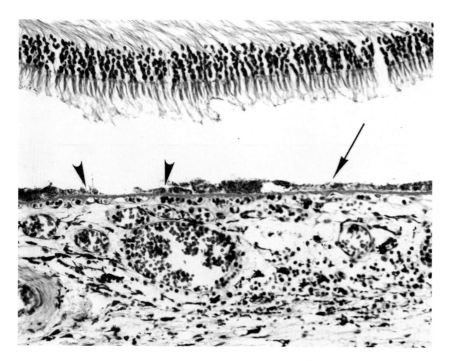

Figure 2.7. Retinal pigment epithelium defect (*between arrowheads*) and depigmentation (*arrow*) associated with choroidal infiltration by leukemic cells (hematoxylin and eosin: ×215). (From: Kincaid MC, Green WR. Ocular and orbital involvement in leukemia. Surv Ophthalmol 1983;27:211–232.)

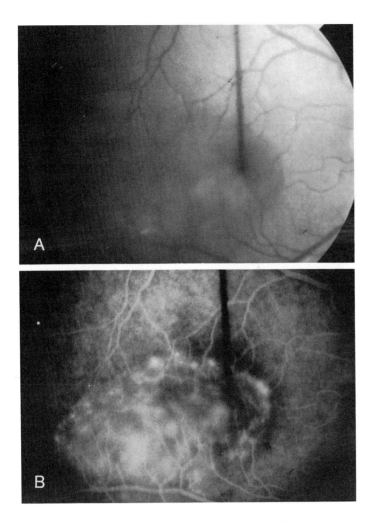

Figure 2.8.
Ophthalmoscopic (**A**) and late-phase fluorescein angiographic (**B**) appearance of retinal detachment in a 12-year-old boy with acute lymphocytic leukemia who presented with decreased vision. (From: Stewart MW, Gitter KA, Cohen G. Acute leukemia presenting as a unilateral exudative retinal detachment. Retina 1989;9:110–114.)

Opportunistic infections with bacteria, viruses, fungi, and other agents may result from the leukemia and from the immunosuppression induced by treatment (28, 42, 49, 50).

Various ophthalmic complications of treatment may occur. Most of the chemotherapeutic agents are toxic to the bone marrow. This toxicity may cause anemia and thrombocytopenia, which may result in hemorrhages and cotton-wool spots. Steroids are known to be cataractogenic. Some patients who have radiation therapy may develop radiation retinopathy or radiation optic neuropathy (51).

In general, leukemic retinopathy is treated indirectly. Systemic chemother-apy is administered to control the underlying disease state; general supportive measures, including blood transfusions, may be utilized. Leukemic infiltrates may respond to systemic chemotherapy, but ocular radiation is usually recommended (28). Subconjunctival steroids and subconjunctival chemotherapeutic agents have been used in rare cases (52). Hyperleukocytic retinopathy may be managed with leukopheresis (53).

Leukopenia

Leukopenia may be seen in patients with bone marrow failure due to any one of numerous causes, including aplastic anemia;

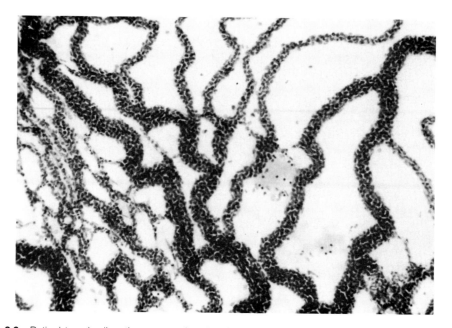

Figure 2.9. Retinal trypsin digestion preparation showing retinal vessels greatly distended by leukemic cells. (Courtesy of Dr. WH Spencer; case presented at Verhoeff Society, Washington, DC, April 1965.)

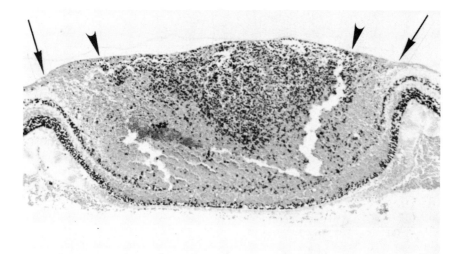

Figure 2.10. Leukemic Roth spot. Retinal hemorrhage (*between arrows*) with central area of leukemic cells (*between arrowheads*) (hematoxylin and eosin: × 100). (Courtesy of Dr. WH Spencer; case presented at Verhoeff Society, Washington, DC, April 1965.)

reversible toxic marrow suppression related to radiation, drugs, or toxins; preleukemic states; the myelophthisic states; myelofibrosis; and various vitamin deficiencies. Relatively specific failure of the neutrophil cell line is seen in patients with congenital cyclic neutropenia, Chédiak-Higashi syndrome, chronic idiopathic neutropenia, drug-induced neutropenias, various immune neutropenias, and Felty's syndrome (54).

Patients with impaired production of granulocytes and monocytes are prone to develop infections, especially with various bacteria and fungi. Ophthalmic manifestations of these infections may be protean.

Chédiak-Higashi Syndrome

Chédiak-Higashi syndrome is transmitted in an autosomal recessive manner. Patients have a partial lack of pigmentation and develop lymphadenopathy and organomegaly from infiltration with abnormal lymphocytes. Ophthalmoscopic features include partial albinism. The retinal pigment epithelium is hypopigmented and contains giant pigment granules. The patients are prone to develop retinal detachment. This may be related to lack of normal development of the photoreceptors (55).

Chronic Granulomatous Disease

Chronic granulomatous disease (CGD) is an example of a disorder characterized by abnormal oxidative killing by phagocytes. In CGD, a failure of the respiratory burst in phagocytic cells causes patients to develop an immunodeficiency syndrome (56). Chorioretinal lesions have been described in familial chronic granulomatous disease of childhood (57, 58). Chorioretinal scars were observed in one case studied postmortem (59).

In a clinicopathological study of a patient with CGD, Grossniklaus et al. (60) observed extensive chorioretinal lesions (Fig. 2.11), poorly formed granulomata in the choroid, and chorioretinal scars (Figs. 2.12, 2.13), all of which were accompanied by retinal pigment epithelial and photoreceptor cell atrophy and variable degrees of retinal pigment epithelial hypertrophy, hyperplasia, and gliosis. No infectious agents were identified.

Patients with acquired immunodeficiency have abnormal function of white blood cells; in these cases the ophthalmic manifestations can be severe. The most common retinal change in these patients is cotton-wool spots. Cytomegalovirus retinitis is the most common ocular infection. (See Chapter 5)

DISEASES OF RED BLOOD CELLS

Anemia

Retinal manifestations of either primary or secondary anemia include hemorrhages, retinal edema, and optic nerve edema, as well as hard and soft exudates. Retinal hemorrhages are primarily seen only in patients who exhibit a profound decrease in hemoglobin concentration; i.e., hemorrhages commonly occur in patients whose hematocrit levels are less than 30% (61).

Additionally, the frequency of hemorrhage appears to depend on whether the anemia coexists with thrombocytopenia. In patients with anemia alone, only 10% will exhibit hemorrhage, but 40% to 70% of patients with anemia and thrombocytopenia will exhibit retinal hemorrhage. Hemorrhage rarely occurs in patients with thrombocytopenia alone.

Polycythemia

Retinal manifestations are common in patients with either primary or secondary polycythemia. These manifestations usually occur when the red blood cell count becomes greater than 6,000,000. Retinal findings include a cyanotic fundus and marked dilation and tortuosity of the retinal vessels. "Severe" stasis is usually accompanied by a marked increase in both superficial and deep intraretinal hemorrhages and swelling of the optic nerve head.

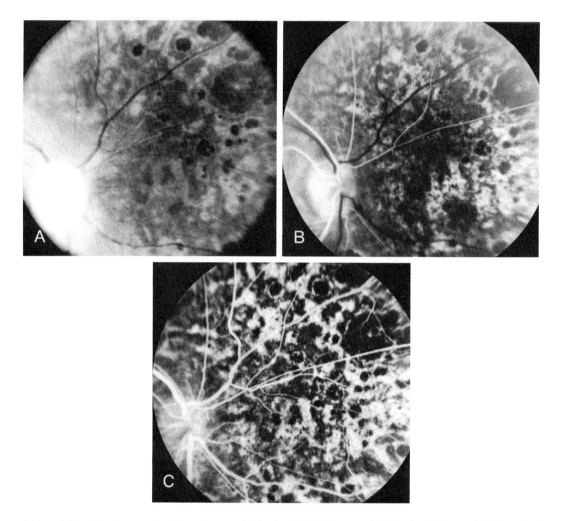

Figure 2.11. Chronic granulomatous disease. **A**. Chorioretinal lesions nasal to disc in right eye exhibiting retinal pigment epithelial hypertrophy and hyperplasia surrounded by atrophy. **B**, Early and **C**, late fluorescein angiograms demonstrating fluorescein blockage surrounded by window defects. (From: Grossniklaus HE, Frank KE, Jacobs G. Chorioretinal lesions in chronic granulomatous disease of childhood: clinicopathologic correlations. Retina 1988;8:270–274.)

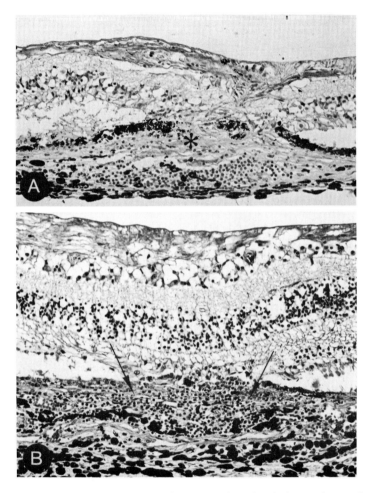

Figure 2.12. Chronic granulomatous disease. **A**. Midperipheral chorioretinal scar characterized by absence of outer retinal layers, retinal pigment epithelium, Bruch's membrane, and glial cell proliferation with extension into the choroid (*asterisk*). **B**. Focal mononuclear choroidal inflammatory cell infiltrate suggestive of poorly formed granuloma (*arrows*) in posterior pole. Inflammatory cells percolate through overlying retinal pigment epithelium; atrophy of the outer retinal layers is also present (hematoxylin and eosin: **A** and **B**, ×175). (From: Grossniklaus HE, Frank KE, Jacobs G. Chorioretinal lesions in chronic granulomatous disease of childhood: clinicopathologic correlations. Retina 1988;8:270–274.)

Figure 2.13. Chronic granulomatous disease. **A**. Area of intact and depigmented retinal pigment epithelium (*between arrows*) and extensive atrophy of the adjacent photoreceptor cell layer corresponds with fluorescein window defects. **B**. Retinal pigment epithelial hypertrophy and hyperplasia; retinal pigment epithelium extends into the choroidal component of the scar (*between arrows*); overlying atrophy of outer retinal layers corresponds with areas of fluorescein blockage (hematoxylin and eosin: **A** and **B**, × 175). (From: Grossniklaus HE, Frank KE, Jacobs G. Chorioretinal lesions in chronic granulomatous disease of childhood: clinicopathologic correlations. Retina 1988;8:270–274.)

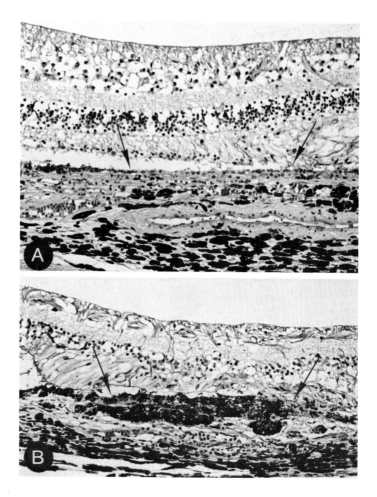

Retinal venous and artery occlusion may occur (61).

Hemoglobinopathies

Of particular interest to ophthalmologists are retinal abnormalities occurring in patients who inherit the sickle cell hemoglobin C gene. Although patients with hemoglobin SS manifest the worst systemic symptomatology, patients with sickle cell hemoglobin C and S-β thalassemia hemoglobinopathies exhibit the most severe ocular complications. The reason for this apparent discrepancy is not completely understood, but it probably relates to the degree of anemia, the rate of sickling, and the viscosity of the blood (62–64). Rarely, retinopathy has been reported with milder forms of the disorder, such as sickle cell trait AS (65).

Approximately 10% of North American blacks of Central and West African origin have abnormal hemoglobins: approximately 8% to 9% have AS hemoglobin; 0.4%, SS disease; 0.1% to 0.3%, SC disease; and 0.5% to 1.0%, S-β thalassemia.

The sickle cell gene results in hemoglobin that has a single substitution of an amino acid—valine for glutamic acid. This gene has been propagated partly because erythrocytes containing sickle-type hemoglobin exhibit resistance to the malaria parasite. Sickling of red cells having abnormal hemoglobin occurs under conditions of decreased oxygen tension, a condition seen more often in organs with more sluggish circulation, i.e., the spleen, intestinal tract, lungs, joints, and bones. Under situations that may induce anoxia, sickling can also occur in other organs. In the reduced state, sickle cell hemoglobin is relatively insoluble, and the molecules accumulate in parallel rows within the red cell, producing a change in cell shape. The stiffened cells become trapped in capillaries and cause occlusions, resulting in ischemia of the affected tissues.

Nonproliferative retinal changes include (62, 66) vascular tortuosity; salmon patches that represent retinal hemorrhages with partially degenerated blood (Fig. 2.14); iridescent spots (Fig. 2.15) that represent old, resolved, subinternal limiting membrane hemorrhage with hemosiderin deposition (Figs 2.16, 2.17) (62, 63); and black sunburst lesions (Fig. 2.18), which result from a retinal hemorrhage that extends to the subretinal space and causes secondary retinal pigment epithelial hyperplasia with migration into the retina in a perivascular location (Fig. 2.19). Additional findings include occlusion of the macular capillaries (Figs. 2.20, 2.21) (67, 68) and remodeling of the parafoveal capillaries (69).

Proliferative sickle cell retinopathy has been classified into five different stages (63). Stage I consists of peripheral arteriolar occlusions. Peripheral AV anastomoses characterize Stage II (Figs. 2.22, 2.23). Stage III consists of neovascularization in a "sea-fan" configuration (Figs. 2.24, 2.25). Stage IV involves vitreous hemorrhage, and Stage V consists of traction or rhegmatogenous retinal detachment (Fig. 2.26). A flow diagram (Fig. 2.27) illustrates the pathogenesis of many of the ocular lesions in sickle cell retinopathy.

Other retinal findings or associations reported in patients with sickle cell hemoglobinopathies include angioid streaks (64) and choroidal vascular infarction (70).

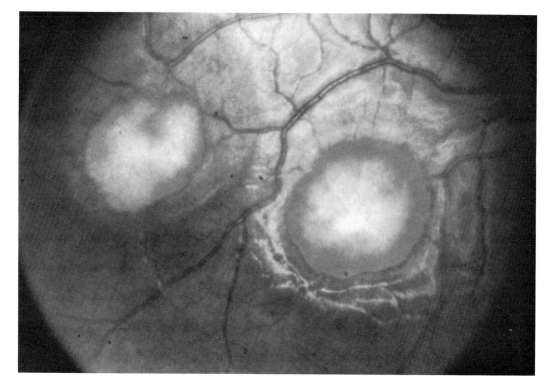

Figure 2.14. Ophthalmoscopic appearance of two salmon patches in patient with SC disease. (Courtesy of KH Packo, MD.)

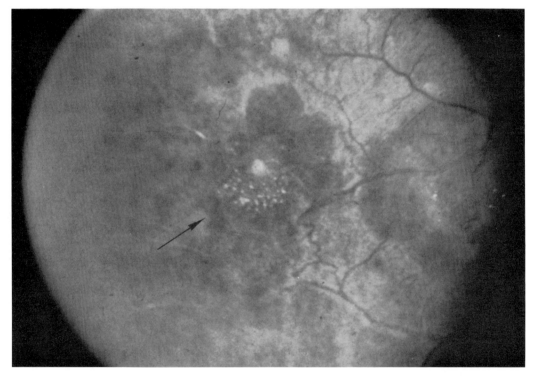

Figure 2.15. Iridescent spot (*arrow*) with slightly glistening and yellowish deposits. (Courtesy of KH Packo, MD.)

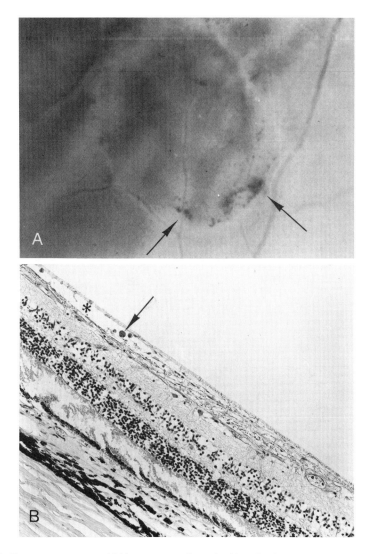

Figure 2.16. **A**. Gross appearance of iridescent spot (*arrow*) with yellowish and slightly glistening, superficial retinal deposits. **B**. Margin of iridescent spot shows an acquired schisis cavity (*asterisk*) located between the internal limiting membrane and the remainder of the retina; the cavity contains hemosiderin-laden macrophages (*arrow*) (hematoxylin and eosin: **B**, ×125). (From: Romayananda N, Goldberg MF, Green WR. Trans Am Acad Ophthalmol Otolaryngol 1973;77:652–676.)

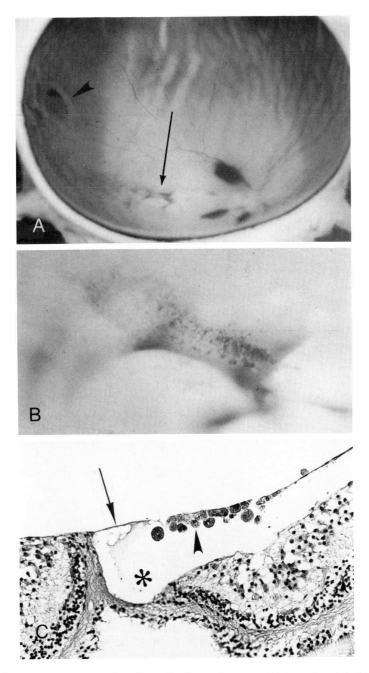

Figure 2.17.   A. Gross appearance of peripapillary retinal hemorrhages and iridescent spots in the macula (*arrow*) and near the equator (*arrowhead*) in a patient who had SC disease. **B**. Closer view of the iridescent spot in the macular area showing rust-colored intraretinal deposits. **C**. Macular iridescent spot consists of an acquired schisis cavity (*asterisk*) located between the internal limiting membrane (*arrow*) and the remainder of the retina and contains a cluster of hemosiderin-laden macrophages (*arrowhead*) (hematoxylin and eosin: **C**, × 130). (From: Romayananda N, Goldberg MF, Green WR. Trans Am Acad Ophthalmol Otolaryngol 1973;77:652–676.)

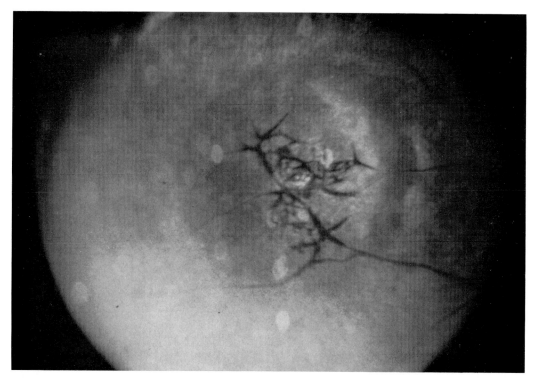

Figure 2.18. Spiculated and pigmented appearance of black sunburst sign. (Courtesy of KH Packo, MD.)

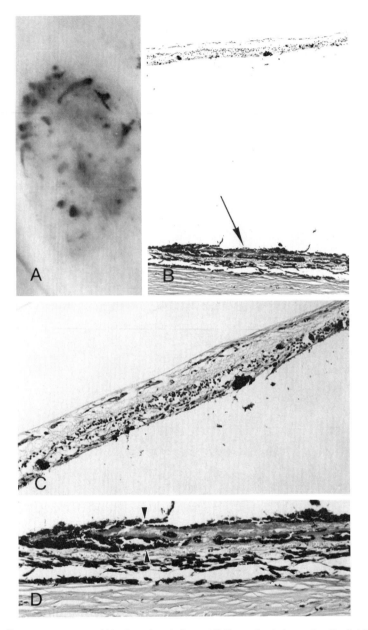

Figure 2.19. **A**. Gross appearance of black sunburst sign exhibiting retinal pigment epithelial (RPE) hyperplasia and migration into retina in perivascular location, giving lesion a spiculated appearance. **B**. Retina (artifactually detached) shows loss of outer nuclear layer and hyperplastic RPE. Corresponding area below (*arrow*) shows laminated hyperplastic RPE (periodic acid Schiff: **B**, ×50). **C**. Higher power view of retina with loss of the photoreceptor cell layer and pigmented cells within the retina (hematoxylin and eosin: **C**, ×130). **D**. Higher power view of hyperplastic RPE arranged in laminated pattern (*between arrowheads*). Choriocapillaris is normal. Special staining of adjacent sections showed hemosiderin deposits in area of hyperplastic RPE and overlying retina (hematoxylin and eosin: **D**, ×135). (From: Romayananda N, Goldberg MF, Green WR. Trans Am Acad Ophthalmol Otolaryngol 1973;77:652–676.)

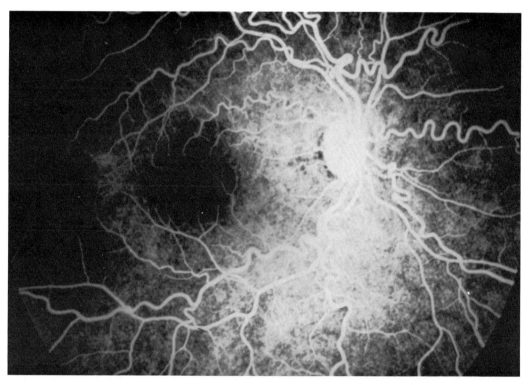

Figure 2.20. Occlusion of parafoveal capillaries with enlargement of the capillary-free zone to about 2.6 mm. (Courtesy KH Packo, MD.)

Figure 2.21. A. Inner retinal ischemic atrophy in sickle cell retinopathy. Section through foveola shows loss of ganglion cell layer in foveal area (*arrows*) (hematoxylin and eosin: **A,** ×100). **B.** Parafoveal area and clivus of macular area. Ganglion cells are totally absent in clivus and inner portion of parafoveal area (*between arrows*) (hematoxylin and eosin: **B,** ×200). (From: Green WR. Retina. In: Spencer WH, ed. Ophthalmic pathology. An atlas and textbook. Philadelphia: WB Saunders, 1985; Vol 2, Ch 8, p 1082.)

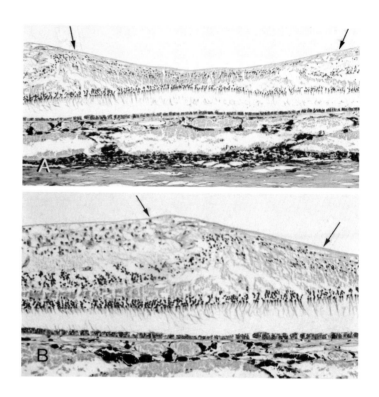

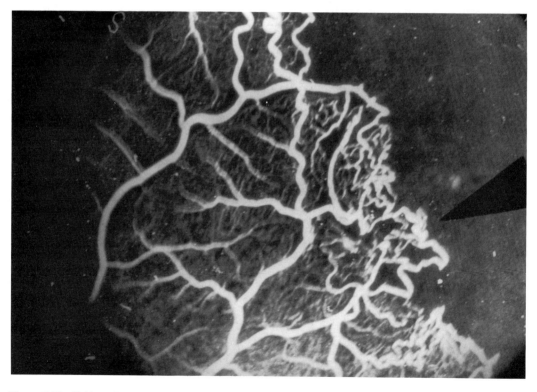

Figure 2.22. Sickle cell retinopathy. Peripheral retinal vascular occlusion and arteriovenous anastomoses. (Courtesy KH Packo, MD.)

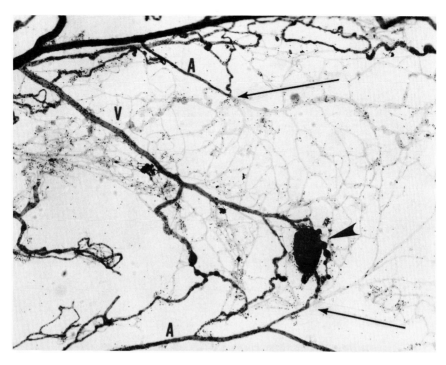

Figure 2.23. Sickle cell retinopathy. Retina, trypsin digestion preparation. Abrupt arteriolar obstruction (*arrows*) with distal vascular hypocellularity. Arteriolar-venular loop with beading is present (*arrowhead*) (A: arterioles; V: venule) (periodic acid Schiff, hematoxylin and eosin: ×29). (From: Romayananda N, Goldberg MF, Green WR. Histopathology of sickle cell retinopathy. Trans Am Acad Ophthalmol Otolaryngol 1973;77:652–676.)

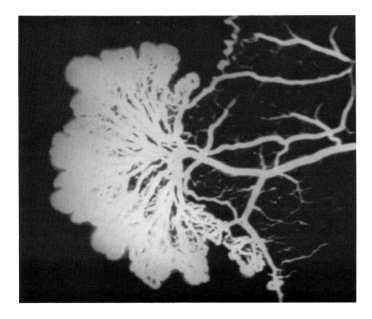

Figure 2.24. Sickle cell retinopathy. Localized retinal neovascularization (sea fan) at junction of perfused and nonperfused retina. (Courtesy KH Packo, MD.)

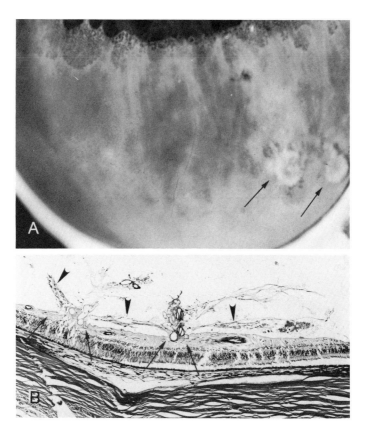

Figure 2.25. Sickle cell retinopathy. **A.** Gross appearance of two "sea-fans" surrounded by hemorrhage (*arrows*). **B**. Section of one of the lesions shows two areas where vessels extend into the vitreous through discontinuities of retinal internal limiting membrane (*between arrows*). Fibroglial tissue (*arrowheads*), a few lymphocytes, and numerous sickled erythrocytes are seen in the vicinity of the sea-fan (hematoxylin and eosin: **B**, ×38). (From: Romayananda N, Goldberg MF, Green WR. Histopathology of sickle cell retinopathy. Trans Am Acad Ophthalmol Otolaryngol 1973;77:652–676.)

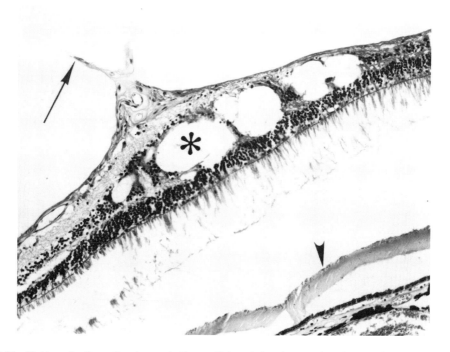

Figure 2.26. Sickle cell retinopathy demonstrating partial posterior vitreous detachment, vitreoretinal adhesion, traction-induced cystic degeneration (*asterisk*), and retinal detachment (*arrowhead*) (hematoxylin and eosin: ×120). (From: Romayananda N, Goldberg MF, Green WR. Histopathology of sickle cell retinopathy. Trans Am Acad Ophthalmol Otolaryngol 1973;77:652–676.)

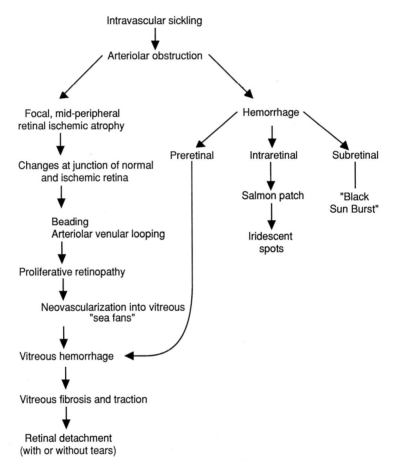

Figure 2.27. Flow diagram representing the pathogenesis of the ocular lesions in sickle cell retinopathy. (From: Romayananda N, Goldberg MF, Green WR. Histopathlogy of sickle cell retinopathy. Trans Am Acad Ophthalmol Otolaryngol 1973;77:652–676.)

Although autoinfarction of retinal neovascularization has been observed (71, 72), progression of proliferative sickle cell retinopathy occurs in a sufficient percentage to warrant therapy in some cases (72, 73). The various modalities and methods of treatment and complications have been reviewed by Stephens (74).

In patients with sickle cell hemoglobinopathy, retinal detachment repair may result in anterior segment and panocular ischemia (64, 75). The risk of this complication can be reduced with pre-, intra-, and post-operative measures to maintain blood pressure, perfusion, and oxygenation (64, 75).

HYPERVISCOSITY RETINOPATHY, HEMOPHILIA, INTRAVASCULAR COAGULOPATHY, AND CIRCULATING AUTOANTIBODIES

Hyperviscosity Retinopathy

Increased amounts of normal or abnormal immunoglobulins and circulating immune complexes in the blood can occur in the plasma cell dyscrasias, including multiple myeloma (IgG or IgΛ), Waldenström's macroglobulinemia (IgM), a variety of other plasma cell disorders, heavy chain disease, and amyloidosis. The paraprotein-induced hyperviscosity leads to the systemic bleeding and neurological ocular disorders characteristic of the hyperviscosity state that is associated with these diseases (76, 77).

The severity of the retinal and choroidal changes appears to be related to the severity of hyperviscosity (78). When serum viscosity becomes mildly elevated to 3 or 4 centipoise (normal is approximately 1.9 centipoise or less), usually no clinical abnormality is detectable. With moderately elevated serum viscosity, small hemorrhages appear in the peripheral retina, and mild venous dilation may occur, accompanied by microaneurysms (Fig. 2.28). With increasing viscosity, venous dilation is more prominent, and compression of the vein at arteriovenous crossings becomes apparent. With in-

creasing severity, there are more numerous and extensive hemorrhages and retinal thickening. Soft exudates appear, and fluorescein angiography shows capillary nonperfusion.

In the more severe stages, the retinal microangiopathy worsens, and there may be disc edema, increasing retinal edema, retinal artery and vein occlusions, and detachment of the sensory retina and the retinal pigment epithelium (Fig. 2.29) (79–81). Although the appearance of the retina is similar to that exhibited in central retinal vein occlusion, the retinopathy of the hyperviscosity state often can be reversed by removing the abnormal blood proteins through plasmapheresis (Fig. 2.30) (78). Other ocular lesions include immunoprotein deposition in the cornea (82, 83) and ciliochoroidal effusion (Fig. 2.31) (79). Ciliary body cysts that become opaque when fixated (Fig. 2.32) may be present and, in rare instances, may be continuous with retinal detachment (Fig. 2.33).

Hemophilia

Ocular complications have been reported in Factor VIII deficiency (hemophilia A), the most common of the congenital coagulopathies, and also in deficiencies of Factors IX and XIII (84–86). Orbital or periorbital hemorrhage is the most commonly reported hemophilic ocular complication followed by subconjunctival hemorrhage. Hemorrhage following ocular surgery has also been reported (84), ranging from mild to severe hyphema and vitreous hemorrhage. Hemorrhage may be controlled with the use of fresh plasma, human antihemophilic factor concentrate, porcine antihemophilic globulin, or cryoprecipitates during elective ocular surgery (87).

Most hemorrhages follow trauma to the eye, but some are spontaneous. In Factor VIII deficiency, bleeding is usually apparent 24 to 36 hours following the trauma. The majority of ocular or periocular hemorrhages are self-limited, but some have required treatment. Severe retrobulbar hemorrhages and those refractory to treat-

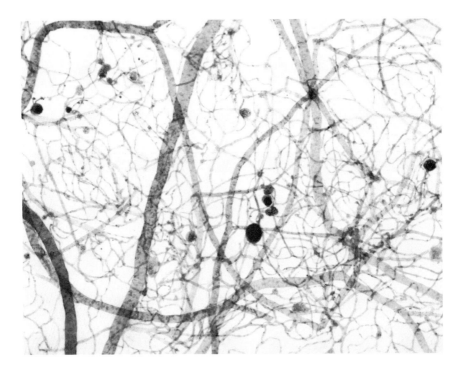

Figure 2.28. Multiple myeloma. Retinal trypsin digest preparation discloses numerous peripheral microaneurysms (periodic acid Schiff: ×40). (From: Khouri GG, Murphy RP, Kuhajda FB, Green WR. Clinicopathologic features in two cases of multiple myeloma. Retina 1986;6:169–175.)

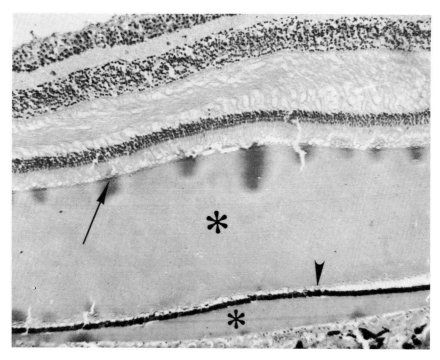

Figure 2.29. Myeloma. Macular area with retinal (*arrow*) and retinal pigment epithelial (*arrowhead*) detachments by a proteinaceous material (*asterisk*) that is rich in IgG (immunoperoxidase: ×90). (From: Khouri GG, Murphy RP, Kuhajda FB, Green WR. Clinicopathologic features in two cases of multiple myeloma. Retina 1986;6:169–175.)

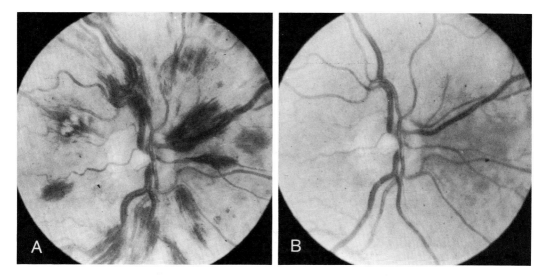

Figure 2.30. Waldenström's macroglobulinemia before (**A**) and after (**B**) plasmapheresis. Before therapy, there is much vascular dilation and tortuosity; flame-shaped hemorrhages and cotton-wool spots are evident. (From: Green WR, Retina. In: Spencer WH, ed. Ophthalmic pathology. An atlas and textbook. Philadelphia: WB Saunders, 1985: Vol 2, Ch 8, p 1083.)

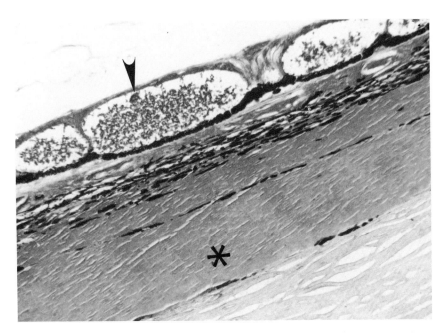

Figure 2.31. Multiple myeloma with positive staining of proteinaceous material for detection of IgG in ciliochoroidal effusion (*asterisk*) and in pars plana cysts (*arrowhead*) (immunoperoxidase: ×135). (From: Khouri GG, Murphy RP, Kuhajda FB, Green WR. Clinicopathologic features in two cases of multiple myeloma. Retina 1986;6:169–175.)

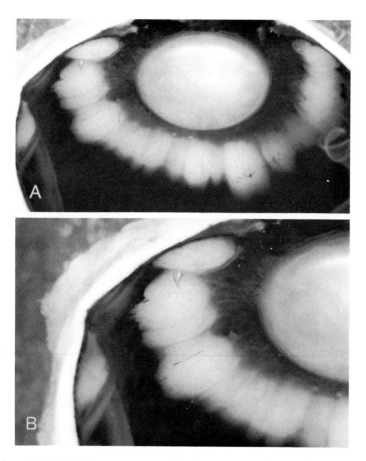

Figure 2.32. Multiple myeloma. Gross appearance of large, opaque cysts around the entire circumference of the pars plana. (From: Khouri GG, Murphy RP, Kuhajda FB, Green WR. Clinicopathologic features in two cases of multiple myeloma. Retina 1986;6:169–175.)

Figure 2.33. Multiple myeloma. **A**. Area illustrates continuity of the proteinaceous material (*asterisk*) under the retina (*to the left*) and in the pars plana cyst (*to the right*). At the ora serrata, there is a 0.8 mm defect in pigment epithelium (*between arrows*) where this layer is detached (*between arrowheads*) along with the nonpigmented ciliary epithelium and the peripheral retina **B**. Higher power shows continuity of pars plana cyst and retinal detachment (periodic acid Schiff **A**, ×40; **B**, ×90).

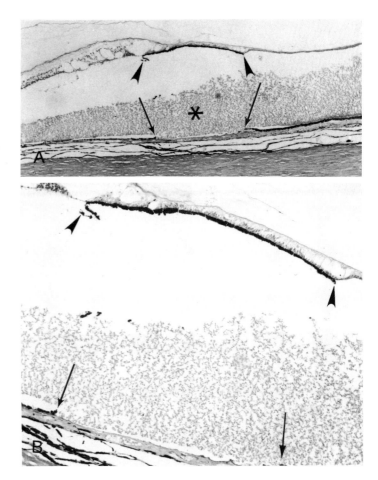

ment may cause central retinal artery occlusion.

Disseminated Intravascular Coagulation

Disseminated intravascular coagulation (DIC) is a syndrome seen in a number of clinical settings, including abruptio placentae, leukemia, malignancy, inflammatory bowel disease, sepsis, and the widespread tissue damage following burns and trauma (88). It is characterized by activation of the coagulation system, consumption of coagulation proteins and platelets, and thrombotic occlusion of small blood vessels, which result in widespread hemorrhage and ischemic tissue damage (89, 90).

Ocular involvement in DIC can include retinal pigment epithelium necrosis and serous retinal detachments resulting from thrombotic occlusion of the choriocapillaris and larger choroidal vessels (Fig. 2.34) (91). Visual loss occurs when the submacular choroid is affected (92, 93). Fluorescein angiography may show leakage at the level of the RPE.

Circulating Autoantibodies

Circulating lupus anticoagulant and antiphospholipid antibodies are circulating antibodies associated with thrombotic vascular disease in both systemic and ocular circulations (94). The circulating lupus anticoagulant (LAC) is a serum immuno-

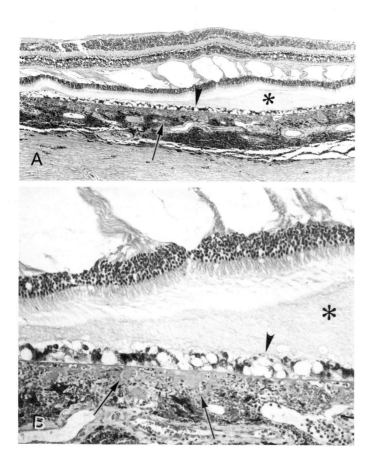

Figure 2.34.
Disseminated intravascular coagulopathy with thrombotic occlusion of the choriocapillaris (*arrows*), mild choroidal hemorrhage, necrosis of the retinal pigment epithelium (*arrowheads*), serous detachment of the macular retina (*asterisks*), and cystoid macular edema that mostly involves the outer plexiform layer (hematoxylin and eosin: **A**, ×40; **B**, ×210). (Courtesy of Dr. HK Leathers.) (From: Green WR. Retina. In: Spencer WH, ed. Ophthalmic pathology. An atlas and textbook. Philadelphia: WB Saunders, 1985; Vol 2, Ch 8, p 1082.)

globulin seen in approximately 10% of lupus cases and in a variety of other systemic disorders (95). Because in vitro it is an antibody that reacts with clotting factors, phospholipid antigens on platelet membranes, and the vascular endothelium to prolong the partial thromboplastin time (PTT), it has been mistakenly called "anticoagulant." Its in vivo behavior is not that of an anticoagulant, because it precipitates thrombosis in both the systemic and cerebral circulations. It can cause thrombocytopenia and spontaneous abortions and may elicit a false-positive VDRL.

Patients with the lupus anticoagulant have had associated branch retinal artery and vein occlusions, ischemic optic neuropathy, transient visual loss, transient diplopia, visual field loss, and vertebrobasilar insufficiency. Some patients with circulating LAC and thrombosis also have anticardiolipin antibodies, which are also antiphospholipid antibodies particularly reactive with cardiolipin, as detected with the use of ELISA. Lupus anticoagulant immunoglobulin should be suspected whenever the PTT is prolonged and unexplained systemic or retinal vascular occlusive disease is present.

Sjögren's syndrome A antigen (SSA) is a protein–ribonucleic acid complex. Patients with mild systemic lupus erythematosus who also exhibit autoantibodies directed against this complex have been described (96). Several of these patients developed severe retinal vasculitis characterized by retinal arteriolitis, progressive irreversible ischemia, and optic disc and retinal neovascularization accompanied by proliferative retinopathy. The presence of retinal arteriolitis should alert the clinician to consider, in the differential diagnosis, autoantibodies to Sjögren's syndrome A antigen. Antibodies directed against Sjögren's syndrome A antigens are found in patients with systemic lupus erythematosus, in those with lupus-like disorders, and in those with Sjögren's syndrome, Waldenström's macroglobulinemia, and progressive systemic sclerosis.

References

Platelet Disorders

1. Handin RI. Hemorrhagic disorders. II. Platelets and purpura. In: Beck WS, ed. Hematology. 4th ed. Cambridge, MA: MIT Press, 1985:433–456.
2. Rubenstein RA, Yanoff M, Albert DM. Thrombocytopenia, anemia, and retinal hemorrhage. Am J Ophthalmol 1968;65:435–439.
3. Adrouny A, Sandler RM, Carmel R. Variable presentation of thrombocytopenia in Graves' disease. Arch Intern Med 1982;142:1460–1464.
4. Ackerman J, Goldstein M, Kanarek I. Spontaneous massive vitreous hemorrhage secondary to thrombocytopenia. Ophthalmic Surg 1980; 11:636–637.
5. Shaw HE, Smith SW, North-Coombes JD. Quinine-induced thrombocytopenia complicating eyelid surgery. Arch Ophthalmol 1987;105:1176.
6. Klepach GL, Wray SH. Bilateral serous retinal detachment with thrombocytopenia during penicillamine therapy. Ann Ophthalmol 1981;13:201–203.
7. Cogan DG. Ocular involvement in disseminated intravascular coagulopathy. Arch Ophthalmol 1975;93:1–8.
8. Percival SPB. Ocular findings in thrombotic thrombocytopenic purpura (Moschcowitz's disease). Br J Ophthalmol 1970;54:73–78.
9. Stefani FH, Brandt F, Pielsticker K. Periarteritis nodosa and thrombotic thrombocytopenic purpura with serous retinal detachment in siblings. Br J Ophthalmol 1978;62:402–407.
10. Wyszynski RE, Frank KE, Grossniklaus HE. Bilateral retinal detachments in thrombotic thrombocytopenic purpura. Graefes Arch Clin Exp Ophthalmol 1988;226:501–504.
11. Lambert SR, High KA, Cotlier E, Benz EJ Jr. Serous retinal detachments in thrombotic thrombocytopenic purpura. Arch Ophthalmol 1985;103:1172–1174.
12. Vaiser A, Hutton WL, Marengo-Rowe AJ, et al. Retinal hemorrhage associated with thrombasthenia. Am J Ophthalmol 1975;80:258–262.
13. Chaudhuri PR, Rosenthal AR, Goulstine DB, et al. Familial exudative vitreoretinopathy associated with familial thrombocytopathy. Br J Ophthalmol 1983;67:755–758.
14. Voaden MJ, Hussain AA, Chan IPR. Studies on retinitis pigmentosa in man. I. Taurine and blood platelets. Br J Ophthalmol 1982;66:771–775.
15. Burch JW, Stanford N, Majerus PW. Inhibition of platelet prostaglandin synthetase by oral aspirin. J Clin Invest 1978;61:314–319.
16. Mortada A, Abboud I. Retinal haemorrhages after prolonged use of salicylates. Br J Ophthalmol 1973;57:199–200.
17. El Baba F, Jarrett WH II, Harbin TS Jr, et al. Massive hemorrhage complicating age-related macular degeneration. Clinicopathologic correlation and the role of anticoagulants. Ophthalmology 1986;93:1581–1592.
18. Crawford JS, Lewandowski RL, Chan W. The effect of aspirin on rebleeding in traumatic hyphema. Am J Ophthalmol 1975;80:543–545.
19. Paris GL, Waltuch GF. Salicylate-induced bleeding problem in ophthalmic plastic surgery. Ophthalmic Surg 1982;13:627–629.
20. Colwell JA, Winocur PD, Haluska PV. Do platelets have anything to do with diabetic microvascular disease? Diabetes 1983;32(Suppl 2):14–19.
21. Borsey DQ, Prowse CV, Gray RS, et al. Platelet and coagulation factors in proliferative diabetic retinopathy. J Clin Pathol 1984;37:659–664.
22. Early Treatment Diabetic Retinopathy Study Research Group. Photocoagulation for diabetic macular edema; Early Treatment Diabetic Retinopathy Study report number 1. Arch Ophthalmol 1985;103:1796–1806.
23. Walsh PN, Kansu T, Savino PJ, et al. Platelet coagulant activities in arterial occlusive disease of the eye. Stroke 1979;10:589–594.
24. Ando F, Kato M, Goto S, et al. Platelet function in bilateral acute retinal necrosis. Am J Ophthalmol 1983;96:27–32.

Abnormalities of White Blood Cells

25. Devita VT Jr, Jaffe ES, Hellman S. Hodgkin's disease and the non-Hodgkin's lymphomas. In: Devita VT Jr, Hellman S, Rosenberg SA, eds. Cancer: principles and practice of oncology. 2nd ed. Philadelphia: JB Lippincott, 1985:1623–1709.
26. Allen RA, Straatsma BR. Ocular involvement in leukemia and allied disorders. Arch Ophthalmol 1961;66:490–508.
27. Nelson CC, Hertzberg BS, Klintworth GK. A histopathologic study of 716 unselected eyes in patients with cancer at the time of death. Am J Ophthalmol 1983;95:788–793.
28. Kincaid MC, Green WR. Ocular and orbital involvement in leukemia. Surv Ophthalmol 1983;27:211–232.
29. Ridgway EW, Jaffe N, Walton DS. Leukemic ophthalmopathy in children. Cancer 1976; 38:1744–1749.
30. Duke-Elder S. System of ophthalmology. Vol 10: Diseases of the retina. St. Louis: CV Mosby, 1967:393–400.
31. Tang RA, Aguirre Vila-Coro A, Wall S, Frankel LS. Acute leukemia presenting as a retinal pigment epithelium detachment. Arch Ophthalmol 1988;106:21–22.
32. Burns CA, Blodi FC, Williamson BK. Acute lymphocytic leukemia and central serous retinopa-

thy. Trans Am Acad Ophthalmol Otolaryngol 1965;69:307–309.

33. Stewart MW, Gitter KA, Cohen G. Acute leukemia presenting as a unilateral exudative retinal detachment. Retina 1989;9:110–114.

34. Rosenthal AR. Ocular manifestations of leukemia; a review. Ophthalmology 1983;90:899–905.

35. Gass JDM. Differential diagnosis of intraocular tumors; a stereoscopic presentation. St. Louis: CV Mosby, 1974:160–176.

36. Clayman HM, Flynn JT, Koch K, Israel C. Retinal pigment epithelial abnormalities in leukemic disease. Am J Ophthalmol 1972;74:416–419.

37. Jakobiec F, Behrens M. Leukemic retinal pigment epitheliopathy, with report of a unilateral case. J Pediatr Ophthalmol 1975;12:10–15.

38. Swartz M, Schumann GB. Acute leukemic infiltration of the vitreous diagnosed by pars plana aspiration. Am J Ophthalmol 1980;90:326–330.

39. Belmont JB, Michelson JB, Bordin GM. Ocular inflammation associated with chronic lymphocytic leukemia. J Ocular Ther Surg 1985;4:125–129.

40. Guyer DR, Schachat AP, Vitale S, et al. Leukemic retinopathy; relationship between fundus lesions and hematologic parameters at diagnosis. Ophthalmology 1989;96:860–864.

41. Duane TD, Osher RH, Green WR. White centered hemorrhages: their significance. Ophthalmology 1980;87:66–69.

42. Green WR. Retina. In: Spencer WH, ed. Ophthalmic pathology. An atlas and textbook. Vol 2. Philadelphia: WB Saunders, 1985:662–668,1058–1064.

43. Brown GC, Brown MM, Hiller T, et al. Cotton-wool spots. Retina 1985;5:206–214.

44. Duke JR, Wilkinson CP, Sigelman S. Retinal microaneurysms in leukemia. Br J Ophthalmol 1968;52:368–374.

45. Jampol LM, Goldberg MF, Busse B. Peripheral retinal microaneurysms in chronic leukemia. Am J Ophthalmol 1975;80:242–248.

46. Frank RN, Ryan SJ Jr. Peripheral retinal neovascularization with chronic myelogenous leukemia. Arch Ophthalmol 1972;87:585–589.

47. Morse PH, McCready JL. Peripheral retinal neovascularization in chronic myelocytic leukemia. Am J Ophthalmol 1971;72:975–978.

48. Leville AS, Morse PH. Platelet-induced retinal neovascularization in leukemia. Am J Ophthalmol 1981;91:640–643.

49. Cogan DG. Immunosuppression and eye disease. Am J Ophthalmol 1977;83:777–788.

50. McDonnell PJ, McDonnell JM, Brown RH, Green WR. Ocular involvement in patients with fungal infections. Ophthalmology 1985;92:706–709.

51. Schachat AP. Radiation retinopathy. In: Ryan SJ, ed. Retina. Vol 2: Medical retina. St. Louis: CV Mosby, 1988:541–545.

52. Rootman J, Gudauskas G. Treatment of ocular leukemia with local chemotherapy. Cancer Treat Rep 1985;69:119–122.

53. Mehta AB, Goldman JM, Kohner E. Hyperleucocytic retinopathy in chronic granulocytic leu-

kemia: the role of intensive leucapheresis. Br J Haematol 1984; 56:661–667.

54. Sesenbrenner LL, Owens AH Jr. Patients with bone marrow failure. In: Harvey AM, Johns RJ, McKusick VA, et al., eds. The principles and practice of medicine. 21st ed. Norwalk, CT: Appleton-Century-Crofts, 1984:529–538.

55. Libert J, Dhermy P, Van Hoof F, et al. Ocular findings in Chediak-Higashi disease: a light and electron microscopic study of two patients. Birth Defects 1982;18:327–344.

56. Babior BM, Crowley CA. Chronic granulomatous disease and other disorders of oxidative killing by phagocytes. In: Stanbury JB, Wyngaarden JB, Fredrickson DS, et al., eds. The metabolic basis of inherited disease. 5th ed. New York: McGraw-Hill, 1983:1956–1985.

57. Martyn LJ, Lischner HW, Pileggi AJ, Harley RD. Chorioretinal lesions in familial chronic granulomatous disease of childhood. Am J Ophthalmol 1972;73:403–418.

58. Palestine AG, Meyers SM, Fauci AS, Gallin JI. Ocular findings in patients with neutrophil dysfunction. Am J Ophthalmol 1983;95:598–604.

59. Rodrigues MM, Palestine AG, Macher AM, Fauci AS. Histopathology of ocular changes in chronic granulomatous disease. Am J Ophthalmol 1983;96:810–812.

60. Grossniklaus HE, Frank KE, Jacobs G. Chorioretinal lesions in chronic granulomatous disease of childhood; clinicopathologic correlations. Retina 1988;8:270–274.

Diseases of Red Blood Cells

61. Cunningham RD. Retinopathy of blood dyscrasias. In: Duane TD, Jaeger EA, eds. Clinical ophthalmology. Philadelphia: JB Lippincott, 1987: Vol 3, Chap 18. 3–5.

62. Goldberg MF. Sickle cell retinopathy. In: Duane TD, Jaeger EA, eds. Clinical ophthalmology. Philadelphia: JB Lippincott, 1979: Vol 3, Chap 17.

63. Goldberg MF. Classification and pathogenesis of proliferative sickle retinopathy. Am J Ophthalmol 1971;71:649–665.

64. Nagpal KC, Goldberg MF, Rabb MF. Ocular manifestations of sickle hemoglobinopathies. Surv Ophthalmol 1977; 21:391–411.

65. Nagpal KC, Asdourian GK, Patrianakos D, et al. Proliferative retinopathy in sickle cell trait; report of seven cases. Arch Intern Med 1977;137:325–328.

66. Romayananda N, Goldberg MF, Green WR. Histopathology of sickle cell retinopathy. Trans Am Acad Ophthalmol Otolaryngol 1973;77:OP652–676.

67. Ryan SJ Jr. Occlusion of the macular capillaries in sickle cell hemoglobin C disease. Am J Ophthalmol 1974;77:459–461.

68. Marsh RJ, Ford SM, Rabb MF, et al. Macular vasculature, visual acuity, and irreversibly sickled cells in homozygous sickle cell disease. Br J Ophthalmol 1982;66:155–160.

69. Asdourian GK, Nagpal KC, Busse B, et al. Mac-

ular and perimacular vascular remodelling in sickling hemoglobinopathies. Br J Ophthalmol 1976;60:431–453.

70. Dizon RV, Jampol LM, Goldberg MF, Juarez C. Choroidal occlusive disease in sickle cell hemoglobinopathies. Surv Ophthalmol 1979;23:297–306.

71. Goldberg MF. Natural history of untreated proliferative sickle retinopathy. Arch Ophthamol 1971;85:428–437.

72. Nagpal KC, Patrianakos D, Asdourian GK, et al. Spontaneous regression (autoinfarction) of proliferative sickle retinopathy. Am J Ophthalmol 1975;80:885–892.

73. Condon PI, Serjeant GR. Behaviour of untreated proliferative sickle retinopathy. Br J Ophthalmol 1980;64:404–411.

74. Stephens RF. Proliferative sickle cell retinopathy: the disease and a review of its management. Ophthalmic Surg 1987;18:222–231.

75. Ryan SJ Jr, Goldberg MF. Anterior segment ischemia following scleral buckling in sickle cell hemoglobinopathy. Am J Ophthalmol 1971;72:35–50.

Hyperviscosity Retinopathy, Hemophilia,
Intravascular Coagulopathy, and Circulating
Autoantibodies

76. Fahey JL, Barth WF, Solomon A. Serum hyperviscosity syndrome. JAMA 1965;192:464–467.

77. Knapp AJ, Gartner S, Henkind P. Multiple myeloma and its ocular manifestations. Surv Ophthalmol 1987;31:343–351.

78. Murphy RP. Treatment of hyperviscosity retinopathy. In: Ryan SJ, Dawson AK, Little HL, eds. Retinal diseases. Orlando: Grune & Stratton, 1985:247–250.

79. Khouri GG, Murphy RP, Kuhajda FP, Green WR. Clinicopathologic features in two cases of multiple myeloma. Retina 1986;6:169–175.

80. Ashton N. Ocular changes in multiple myelomatosis. Arch Ophthalmol 1965;73:487–494.

81. Foos RY, Allen RA. Opaque cysts of the ciliary body (pars ciliaris retinae). Arch Ophthalmol 1967;77:559–568.

82. Miller KH, Green WR, Stark WJ, et al. Immunoprotein deposition in the cornea. Ophthalmology 1980;87:944–950.

83. Bourne WM, Kyle RA, Brubaker RF, Greipp PR. Incidence of corneal crystals in the monoclonal gammopathies. Am J Ophthalmol 1989;107:192–193.

84. Rubenstein RA, Albert DM, Scheie HG. Ocular complications of hemophilia. Arch Ophthalmol 1966;76:230–232.

85. Zimmerman A, Merigan TC. Retrobulbar hemorrhage in a hemophiliac with irreversible loss of vision. Arch Ophthalmol 1960;64:949–950.

86. Wong GY, Fisher LM, Geeraets WJ. Ocular complications of factor XIII deficiency. Am J Ophthalmol 1969;67:346–351.

87. Richard RD, Spurling CL. Elective ocular surgery in hemophilia. Arch Ophthalmol 1973;89:167–168.

88. Martin VAF. Disseminated intravascular coagulopathy. Trans Ophthalmol Soc UK 1978;98:506–507.

89. Samples FR, Buettner H. Ocular involvement in disseminated intravascular coagulation (DIC). Ophthalmology 1983;90:914–916.

90. Azar P, Smith RS, Greenberg MH. Ocular findings in disseminated intravascular coagulation. Am J Ophthalmol 1974;78:493–496.

91. Hoines J, Buettner H. Ocular complications of disseminated intravascular coagulation (DIC) in abruptio placentae. Retina 1989;9:105–109.

92. Cogan DG. Ocular involvement in disseminated intravascular coagulopathy. Arch Ophthalmol 1975;93:1–8.

93. Patchett RB, Wilson WB, Ellis PP. Ophthalmic complications with disseminated intravascular coagulation. Br J Ophthalmol 1988;72:377–379.

94. Levine SR, Crofts JW, Lesser GR, et al. Visual symptoms associated with the presence of lupus anticoagulant. Ophthalmology 1988;95:686–692.

95. Harris EN, Gharavi AE, Hughes GRV. Anti-phospholipid antibodies. Clin Rheum Dis 1985;11:591–609.

96. Farmer SG, Kinyoun JL, Nelson JL, Wener MH. Retinal vasculitis associated with autoantibodies to Sjögren's syndrome A antigen. Am J Ophthalmol 1985;100:814–821.

CHAPTER 3

Hypertensive Retinopathy, Choroidopathy, and Optic Neuropathy: A Clinical and Pathophysiological Approach to Classification

Mark O.M. Tso, Gary W. Abrams, and Lee M. Jampol

INTRODUCTION

Systemic hypertension accounts for the greatest number of physician visits for any disease (1). The Third Joint National Committee classifies hypertension as a minimum diastolic blood pressure of 90 mm Hg or a minimum systolic blood pressure of 160 mm Hg (2). With this classification, 57 million Americans are estimated to have hypertension. Any degree of hypertension increases the risk of cardiovascular disease, but higher levels of blood pressure intensify that risk. The Third Joint National Committee classification of blood pressure is presented in Table 3.1. This classification categorizes blood pressure into several grades of severity. Blood pressure values are based on an average of two or more blood pressure recordings taken on two or more visits. Hypertension can result from many causes (Table 3.2), but 90% or more of cases are due to essential hypertension. The majority of the remainder are due to congenital or acquired renal diseases such as dysgenesis, renal artery stenosis, or glomerulonephritis.

Because the arteries and veins within the human body are mostly covered by skin or mucous membrane, the vascular constriction and sclerosis induced by hypertension cannot be visualized noninvasively. However, there are several methods or techniques for viewing arteries and veins

of the retina, choroid, and optic nerve, the important ocular structures affected by systemic hypertension. The retinal arteries and veins can be directly examined in vivo by ophthalmoscopy, and, in patients with retinal vascular diseases, the changes in the tissues of the retina and the optic nerve head can be seen. Although the ophthalmoscope cannot present an unobstructed view of the choroidal vasculature

Table 3.1. Third Joint National Committee Classification of Blood Pressure[a,b]

Range (mm Hg)	Category
Diastolic	
< 85	Normal BP
85–89	High normal BP
90–104	Mild hypertension
105–114	Moderate hypertension
≥ 115	Severe hypertension
Systolic, when diastolic BP<90	
< 140	Normal BP
< 140–159	Borderline isolated systolic hypertension
≥ 160	Isolated systolic hypertension

[a]A classification of borderline systolic hypertension (systolic BP 140 to 159 mm Hg) or isolated systolic hypertension (systolic BP ≥ 160 mm Hg) takes precedence over a classification of high normal BP (diastolic BP 85 to 89 mm Hg) when both occur in the same person. A classification of high normal BP (diastolic BP 85 to 89 mm Hg) takes precedence over a classification of normal BP (systolic BP < 140 mm Hg) when both occur in the same person.
[b]From Kaplan NM. Clinical hypertension, 4th edition. Baltimore: Williams & Wilkins, 1986.

Table 3.2. Types of Hypertension

I. Systolic and diastolic hypertension
  A. Essential
  B. Secondary
    1. Renal
    2. Endocrine
    3. Coarctation of the aorta
    4. Pregnancy-induced hypertension
    5. Neurological disorders
    6. Acute stress, including surgery
    7. Increased intravascular volume
    8. Alcohol, drugs, etc.
II. Systolic hypertension
  A. Increased cardiac output
    1. Aortic valvular insufficiency
    2. Arteriovenous fistula, patent ductus arteriosus
    3. Thyrotoxicosis
    4. Paget's disease of bone
    5. Beriberi
    6. Hyperkinetic circulation
  B. Rigidity of aorta

because this vasculature is located behind the retinal pigment epithelium, a disturbance in the choroidal circulation may cause secondary alterations in the retinal pigment epithelium and retina that can be seen ophthalmoscopically. Similarly, vascular disturbance of the posterior optic nerve cannot be visualized ophthalmoscopically, but optic nerve head changes induced by posterior vascular alterations can be. These changes include ischemia, edema, or atrophy of the optic disc. Because the eye findings reflect the severity and the adequacy of control of hypertension, monitoring ophthalmoscopic changes in hypertensive retinopathy, choroidopathy, and optic neuropathy has guided physicians in caring for their hypertensive patients.

In recent years, the development of angiography has enabled the physician to study the dynamic circulations of the retina, choroid, and optic nerve head. Retinal capillaries, which are not normally visible when ophthalmoscopy is performed, may be visualized with fluorescein angiography. Leakage, occlusion, dilation, microaneurysm formation, and other pathological alterations of the retinal capillaries also may be observed (Fig. 3.1). The choroidal circulation can be examined by performing angiographic studies that use indocyanine green, although current techniques provide poor resolution of the vascular details. Angiography of the posterior portion of the eye in patients with hypertension has provided physicians with new information, unavailable by other methods of study, about the pathology of hypertensive retinal vascular diseases.

The alterations in the retinal vasculature may reflect the status of the vasculature of other organs of the body, especially the central nervous system, the cardiovascular system, the hemopoietic system, and the kidneys. The structure and function of elements of these organ systems are biologically related to those of ocular elements. For example, striking similarity exists between the structure and function of the retina and optic nerve and those of the brain. All three tissues exhibit blood-tissue barriers. The optic nerve is not a peripheral nerve but a white fiber tract of the central nervous system. The axons of the optic nerve are enveloped by the plasmalemma and cytoplasm of oligodendrocytes, as are those found in the central nervous system (3). The retina is not a peripheral sensory organ but an organized group of neurons that originate in the central nervous system and that receive, analyze, synthesize, and transmit impulses to other parts of the brain for correlation and signal interpretation. When various vascular changes occur, the tissues of the retina and the optic nerve react similarly to those of the central nervous system. Ischemia, edema, and infarction such as those seen in the retina and optic nerve are also found in the central nervous system. Any changes in the cardiovascular system that affect perfusion pressure may be reflected by changes in the retinal vasculature. In addition, changes in the blood such as anemia, polycythemia, or changes in blood viscosity may be manifest in the retinal circulation. The microcirculations of the kidneys and the eyes are often affected by systemic diseases in a similar fashion. Hypertension, which can be induced by a number of renal diseases, may produce

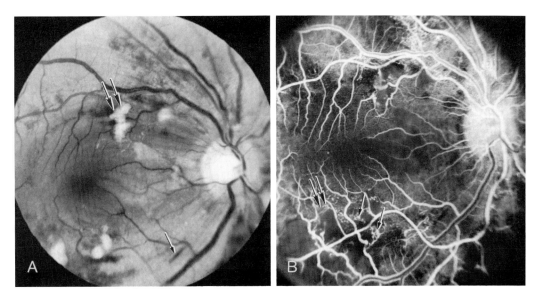

Figure 3.1. A. Exudative phase of hypertensive retinopathy, showing linear or flame-shaped hemorrhage (*single arrow*) and cotton-wool spots (*double arrows*), which are arranged at a right angle to the direction of the nerve fibers, lying anterior to retinal vessels. Moderate narrowing of the retinal arteries and engorgement of retinal veins are seen. **B.** Fluorescein angiogram of exudative phase of hypertensive retinopathy showing focal areas of nonperfusion (*double arrows*), dilation of retinal capillaries and capillary microaneurysm (*single arrow*) around the cotton-wool spots.

similar ocular and renal vascular changes.

Nutrition to the retina is supplied by both the retinal and choroidal circulations. Of the total volume of blood flowing through the ocular tissues, only 2% passes through the retinal circulation (4); more than 70% passes through the choroid, and approximately 28% flows through the iris and ciliary body. Anatomically, the retinal and choroidal circulations are separated by the retinal pigment epithelium and photoreceptor cells. The structure and physiology of these circulations are very different. The circulatory dynamics of the optic nerve also differ from those of the choroid and retina. Retinal vessels are similar to the blood vessels of the central nervous system, with cell junctions that maintain a blood-retinal barrier. Retinal vessels autoregulate flow in response to changes in blood pressure, ocular pressure, and oxygenation of the blood. In contrast, the choroidal blood vessels are similar to other systemic blood vessels. The choroidal vessels lack tight junctions, and vascular tone is regulated by the sympathetic

nervous system. The optic nerve vasculature, supplied by branches from the central retinal artery, the choroid, and the pia mater, exhibits characteristics of both the retinal and choroidal circulations. Various forms and stages of hypertension affect these three circulations differently. Most attention has been focused on alterations of the retina induced by hypertension, because these changes are the most easily observed.

As early as 1898, retinal vascular changes had been reported in patients with cerebrovascular insufficiency and renal disease (5). Subsequently, a number of physicians described the retinal vascular changes of systemic hypertension (6–19). Several classifications of hypertensive retinopathy have been proposed; these classifications have been modified and improved. In the last 20 years, the unique anatomical and physiological characteristics of the retinal, choroidal, and optic nerve circulations have been described, and the descriptions have expanded the understanding of hypertensive retinopathy, choroidopathy, and optic neuropathy. Furthermore, the development of new classes of pharmacological agents used in the treatment of systemic hypertension has greatly altered the clinical course of hypertensive retinopathy, which had no effective treatment as recently as 40 years ago. In the past, a classification such as that of Keith, Wagener, and Barker had prognostic significance (6), but in recent decades, the survival rate of patients has depended more on the efficacy of treatment and the promptness of its initiation than on the classification of the retinopathy. In this chapter, we present some of the recent information on the anatomy and physiology of the retinal, choroidal, and optic nerve circulations, a brief overview of previously used classifications of hypertensive retinopathy, and a new approach to the classification of hypertensive ocular disease.

STRUCTURE AND PHYSIOLOGICAL REGULATION OF THE RETINAL VASCULATURE

The retinal circulation is supplied by the central retinal artery, which is a branch of the ophthalmic artery. The central retinal artery runs anteriorly in the connective tissue of the orbit, pierces the dural and arachnoid sheaths approximately 10 mm behind the lamina cribrosa, turns forward for a short distance in the subarachnoid space, and penetrates the pia mater to enter the optic nerve. The central retinal artery divides into four retinal arteries after piercing the lamina cribrosa in the optic nerve head. Sympathetic nerve endings are found in the extraocular portion of the central retinal artery but are absent anterior to the lamina cribrosa (20). Histologically, the central retinal artery has the architecture of a small muscular artery because it is lined by distinct tunicae intima, media, and adventitia. A well-developed internal elastic lamina is seen. In contrast, the retinal arteries in the posterior pole do not have an internal elastic lamina but have 5 to 7 layers of smooth muscle cells in the

tunica media; these are reduced to 2 to 3 layers at the equator and only 1 or 2 layers in the periphery. The absence of the internal elastic lamina in the retinal arteries is balanced by a well-developed tunica media, which responds vigorously to elevated blood pressure. Whether the retinal arteries should be called small muscular arteries or arterioles is controversial (3, 21). In this chapter, we use the term retinal "artery" instead of "arteriole" for the retinal vascular tree. Discussion of hypertensive retinopathy focuses upon the arteries because the pathological process most prominently affects the small muscular arteries.

The adventitia of the extraocular portion of the central retinal artery is continuous with the pia mater. Within the eye, a narrow perivascular space surrounds the retinal vessels and is lined externally by a layer of Müller cells or glial cells separating the vessels from surrounding neural elements. This perivascular space is very narrow in the young, but it enlarges with age. This space accumulates a growing amount of basement membrane material of smooth muscle cells and glial cells (Fig. 3.2) as the individual ages; the accumulation partially accounts for the increased light reflex of sclerosis of the retinal arteries in the aging patient and in the chronic hypertensive patient. In individuals with papilledema, this space becomes even more prominent, filling with debris of various cells, basement membrane material, and even macrophages; this condition presents clinically as perivascular sheathing (22).

The retinal capillary bed is a complex network arranged in distinct layers. For example, a superficial capillary network is thought to lie in the nerve fiber layer, with a deep capillary network set in the inner nuclear layer (23, 24). Another view depicts the retinal capillary system as a three-dimensional plexus with capillaries suspended like a hammock between the retinal arteries and veins (25). Shimizu and Ujiie studied the retinal capillaries in three-dimensional vascular casts and observed a well-defined, layered pattern with an outer capillary layer, an inner capillary

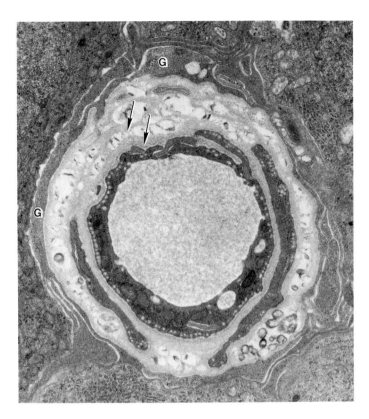

Figure 3.2. An electron micrograph of a retinal arteriole showing increase in perivascular space filling with basement membrane-like material (*arrows*). The perivascular space is surrounded by an encircling layer of glial processes (*G*), separating the retinal vasculature from the retinal neural elements. This widening of the perivascular space increases the light reflex in the wall of the arteriole on ophthalmoscopy and gives a copper wiring appearance.

layer, and a radial peripapillary layer around the optic nerve head (26).

Specific retinal vascular disorders seem to preferentially affect the superficial or deep capillaries. For example, the exudative retinopathy manifested in diabetes tends to affect the deep capillaries, and the hemorrhages accumulate in the outer plexiform and inner nuclear layers. On the other hand, the hemorrhages due to hypertension frequently arise from the superficial capillaries in the nerve fiber layer.

Unique features of the retinal vasculature are the presence of a blood-retinal barrier and specialized pericytes around the retinal capillaries (27). The pericytes are approximately equal in number to endothelial cells and are encased within the basement membrane of the retinal capillaries. Their functions are subject to speculation, but they may control the tone of the capillaries, regulating flow throughout the capillary bed. The blood-retinal barrier is present at two sites: the inner blood-retinal barrier at the retinal vasculature and the outer blood-retinal barrier at the retinal pigment epithelium. The retinal capillary wall is of the continuous type, in contrast to the discontinuous wall of the choriocapillaris. The endothelial cells of the retinal capillaries are joined by a zonula occludens type of cell junction. The blood-retinal barrier appears to lie in these specialized cell junctions and in the integrity of the plasmalemma of the endothelial cells. The endothelial cells of the retinal capillaries are noncycling cells that, under normal circumstances, show no proliferation or replacement, as shown by the absence of thymidine uptake in normal endothelial cells (28). However, when the eye becomes diseased or injured, endothelial cells may proliferate; this multiplication of cells seems to be limited to endothelial cells of postcapillary venules.

The blood-retinal barrier may be broken in various disease states. In these pathological states, either the cell junction or the plasmalemma of the endothelial cells is impaired. Five categories of pathological alterations may take place (27): (a) Necrosis of the cytoplasm of endothelial cells may allow intravascular components to leak into the extravascular space. For example, in cases of malignant hypertension, necrosis of endothelial cells and inundation of plasma proteins from retinal vessels have been found (10). (b) Disruption of the cell junctions between the endothelial cells may cause macromolecules to leak into the extracellular space. In cystoid macular edema due to malignant hypertension, retinal vessels may be seen to leak fluorescein dye. In an experimental study of hypertension using a horseradish peroxidase tracer, extravascular leakage without endothelial cell necrosis was seen; the leakage was presumably due to the opening of the endothelial cell junctions. In experimental studies of diabetes in the dog, the opening of the endothelial cell junctions of retinal blood vessels was observed, and horseradish peroxidase tracer was demonstrated to pass from the intravascular compartment through the open cell junctions into the perivascular space (29). (c) Increase in endothelial cell pinocytotic activity and vascular transport may account for some of the examples of disruption of the blood-retinal barrier. This form of transport is uncommon across the endothelium of normal retinal capillaries, even though it is commonly seen in the endothelium of the capillaries of skeletal muscles. Increased numbers of pinocytotic vesicles were noted in endothelial cells of leaking retinal capillaries in monkeys that had undergone lens extraction associated with vitreous loss or that had ocular hypotony. However, the extent to which the increase in pinocytotic activity contributes to the disruption of the blood-retinal barrier is not known. (d) Focal attenuation of the cytoplasm of endothelial cells is seen in some pathological states. For example, in patients with diabetic retinopathy, new vessels form and develop fenestrations in the cytoplasm of the endothelial cells, accounting for the leakage from the retinal or vitreous neovasculari-

zation. (e) Failure of formation of tight cell junctions of retinal capillaries is rare but has been observed in retinopathy of prematurity. It is difficult to differentiate faulty formation of cell junctions from disruption of cell junctions.

The retinal vasculature contains no autonomic nerves, and the vascular tone is autoregulated by at least two mechanisms (30–32), a myogenic mechanism and a metabolic mechanism. In the myogenic mechanism, the vascular tone is believed to be regulated by pacemaker cells in the vessel wall, which are influenced by the transmural pressure or intraocular pressure. In a study of blood flow using the microsphere impaction method, it was demonstrated that autoregulation of the retinal circulation takes place when perfusion pressure changes (33). It was shown that an elevation of intraocular pressure resulted in dilation of retinal vessels (34, 35). Riva et al. demonstrated that the retinal circulation autoregulates within physiological variations of intraocular pressure (36). These and other experiments showed that the muscle tone of the retinal vasculature varies in response to changes in perfusion pressure and intraocular pressure to provide a constant blood flow. In systemic hypertension, which stimulates this myogenic mechanism in the retinal vasculature, the retinal arteries become narrower.

In the metabolic mechanism, the retinal blood vessels alter their vascular tone and resistance so that the concentration of important metabolites and nutrients are maintained at a physiological level (30–32). It was found that a marked retinal vasoconstriction occurs in response to oxygen breathing (37–39). An elevation in the partial pressure of carbon dioxide, a decrease in blood pH, and an accumulation of metabolites tend to decrease vascular tone (39–43).

The reactivity of the retinal vasculature to pressure or metabolic changes is influenced by aging and by many systemic conditions (31, 37, 42, 43). Aging leads to a mild loss of autoregulation. Hyperglycemia impairs vascular reactivity; thus, diabetic patients have decreased vascular reactivity and show various levels of inability to adapt to normal changes in intraocular pressure and oxygen partial pressure. Patients with hypertensive retinopathy have a similar decrease in vascular reactivity. In retinopathy of prematurity, the retinal vessels of the newborn shown an exaggerated vasoconstrictive response to increased partial pressure of oxygen. This response may result in retinal ischemia. The retinal circulation of a normal adult will respond to the same stimulus with only mild vasoconstriction and produce no retinal infarction. Autoregulation of the retinal vasculature plays an important part in hypertensive retinopathy, as demonstrated by the retinal vascular response to elevation or lowering of the systemic blood pressure. Ophthalmoscopic study of the retinal vasculature indicates rather accurately the vascular reactivity and also the perfusion pressure in the retinal vessels.

STRUCTURE AND PHYSIOLOGICAL REGULATION OF THE CHOROIDAL VASCULATURE

The choroidal vasculature consists of multiple layers of interwoven blood vessels lying between the retinal pigment epithelium and the sclera. The volume of blood flowing throughout the choroid per minute is one of the highest in the body: 809 ± 73 ml/minute in rabbits, 734 ± 94 ml/minute in cats, and 677 ± 67 ml/minute in monkeys (33). Although the function of this extremely high blood flow is not clearly understood, the structure of the choroidal vessels facilitates this flow velocity.

The choroidal vasculature is primarily perfused by the short posterior ciliary arteries, with a minor supply of blood received from the peripapillary blood vessels of the optic nerve and sheath. At the posterior pole of the globe, the large choroidal arteries temporal to the macula run relatively straight toward the equator. A layer of medium-sized arteries and veins forms interarterial and intervenous shunts (Fig. 3.3) (44). It has been speculated that these

shunts help to distribute blood in the choroid. The medium-sized choroidal arteries are not end arteries, and occlusion of these arteries and veins will produce only patchy choroidal ischemia. The arterioles branching off these arteries run a short course in the macular area, turning at right angles to supply the center of a lobular arrangement of the choriocapillaris (a choroidal lobule) (Figs. 3.4–3.7) (44–46). The choriocapillaries radiate from the central arteriole and are drained by slightly dilated choriocapillaries at the periphery of the lobule to the ampullae of the postcapillary venules. The postcapillary venules vary in diameter and are joined together to form choroidal veins, which drain to the vortex veins.

The equator and the periphery of the eye do not exhibit the distinct lobular structure of the choriocapillaris of the posterior pole (44). The medium-sized arteries run anteriorly from the posterior pole, and veins drain anteriorly into the vortex veins. As a result, the choriocapillaris runs a direct course in spindle segments, joining the precapillary arterioles to the postcapillary venules (Figs. 3.6B, 3.7B). The venules, however, are more tortuous, making more angular turns than the arterioles.

In the periphery of the eye anterior to the equator, the choroidal arteries and veins run perpendicular to the ora serrata. The choriocapillaries tortuously join the precapillary arterioles to the postcapillary venules at right angles, resembling a ladder (Figs. 3.6C, 3.7C). The regional variation of the structure of the choroidal vasculature observed in humans is supported by the observation that the choroidal blood flow in nonhuman primates has marked regional variations. In the monkey, the blood flow in the macular area is 6.5 ml/minute/mm^2, 5 to 10 times that of the equatorial and peripheral regions (33). The lobular pattern of the posterior pole provides a more efficient system of blood flow than do the spindle and ladder patterns in the equatorial and peripheral choroid. Choroidal ischemia in the posterior pole gives a patchy whitening of the outer retina corresponding to the lobular pattern

Figure 3.3. Scanning electron micrographs of the choroidal vasculature after large choroidal arteries and veins were dissected away. **A.** Medium-sized choroidal arteries and veins appear in haphazard pattern. Interarterial shunts (*broken line*) occur between two systems of arterial trees (*A* to *A*) (×75). **B.** Medium-sized choroidal veins are tortuous and branch frequently. Shunts (*broken line*) are noted between adjacent veins (*v*) (×75).

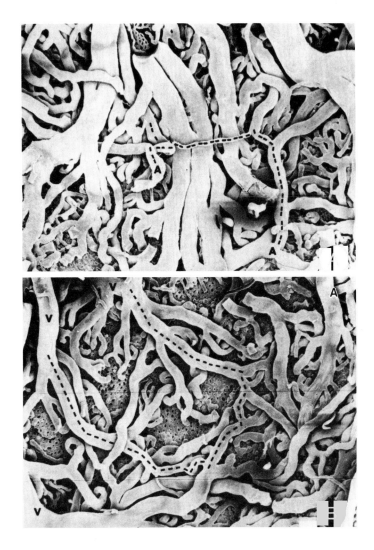

of the choriocapillaris, while choroidal ischemia in the periphery produces a triangular whitening of the outer retina with the base of the triangle toward the ora serrata (47, 48).

The endothelial wall of the choriocapillaris is discontinuous (27). The cell body of the choriocapillary endothelial cell lies in the posterior aspect of the blood vessel, while the anterior capillary wall shows a number of endothelial fenestrations. The cell junctions between adjacent endothelial cells are mostly zonula adherens. Zonula occludens are poorly formed or lacking (3). A pericyte surrounds a choriocapil-

lary, and the cell body is always on the posterior aspect of the capillary. The anterior aspect of the normal choroidal capillary has no pericytic process, and the anterior endothelial fenestrations face Bruch's membrane and the retinal pigment epithelium. Since the choriocapillaris is fenestrated, no blood-choroidal barrier exists, so that plasma proteins as large as serum albumin are able to escape into the choroidal stroma. The outer blood-retinal barrier lies in the plasmalemma of the retinal pigment epithelium and the zonula occludens between these cells. Choroidal vascular occlusion causes dis-

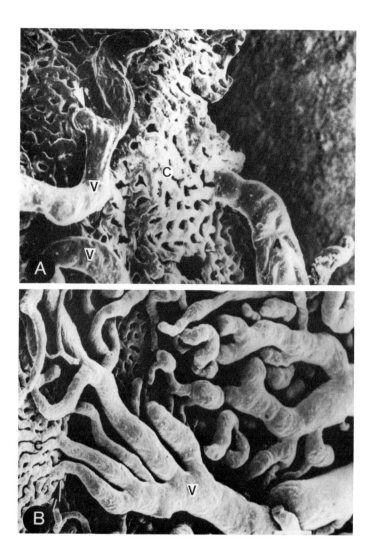

Figure 3.4. Scanning electron micrographs of choroidal vasculature. **A.** Oblique view showing relationship of choroidal precapillary arterioles, choriocapillaris, and choroidal postcapillary venules in posterior pole. Precapillary arteriole (A) makes sharp turn foward and assumes narrower diameter to supply choriocapillaris (C). Venule (V) exhibits small ampullae (arrow) on leaving choriocapillaris (×200). **B.** Short venules emerge to form a medium-sized vein of irregular diameter. One postcapillary venule (V) shows ampullar enlargement (arrow) on leaving choriocapillaris (C) (original magnification ×200).

ruption of the retinal pigment epithelial cells and their cell junctions, resulting in leakage of tracer from the choroidal stroma into the subretinal space and retina.

The physiological control displayed by the choroidal vasculature is very different from that displayed by the retinal vasculature (30, 32, 49–55). Four theories have been advanced to explain the regulatory pathway.

First, the sympathetic nervous system plays an important role in the regulation of the choroidal blood flow. Stimulation of the cervical sympathetic chain decreases choroidal blood flow, and sym-

pathetic denervation increases choroidal circulation (51). In rhesus monkeys, induced systemic hypertension followed by sympathectomies (31) resulted in multifocal choroidal leakage through the retinal pigment epithelium into the subretinal space and an associated leakage from retinal capillaries in the macula. In normal eyes, the sympathetic nervous system seems to protect the choroidal circulation from a sudden rise in systemic blood pressure.

A second possible regulatory pathway of the choroidal vasculature is by way of the porous choriocapillaris. The choriocapillaris has fenestrations in the capillary

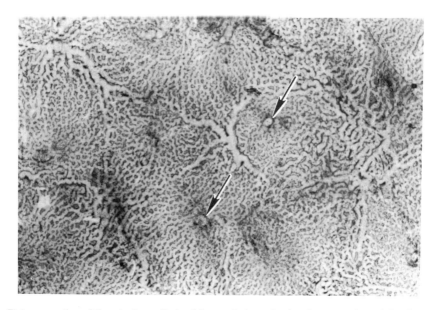

Figure 3.5. Flat preparation of the choriocapillaris of the posterior pole showing central arterioles (*arrows*) and radiating capillary channels, which are drained by circumferential peripheral venules (×40).

wall so that proteins and polypeptides may pass through these pores and leak into the choroidal stroma. In renal hypertension, the powerful vasoconstrictor angiotensin II may pass through the porous choriocapillaris into the choroidal stroma and act on the choroidal arteriolar muscular wall to produce vasoconstriction (52).

Third, it has also been postulated but not confirmed that the choroidal circulation is partially regulated by heat or light received indirectly through the retina in the visual process (31, 49).

Last, intraocular pressure also affects the choroidal circulation (4, 31, 53). An inverse, but not perfectly linear, relationship was reported to exist between choroidal blood flow and intraocular pressure (4, 31). Using the microsphere impaction method, nonlinearity could be shown in the middle range of ocular hypertension. Using indocyanine dye clearance, it was found that elevating intraocular pressure increased choroidal vascular resistance, probably due to pressure-induced obstruction of the vortex vein as it runs through the oblique scleral canal (31).

PREVIOUS CLASSIFICATIONS OF HYPERTENSIVE RETINOPATHY

Whereas the classification system we will describe is based on pathophysiological changes in the retinal, choroidal, and optic nerve vasculature, previous classifications of hypertensive eye disease have focused on the clinical manifestations and degrees of changes found to occur in the retinal vasculature. The first major attempt to classify the retinal vascular changes of systemic hypertension was made in 1939 (6). A number of modifications and revisions to this classification have been proposed (7–9, 15, 16).

In a 1939 study, Keith et al. observed 219 hypertensive patients for a minimum of 5 years (6). The patients were divided into four groups (Table 3.3), and their blood pressure, symptoms, survival, and ophthalmoscopic findings were correlated. The major contribution of this classification was that it recognized distinct groups of patients with differential retinal changes, which were correlated with survival.

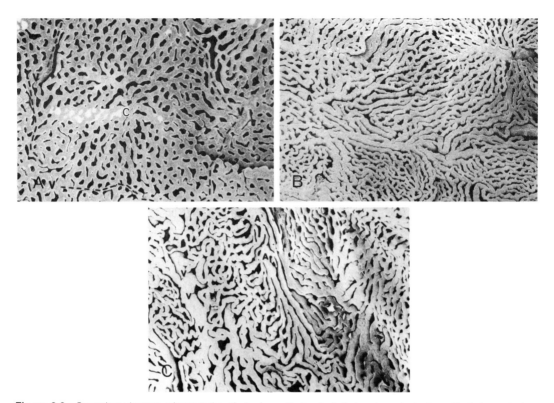

Figure 3.6. Scanning electron micrographs of choriocapillaris. **A.** Anterior view of choriocapillaris in posterior pole. Precapillary arteriole (C) is localized by comparing anterior and posterior views of vascular cast. Choriocapillaries radiate from the central arteriole in anastomosing channels and are drained by peripheral venules (V). Broken line indicates lobular segment of choriocapillaris fed by an arteriole (× 135). **B.** Choriocapillaris at equator seen anteriorly. Segment of choriocapillaris (C) is fed by precapillary arteriole (A) and drained by postcapillary venule (V). Arterioles and venules come forward to lie in same plane as choriocapillaris. Note that venules have larger diameter than arterioles. Segment of capillaries is spindle shaped (× 75). **C.** Choriocapillaris at periphery seen anteriorly. Precapillary arterioles (A) run parallel to postcapillary venules (V). Choriocapillaris between them takes tortuous course at right angles to other vessels (× 100).

The 1939 study did not, however, give objective criteria to quantitate arterial narrowing. In 1947, better defined criteria for the classification of hypertensive retinopathy were reported, and well-illustrated retinal fundus changes were described by Wagener et al. (7) (Tables 3.4, 3.5). Hypertensive retinopathy was classified into acute, chronic, and terminal (malignant) phases. Three distinct alterations in the retinal arteries were recognized: (a) generalized narrowing, (b) sclerosis, and (c) focal constriction due to spasm. Also, sclerosis of choroidal arterioles was reported to be a component of hypertensive retinopathy. In order to better quantitate narrowing of arteries, two methods were proposed: (a) comparison of the caliber of retinal arteries of hypertensive patients with the average caliber of retinal arteries of individuals who had no hypertension, and (b) estimation of the ratio of diameters of arteries to veins in the retina.

In 1953, the coexistence of hypertensive and arteriosclerotic retinal arterial changes was recognized, and an attempt was made to differentiate hypertensive from arteriosclerotic changes (8) (Table 3.6). However, it was not recognized until 1957 that the changes in the fundus in systemic hypertension depended on the degree of arteriosclerosis of the retinal arteries at the onset

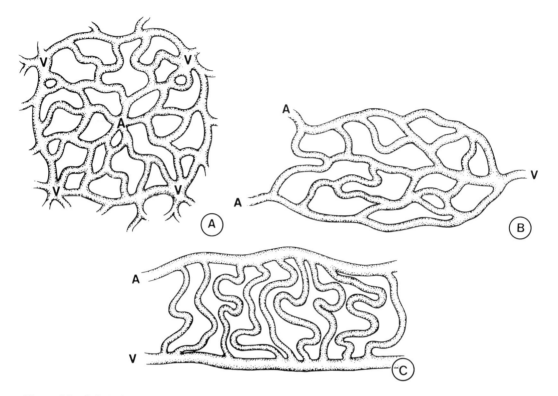

Figure 3.7. **A.** Lobular pattern of posterior choriocapillaris. **B.** Spindle pattern of equatorial choriocapillaris. **C.** Ladder pattern of peripheral choriocapillaris. *A* indicates arterioles; *V*, venules.

of hypertension (9). It was stated that arteriosclerosis often occurs with aging, traumatic retinopathy, uveal inflammation, and systemic diseases. For example, patients with diabetes mellitus may develop arteriosclerosis more readily. Hypertension accelerates the arteriosclerotic process, and arteriosclerosis modulates the appearance of hypertensive retinopathy. Arteriosclerosis has a "protective effect" on the retinal arteries, and a level of blood pressure that may cause fulminating retinopathy in a young, nonarteriosclerotic patient may cause minimal change in the arteriosclerotic patient. When hyperten-

Table 3.3. Keith-Wagener-Barker's Classification of Hypertensive Retinopathy

Group 1	Mild narrowing or sclerosis of retinal arteries
Group 2	Generalized and localized narrowing of the arteries, moderate or marked sclerosis of retinal arteries with exaggeration of arterial reflex and arteriovenous compression; thrombosis of retinal veins and "retinitis of the arteriosclerotic type"
Group 3	"Angiospastic retinitis" characterized by retinal edema, cotton-wool patches, and hemorrhages, superimposed on sclerotic and spastic arterioles
Group 4	Diffuse retinal and optic disc edema with narrowing of the arteries

Table 3.4. Wagener-Clay-Gibner's Classification of Generalized Narrowing of Arteries

Grade 1	Reduction of caliber of arteries to $\frac{3}{4}$ average caliber of normal arteries or $\frac{1}{2}$ caliber of veins
Grade 2	Reduction of caliber of arteries to $\frac{1}{2}$ average caliber of normal arteries or $\frac{1}{3}$ caliber of veins
Grade 3	Reduction of caliber of arteries to $\frac{1}{3}$ average caliber of normal arteries or $\frac{1}{4}$ caliber of veins
Grade 4	Arteries thread-like or invisible

Table 3.5. Wagener-Clay-Gibner's Classification of Sclerosis of Arteries

Grade 1	Brightening of arterial wall with mild depression of the veins at arteriovenous crossing
Grade 2	Copper color of artery with definitive depression of underlying veins
Grade 3	Silver color of artery and widening of arteriovenous crossing
Grade 4	Artery visible as a fibrous cord without blood stream

sion persists for a long period, the young, hypertensive patient will develop arteriosclerotic changes. The 1957 classification features seven categories, based on the state of retinal arteries at the onset of hypertension (9) (Table 3.7). The advantage of this system over previous classifications was its ability to explain the variable presentation and course of hypertensive retinopathy.

PATHOPHYSIOLOGICAL APPROACH TO HYPERTENSIVE OCULAR DISEASE

The retina, choroid, and optic nerve are supplied by different systems of blood vessels, each having distinct anatomical and physiological properties. The tissues supplied by each of these vascular systems respond differently to systemic hypertension. Therefore, an appropriate approach

Table 3.6. Modified Scheie's Classification of Hypertensive Retinopathy

Hypertension

Grade 0	No changes
Grade 1	Barely detectable arterial narrowing
Grade 2	Obvious arterial narrowing with focal irregularities
Grade 3	Grade 2 + retinal hemorrhages and/or exudate
Grade 4	Grade 3 + papilledema

Arteriolar Sclerosis

Grade 0	Normal
Grade 1	Barely detectable light reflex changes in arterial wall
Grade 2	Obvious increased light reflex changes in arterial wall
Grade 3	Copper wire arteries
Grade 4	Silver wire arteries

to hypertensive retinopathy is to designate the categories (a) hypertensive choroidopathy, (b) hypertensive retinopathy, and (c) hypertensive optic neuropathy (Table 3.8).

The clinical manifestations of each of these categories of hypertensive eye disease depend on the age and vascular status of the patients at the onset of hypertension. Furthermore, because effective medical and surgical treatment regimens have been developed, the appearance of hypertensive ocular changes may be modulated. More hypertensive patients are surviving, and their life expectancy is increasing. Therefore, classification of hypertensive retinopathy depends upon the efficacy of the treatment regimen.

Hypertensive Choroidopathy

Clinical Findings

Hypertensive choroidopathy is seen in patients suffering from acute hypertension. Typically, it occurs in relatively young individuals whose vessels are pliable, not sclerotic, and whose vessels respond by constricting when the sympathetic vascular tone is increased. Hypertensive choroidopathy is seen in patients with pregnancy-induced hypertension (preeclampsia and eclampsia), renal diseases, pheochromocytoma, acquired diseases of connective tissue, and accelerated essential hypertension. The patients may manifest other signs of acclerated hypertension, including hypertensive encephalopathy. The early ocular manifestations include disturbances of the retinal pigment epithelium and the choroid. Some accompanying retinal vascular manifestations are frequently seen. If the disease is allowed to progress without appropriate therapy, the vasoconstrictive phase of hypertensive retinopathy may occur, followed by the exudative phase.

In the early phase of choroidopathy, the fundus exhibits pale white or reddish patches of outer retina (Elschnig's spots) corresponding to areas of hypoperfusion of the underlying choriocapillaris, as seen

Table 3.7. Leishman's Classification of Hypertensive Retinopathy

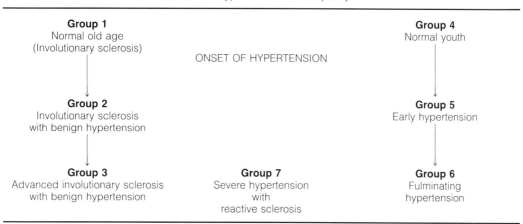

by fluorescein angiography (Fig. 3.8). In the late phase of angiography, these pigment epithelial lesions leak fluorescein dye diffusely (Fig. 3.9). Focal serous detachment of the retina in the posterior pole may be observed (Fig. 3.10). A macular star due to accumulation of the hard exudate in Henle's nerve fiber layer may be observed in the perifoveal region. The retinal arteries may show only focal constriction, with mild congestion of the retinal veins. At the equatorial regions, lesions similar to Elschnig's spots (Siegrist spots) may be arranged in a linear fashion along the course of a choroidal vessel.

If the blood pressure is controlled, chronic Elschnig's spots (Fig. 3.11) develop and show a pigmented center with a depigmented halo. The fluorescein an-

Table 3.8. A Pathophysiological Approach to Hypertensive Ocular Disease

1. Hypertensive choroidopathy

2. Hypertensive retinopathy

   A. Vasoconstrictive phase
   B. Sclerotic phase
   C. Exudative phase
   D. Complications of the sclerotic phase

3. Hypertensive optic neuropathy

   A. Optic disc edema
   B. Optic atrophy
   C. Ischemic optic neuropathy

giogram shows that the pigment epithelium heals with no further leakage of fluorescein into the subretinal space, though a window defect of hyperfluorescence still exists.

Pathophysiological Mechanism of Hypertensive Choroidopathy

There are several possible theories for explaining why the choroidal vasculature is more severely affected than the retinal vasculature when the abrupt onset of severe hypertension occurs in young patients. Anatomically, the choroidal arteries run a short course without much branching and supply the choriocapillaris at right angles (Fig. 3.5). The systemic blood pressure is thus transmitted directly to the choriocapillaris. In order to protect the choriocapillaris from elevated blood pressure, the choroidal arteries and arterioles, which are regulated by sympathetic control, constrict vigorously, which may limit blood flow in the choriocapillaris and cause ischemic changes in the overlying retinal pigment epithelium (fibrinoid necrosis). The lobular arrangement of the choriocapillaris in the posterior pole of the eye explains the scattered arrangement and shape of the Elschnig's spots.

In some patients with hypertension, the plasma level of angiotensin II may be elevated. It has been postulated that, since

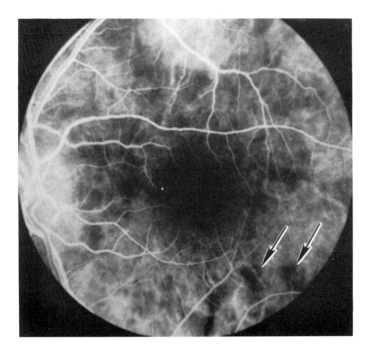

Figure 3.8. Fluorescein angiogram of a 24-year-old patient with Goodpasture's syndrome, renal failure, and a blood pressure of 200/120 mm Hg. Noteworthy is the choroidopathy with areas of hypoperfusion (*arrows*), which correspond to the lobular pattern of posterior choriocapillaris.

the choriocapillaris is fenestrated, angiotensin II may be passed into the choroidal stroma and act directly on the external choroidal arteriolar wall, producing severe constriction and ischemia (52).

In contrast, the retinal circulation is largely under the influence of autoregulatory mechanisms. In the early stages of severely elevated blood pressure, the retinal vessels may be able to maintain their vascular tone by focal constriction and thereby preserve an appropriate physiological environment for the inner retina.

While previous studies partially characterized the pathophysiological processes of hypertensive choroidopathy, none gave a complete description of all phases of hypertensive choroidopathy (55–61). A recent experimental pathological study of hypertension in nonhuman primates has more clearly defined the pathological process and pathophysiological mechanisms (52). The hypertensive choroidopathy in these animals could be divided into three phases: acute ischemic phase, chronic occlusive phase, and chronic reparative phase. In the acute ischemic phase, the choriocapillaris and choroidal arteries ap-

peared patent, but the choroidal arterioles were severely constricted and exhibited very narrowed lumina (Fig. 3.12). The absence of pericytes in the inner aspect of the fenestrated choriocapillaris made it unlikely that the choriocapillaris constricts effectively in the hypertensive state, accounting for the initial patency of the choriocapillaris. The choroidal arterioles, however, had extremely narrow lumina, lined by endothelial cells with convoluted nuclei (Fig. 3.13). The cytoplasm of the smooth muscle cells showed hydropic swelling and scattered, disarranged bundles of myofilaments. Vasoconstriction of the choroidal arterioles appeared to be the initial primary response of the choroidal vasculature to severe hypertension, probably influenced by sympathetic tone and by angiotensin II.

Some of the choriocapillaries distal to the occluded arterioles had necrotic endothelial cells, which were desquamated into the lumina (Fig. 3.14). The overlying retinal pigment epithelial cells exhibited intracellular edema, vacuolation of endoplasmic reticulum, and loss of basal enfolding. These degenerative changes of the

Figure 3.9. A. Elschnig's spots (*arrows*). Patchy yellow lesions of retinal pigment epithelium are seen. **B.** Lesions leak fluorescein diffusely (*arrows*).

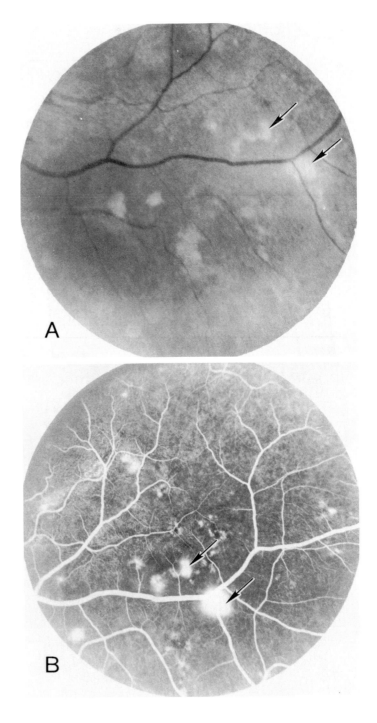

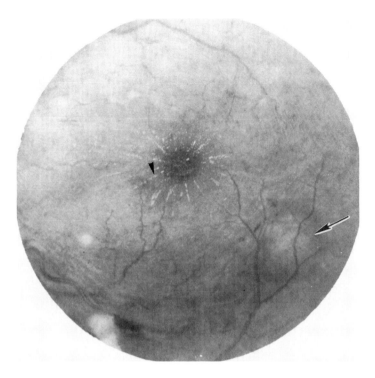

Figure 3.10. Hypertensive choroidopathy in a 37-year-old woman with blood pressure of 236/140 mm Hg. Focal serous detachment of retina is present (*arrow*). Macular star with leakage of hard exudate is seen (*arrowhead*).

retinal pigment epithelium represent the early histological findings of acute Elschnig's spots.

In the chronic occlusive phase of hypertensive choroidopathy, the choroidal arteries and arterioles showed hyperplastic changes, accompanied by fibrinoid necrosis. In the tunica intima, proliferated intimal cells surrounded by internal elastic membrane assumed an onionskin appearance, and the lumen was largely occluded (Figs. 3.15, 3.16). Fibrin deposits were seen in the vessel wall. In the tunica media, concentric lamellae of basement membrane material and cellular debris exhibiting fragments of degenerative smooth muscle cells were observed. The choriocapillaris was diffusely occluded by thrombus. The endothelial cells and pericytes of the choriocapillaris were denuded, and the overlying retinal pigment epithelium was necrotic. A tracer study with horseradish peroxidase revealed leakage of the tracer into the subretinal space corresponding to the leakage of fluorescein noted in the fluorescein angiogram.

In the chronic reparative phase, recanalization of the occluded choroidal arteries began. Tufts of proliferative endothelial cells were introduced into the occluded lumina of blood vessels, forming recanalized choroidal arteries that had small lumina. Also seen were ghost choriocapillaries, which consisted of vascular basement membrane without endothelial cells (Fig. 3.17). Other choriocapillaries were replaced by new vessels, which had cuboidal, nonfenestrated endothelial cells. Occasionally, an added layer of smooth muscle cells was present around the choriocapillaries. As a result of increased connective tissue deposited between choriocapillaries, there was histological widening of the connective tissue pillars between choriocapillaries. The retinal pigment epithelium overlying these lesions was depigmented and attenuated and at times showed reactive proliferation. In the chronic reparative phase, reestablishment of the choroidal circulation resulted in reabsorption of the subretinal fluid, which brought about reattachment of the retina.

The formation of Elschnig's spots is re-

Figure 3.11. **A.** Elschnig's spots of hypertensive choroidopathy in the "healed" stage. Lesions (*arrow*) have a pigmented center and a hypopigmented halo. This 48-year-old man was hospitalized 6 months earlier for hypertensive encephalopathy. **B.** Fluorescein angiogram shows no leakage at the retinal pigment epithelium (*arrow*).

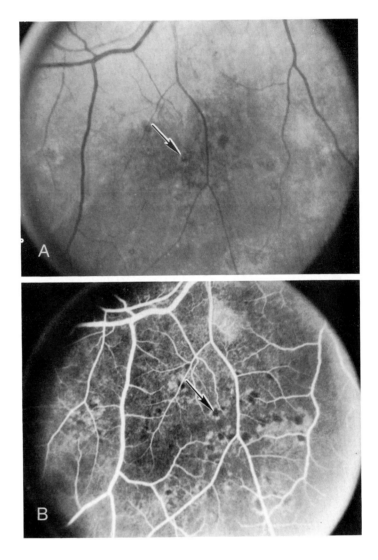

lated to the lobular arrangement of the choriocapillaris, whereby each lobule is fed centrally by a small arteriole and drained peripherally by a system of venules. The severely constricted central arteriole causes focal necrosis of overlying pigment epithelium. This observation further supports the theory that each lobule of choriocapillaris functions as an independent circulatory unit.

Focal retinal detachment is an important feature in accelerated hypertension (61). In patients with preeclampsia, it was noted that retinal detachment was accompanied by areas of choroidal nonperfusion and a lobular pattern of leakage of fluorescein through the retinal pigment epithelium (62–64). All of these changes could be explained by the pathological events seen in the chronic occlusive phase of hypertensive choroidopathy.

Hypertensive Retinopathy

Clinical Findings

Hypertensive retinopathy can be conveniently divided into four phases: 1) vaso-

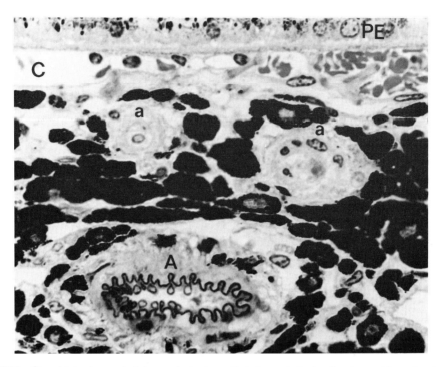

Figure 3.12. Choroidal artery, arterioles, and choriocapillaris in acute ischemic phase of hypertensive choroidopathy. Choroidal artery (*A*) is unremarkable, showing single layer of endothelium surrounded by corrugated internal elastic lamina. In contrast, choroidal arterioles (*a*) are obliterated. Choriocapillaris (*C*) appears patent. *PE* indicates retinal pigment epithelium (toluidine blue: ×800).

constrictive phase, 2) sclerotic phase, 3) exudative phase, and 4) complications of the sclerotic phase. While each phase may have distinct clinical features, the phases often merge into one another. Furthermore, the order of these four phases may not be sequential. For example, a patient who has long standing hypertension and is in the sclerotic phase of hypertensive retinopathy may inadvertently discontinue his medication, which may result in a sudden rise of blood pressure and development of the exudative phase. Conversely, a patient who has markedly elevated blood pressure may receive adequate treatment and move from the exudative to the sclerotic phase.

The vasoconstrictive and sclerotic phases are relatively asymptomatic. Loss of vision comes most frequently with complications of the sclerotic phase (phase 4) or, less commonly, during the exudative phase (phase 3). Some patients may not be aware of their hypertensive retinopathy until the late stages of the disease. The division of hypertensive retinopathy into four phases gives physicians an indication of the efficacy of treatment and offers some prognostic guides. The prognosis and the categorization of the phases of the disease will be affected by antihypertensive therapy.

Vasoconstrictive Phase. The caliber and regularity of retinal vessels is best appreciated using red-free light. Examination is best done with slit-lamp biomicroscopy using a contact lens, but, alternatively, slit-lamp indirect biomicroscopy with the 60-diopter or 90-diopter lens is helpful. Direct ophthalmoscopy remains useful, but the other methods provide a wider field of view, so examination and comparison of vessels in all quadrants is made easier.

In the vasoconstrictive phase, the elevated blood pressure stimulates pliable and nonsclerotic retinal blood vessels to increase their tone by autoregulation. The

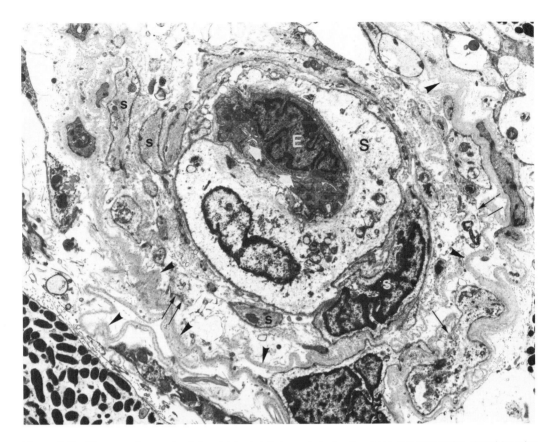

Figure 3.13. Electron micrograph of choroidal arteriole in acute ischemic phase of hypertensive choroidopathy. Lumen of choroidal arteriole is extremely narrow (*white arrows*) and lined by endothelial cells (*E*) with convoluted nuclei. Some cytoplasm of smooth muscle cells (*S*) shows hydropic swelling and scattered bundles of myofilaments. Other muscle cells (*thin black arrows*) exhibit stages of degeneration and disintegration. Fragments of still others (*s*) show bundles of relatively normal myofilaments. Remnants of basement membrane (*arrowheads*) of degenerated smooth muscle form corrugated concentric rings (×4000).

more youthful and elastic the retinal blood vessels are, the greater the response will be. Diffuse constriction of the arteries in the young patient with normal vessels has been described (9). Also noted was the presence of focal constrictions in young patients (17, 18). Both diffuse and focal constrictions of arteries were found in newborn infants with hypertension (65). In patients with preexisting sclerosis, the vasoconstrictive phase is manifested differently than in patients without sclerosis. Focal constriction of nonsclerotic segments of vessels in hypertensive patients was described, but there was adjacent dilation of sclerotic segments due to long-standing elevation of intraluminal pressure (9).

The primary site of vasoconstriction is in the precapillary arterioles. Clinically, vasoconstriction is most prominently seen in the second and third order arteries and less commonly in vessels within 1 disc diameter of the disc. The degree of vasoconstriction is influenced by preexisting sclerosis of the retinal arteries, and vasoconstriction due to hypertension is most prominent in young patients with pliable, nonsclerotic vessels. Comparison of arterial and venous calibers is not an accurate method of detecting vasoconstriction, because venous caliber can vary greatly. The

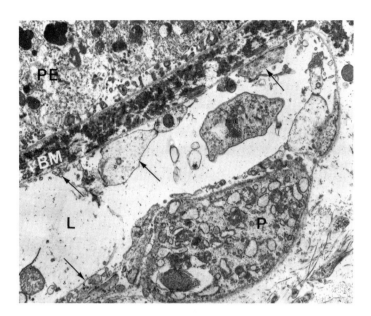

Figure 3.14. Electron micrograph of choriocapillaris of acute ischemic phase in hypertensive choroidopathy. Choriocapillary adjacent to occluded arterioles shows necrosis of endothelial cells (*arrows*) that desquamate into lumen. Hydropic degeneration of pericyte (*P*) is noted. Lumen of capillary (*L*) is still patent. Fibrinous deposits appear at Bruch's membrane (*BM*). Overlying retinal pigment epithelium (*PE*) exhibits loss of basal infoldings (×9330).

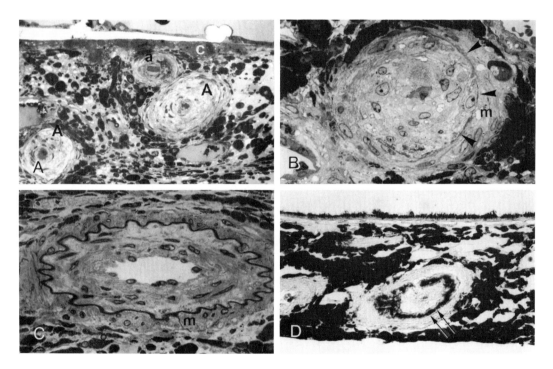

Figure 3.15. Choroidal arteries in chronic occlusive phase of hypertensive choroidopathy. **A.** Choroidal arteries (*A*) and arterioles (*a*) show marked hyperplastic arteriosclerosis. Lumina are extremely narrowed by thickened and laminated vessel wall. Choriocapillaris (*C*) is occluded by thrombus (toluidine blue: original magnification ×200). **B.** Intimal cells proliferated within internal elastic lamina (*arrowheads*) have occluded lumen. Tunica media (*m*) is attenuated and stretched around thickened intima (toluidine blue: original magnification ×420). **C.** Proliferated intimal cells surrounded by internal elastic lamella show onionskin appearance (toluidine blue: ×520). **D.** Fibrin deposit (*arrows*) is seen in choroidal arterial wall (phosphotungstic acid-hematoxylin: ×280).

Figure 3.16. Electron micrograph of choroidal arteriole in chronic occlusive phase of hypertensive choroidopathy. Wall of occluded choroidal arteriole is composed of multiple, concentric laminae of basement membrane material (*arrows*) and cell debris with fragments of smooth muscle cells (*arrowheads*). C indicates choriocapillaris (×3870).

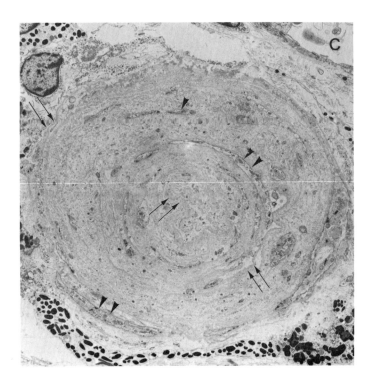

best method of estimating arterial constriction is to take photographs of the fundus and compare them with those of standard fundi demonstrating a similar degree of sclerosis (see the following section).

Sclerotic Phase. If elevated blood pressure in the vasoconstrictive phase is controlled promptly with medication or surgery, the retinal vessels may return to a normal state with no permanent pathological changes. On the other hand, if the blood pressure remains elevated over a period of time, sclerotic changes will develop. An attempt was made to separate the hypertensive features from the arteriosclerotic features of the retinal vasculature (8) (Table 3.6). It was proposed that, while the hypertensive changes indicate the severity of the hypertensive processes, the arteriosclerotic alterations reflect organic damage to the arterioles by the wear and tear of hypertension.

Previous attempts have been made to qualitatively and quantitatively define sclerotic changes of the retinal vasculature

(6–9, 11, 12, 16, 18). Clinically, features of the sclerotic vessels may include (a) narrowing of the arteries, (b) arteriovenous nicking, (c) sclerosis of the vessel wall resulting in alteration in the light reflex of the vessel wall, (d) vascular tortuosity, and (e) an increased angle of branching of the arteries and arterioles. Some of these vascular changes in the retina can be found in the "normal" population, but they are found more frequently in hypertensive patients. In both populations, these changes are age-dependent. One study using multivariate statistical analysis of the ophthalmoscopic findings showed a weak but significant correlation between retinal arteriolar changes and both blood pressure and mortality (66). There was, however, considerable overlap between normal subjects and hypertensive subjects, as well as notable variations in interobserver and intraobserver observations (67). It was concluded that the clinical signs such as "straightening of the arteries, arterial narrowing, arteriovenous crossing changes, and widening of the light

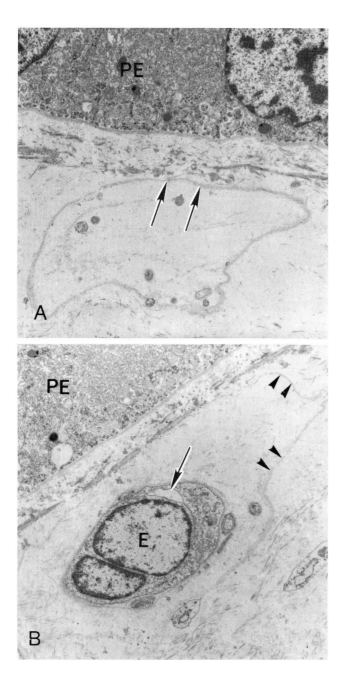

Figure 3.17. Electron micrographs of choriocapillaris in chronic reparative phase of hypertensive choroidopathy. **A.** Ghost choriocapillary is noted with basement membrane remnant (*arrows*). Endothelial cells are gone. Overlying retinal pigment epithelium (*PE*) appears intact (×8170). **B.** Recanalized capillary with small lumen (*arrow*) is lined by endothelial cells (*E*) in ghost capillary with remnants of basement membrane (*arrowheads*). *PE* indicates retinal pigment epithelium (×7000).

reflex'' are unreliable indices of hypertensive vascular disease because of their variability and common occurrence in older, normotensive individuals (14, 17, 18, 67, 68) (Figs. 3.18–3.21). A simplified grading system with reference photographs is presented to illustrate the graded vascular alterations and to chart the progress of hypertensive patients and their response to therapy (69) (Table 3.9).

Narrowing of Arteries (Fig. 3.18). Generalized arterial narrowing, with or without localized constriction, is a good indicator of hypertension, although nar-

Table 3.9.   Grading of the Retinal Vasculature in Hypertensive Retinopathy with Reference Photographs of the Fundus[a]

1. Arterial	a. Mild
	b. Moderate
	c. Severe
2. Arteriovenous nicking	a. Mild
	b. Moderate
	c. Branch venous occlusion
3. Arterial sclerosis	a. Mild
	b. Copper wiring
	c. Silver wiring
4. Arterial tortuosity	a. Mild
	b. Moderate
	c. Severe
5. Branching angle of arteries	a. Mild = 45–60°
	b. Moderate = 60–90°
	c. Severe = > 90°

[a]Modified from Bock KD. Regression of retinal vascular changes by antihypertensive therapy. Hypertension 1984; 6 (6pt2):III158–162. See Figures 3.18–3.21.

rowing is notoriously difficult to quantitate. Some investigators have compared the arterial diameter with that of the veins, but the veins are frequently dilated and are an inappropriate reference standard. Early narrowing most commonly occurs in the smaller branches of the arterial tree after the second or third branching of the retinal arteries. Because retinal vascular narrowing is found in many ocular diseases such as high myopia, uveitis, and retinal dystrophies, the examiner must apply clinical judgment in evaluating arterial narrowing. In grading of the arterial caliber, the following three grades are suggested: (a) mild narrowing, (b) moderate narrowing, and (c) severe narrowing. The diameter of the arteries should be judged in the overall setting of the structure of the fundus and compared with the "average" caliber of retinal vessels in a normal fundus (Fig. 3.18).

Arteriovenous Crossing Changes (Fig. 3.19).   Changes at the arteriovenous crossing can be more objectively defined than arterial narrowing can be. Statistically significant relationships have been noted between the severity of arteriovenous crossing and left ventricular hypertrophy (16). Arteriovenous nicking can be evaluated when

an artery passes anteriorly over a vein but not vice versa. This physical sign is classified in three grades: (a) mild arteriovenous nicking, (b) moderate arteriovenous nicking, and (c) branch venous occlusion (Fig. 3.19). In mild arteriovenous nicking, there is a slight deflection of the vein beneath the artery and early concealment of the vein. In moderate arteriovenous nicking, the vein tapers under the artery; apparent constriction and deflection (Gunn's sign) are also present. The vein may be mildly distended for some distance peripheral to the crossing, a condition known as "banking" of the veins. In venous occlusion, hemorrhage and exudate are seen distal to the arteriovenous crossing.

Arteriovenous nicking may be exaggerated in a patient whose diffuse arteriosclerosis is secondary to aging. One study of hypertensive retinopathy in the newborn infant surprisingly noted that three of the patients had abnormal tortuosity and arteriovenous nicking (65).

Sclerosis (Fig. 3.20).   Sclerosis of the arterial wall is frequently gauged by the light reflex of the vessel wall. Although this change may be seen with aging, it is useful as an additional parameter for evaluation. Sclerosis may be divided into three grades: (a) mildly increased light reflex, (b) copper wiring, and (c) silver wiring (Fig. 3.20). In the early stage of the sclerotic process, widening of the light reflex from the wall of the arteries is seen. As the reflex increases, it eventually covers the entire anterior surface of the artery. The blood vessels assume a burnished copper appearance, termed "copper wiring" (5). In the most severe form of arteriosclerosis, the vessel wall becomes so thick and hyalinized that the arteries appear as whitish, silvery cords, even though there may still be blood flow.

Arterial Tortuosity (Fig. 3.21).   Tortuosity of the arteries is observed in prolonged hypertension. Because of the increased intraluminal pressure, fibrosis of muscle fibers occurs, resulting in an increase in the length of the arteries, such that the retinal arteries assume a winding course in the retina. This condition must

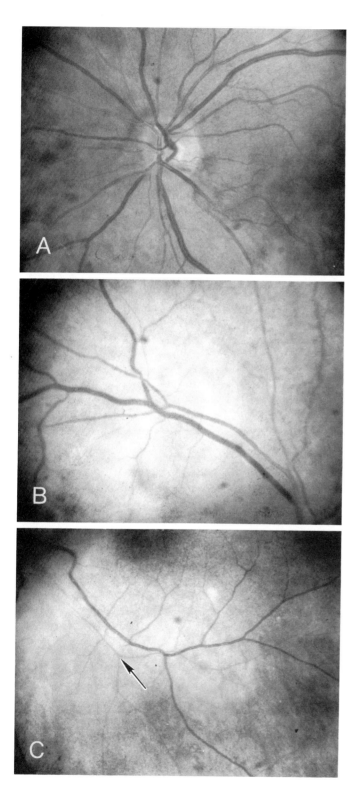

Figure 3.18. Reference photographs for rating of retinal arterial narrowing in sclerotic phase of hypertensive retinopathy. **A.** Mild narrowing of retinal arteries. **B.** Moderate narrowing of retinal arteries. **C.** Severe narrowing of retinal arteries. *Arrow* indicates moderate branching of arteries at 60–90°.

Figure 3.19. Reference photographs for rating of arteriovenous crossing in sclerotic phase of hypertensive retinopathy.
A. Mild arteriovenous crossing. Noteworthy is a slight deflection (*arrows*) and early concealment of the vein behind the artery.
B. Moderate arteriovenous crossing. The vein (*arrow*) tapers behind the artery with apparent constriction and deflection.
C. Branch retinal vein occlusion (*arrow*) showing congestion of the vein with hemorrhage in the nerve fiber layer and severe arteriovenous crossing.

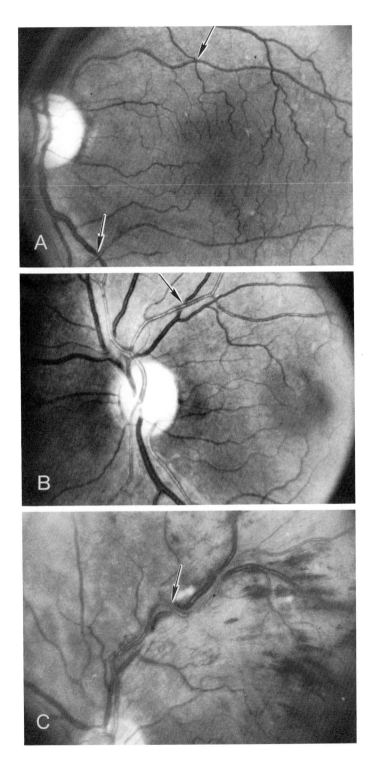

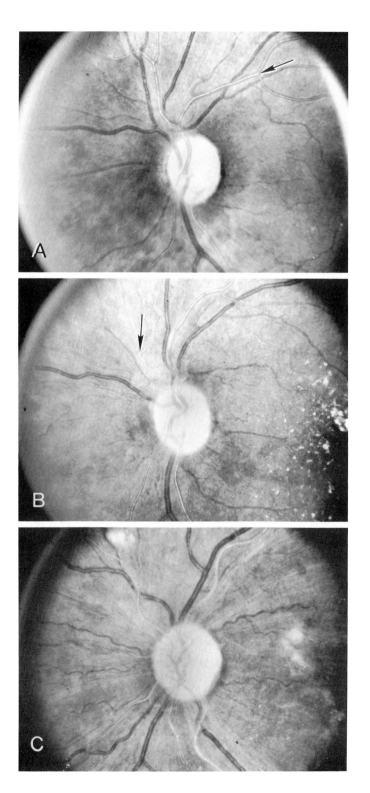

Figure 3.20. Reference photographs for rating of sclerosis of arterial wall in hypertensive retinopathy. **A.** Mild increase in light reflex. *Arrow* indicates severe arterial branching angle of over 90°. **B.** Copper wiring. Note that the blood vessels assume a burnished copper appearance. *Arrow* indicates mild arterial branching angle of 45–60°. **C.** Silver wiring. The arterial wall is so thick and hyalinized that the arteries appear as whitish, silvery cords, even though there is still blood flow within the vessels.

Figure 3.21. Reference photographs for rating of tortuosity of arteries in sclerotic phase of hypertensive retinopathy. **A.** Mild tortuosity. *Arrow* indicates severe arterial branching angle of over 90°. **B.** Moderate tortuosity. **C.** Severe tortuosity.

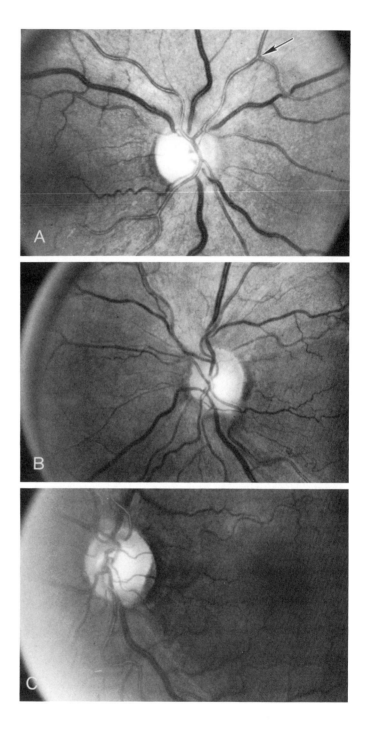

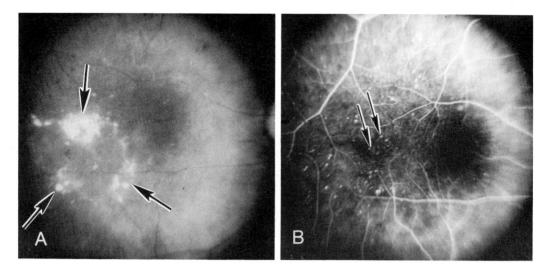

Figure 3.22. A. Exudative phase of hypertensive retinopathy showing circinate hard exudate (*arrows*) in the perimacular area. Note that there is marked narrowing of the entire retinal vasculature. **B.** Fluorescein angiogram shows clusters of microaneurysms (*arrows*) in the center of the area ringed by hard exudates.

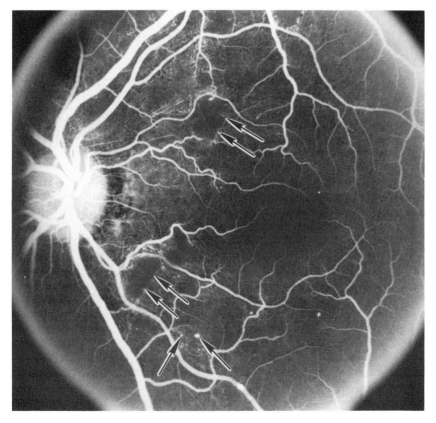

Figure 3.23. Exudative phase of hypertensive retinopathy. Noteworthy are the multiple areas of nonperfusion (*double arrows*) and capillary dilation with microaneurysms (*single arrows*) around cotton-wool spots.

Figure 3.24. A. Fundus photo of a 26-year-old hypertensive patient with a blood pressure of 160/100 mm Hg, showing focal areas of inner retinal thinning. **B.** The same patient omitted medication and the blood pressure rose to 250/190 mm Hg. Hemorrhages (*arrows*) and cotton-wool spots (*arrowhead*) are seen.

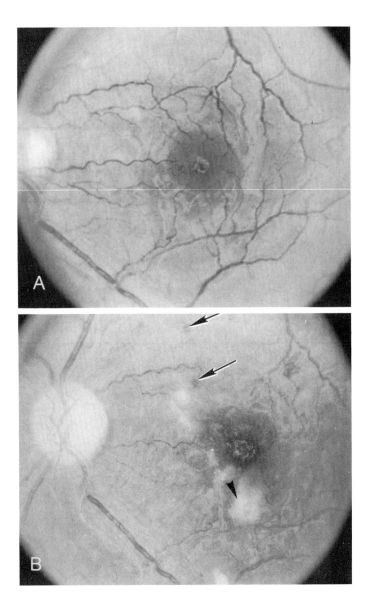

be differentiated from congenital tortuosity of retinal vessels, a common, benign condition of the eye. We classify vascular tortuosity into three grades: (*a*) mild, (*b*) moderate, and (*c*) severe (Fig. 3.21).

Angle of Arterial Branching. Another sign of hypertensive vascular disease is the angle assumed by the large branching arteries, particularly in the second or third order of branching. The greater the blood pressure, the wider the angle of branching: a mild branching angle between the

branching arteries is from 45° to 60° (Fig. 3.20B); a moderate branching angle is from 60° to 90° (Fig. 3.18C); and a severe branching angle is over 90° (Figs. 3.20A, 3.21A).

Exudative Phase. The exudative phase of hypertensive retinopathy may accompany or follow hypertensive choroidopathy or the vasoconstrictive or sclerotic phases of hypertensive retinopathy. In the sclerotic phase of hypertensive retinopathy, there may be no disruption of the blood-retinal barrier, as measured by fluorescein

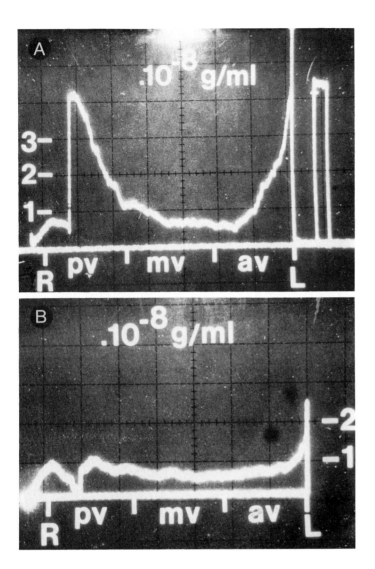

Figure 3.25. A. Vitreous fluoro-photometric tracings of hypertensive patients. Tracing of a patient in the exudative phase of hypertension showing increased accumulation of fluorescein in posterior vitreous 1 hour after injection of sodium fluorescein. **B.** Vitreous fluorophotometric tracing of another patient in the sclerotic phase of hypertension showing normal level of fluorescein accumulation in vitreous 1 hour after intravenous fluorescein injection. *R* indicates retina; *L*, lens; *pv*, posterior vitreous; *mv*, midvitreous; *av*, anterior vitreous.

angiography and vitreous fluorophotometry (70). However, when the blood pressure is suddenly or progressively elevated, the patient may pass into the exudative phase of hypertensive retinopathy. Following the onset of acute, severe hypertension, the patient may rapidly progress from the vasoconstrictive phase directly to the exudative phase of retinopathy. Its onset indicates that the perfusion pressure has overcome physiological autoregulatory mechanisms of the retinal arteries, resulting in disruption of the blood-retinal barrier, leakage of fluid and blood cells from the circulatory system, disruption of the vessel walls, and impairment of blood flow, which often produces ischemia (Fig. 3.1).

One of the early signs of exudative retinopathy is the appearance of small *linear or flame-shaped hemorrhages*, mostly in the nerve fiber layer in the peripapillary region. These retinal hemorrhages are linear because the bleeding occurs in the nerve fiber layer of the retina and the extravasated blood extends along the axons of the ganglion cells. When bleeding develops in the deeper layers of the retina, the hemorrhage assumes an oval outline because the spread of extravasated blood is limited by the processes of the Muller cells and is exhibited in the forms of blots or dots. Occasionally, the hemorrhage may break through the internal limiting membrane and occupy a subhyaloid location, presenting as a boat-shaped hemorrhage in the posterior pole.

Hard, waxy exudates represent extravasated plasma lipoproteins, phospholipids, cholesterol, and triglycerides. These exudates assume a brilliant yellow color and are most frequently seen scattered in the posterior pole. Exudates may appear in the foveal area in a star-shaped configuration radiating from the macular area along Henle's nerve fiber layer. In other patients, hard exudates may form a halo around a macroaneurysm or a cluster of leaking capillary microaneurysms. This ring presentation of hard exudate is known as circinate retinopathy (Fig. 3.22).

Cotton-wool spots are whitish-gray or yellow patches with grayed edges in the nerve fiber layer of the retina, mostly in the posterior pole, particularly around the peripapillary region (Fig. 3.1). Most frequently, the longitudinal axes of the cotton-wool spots are seen at right angles to the direction of the nerve fiber layers. They are most frequently located superficial to the retinal blood vessels. Fluorescein angiography frequently reveals nonperfusion of the cotton-wool spots. Surrounding these spots, dilated retinal capillaries, capillary telangiectasis, and capillary nonperfusion are seen (Figs. 3.1, 3.23). Collaterals with beaded vascular channels and staining of the retinal tissue by extracellular fluorescein may also be noted. With time, the cotton-wool spots may develop a granular appearance (Fig. 3.24) and eventually disappear. However, when they disappear, the retina may appear thinned, and a shiny, irregular appearance of the internal limiting membrane may develop. These areas are called "macular depressions" and represent focal loss of the inner retinal elements due to infarction.

Disruption of the blood-retinal barrier in the exudative phase of hypertensive retinopathy can be quantitated by vitreous fluorophotometry (70). Sodium fluorescein is injected intravenously, and, 1 hour later, the accumulation of fluorescein in the vitreous is measured by vitreous fluorophotometry. Patients in the exudative phase of hypertensive retinopathy will have an increased fluorescein concentration in the vitreous (Fig. 3.25). When the blood pressure of patients with exudative retinopathy is controlled and the exudative changes resolve, the vitreous fluorophotometric readings return to normal. Patients in the vasoconstrictive or sclerotic phase may have normal vitreous fluorescein concentrations. It should be noted that the increased vitreous fluorescein concentration may result from leakage through the retinal pigment epithelium or from the retinal vasculature. Vitreous fluorophotometric study cannot pinpoint the source of leakage.

Complications of the Sclerotic Phase. Complications of retinal hypertensive arteriosclerosis include central or branch retinal artery occlusion (Fig. 3.26), central or branch retinal vein occlusion (Fig. 3.27), macroaneurysm (Fig. 3.28), and epiretinal membrane. Retinal neovascularization and proliferative vascular retinopathy (vitreous hemorrhage, traction retinal detachment) may result from retinal ischemia. Cystoid macular edema may develop secondary to ischemic changes. After vascular occlusion, vascular remodeling may be seen, especially if the blood pressure has been controlled. However, visual function may not return because of the previous ischemic necrosis that occurred during the acute phase.

The visual acuity of a patient with hypertensive retinopathy is frequently minimally affected, because most of the changes are scattered about within the posterior pole. However, central vision will be affected when hypertensive retinopathy is complicated by branch artery or vein occlusion, macular edema, macular hemorrhage or exudates, macular capillary dropout, or the development of an epiretinal membrane in the macular area with wrinkling of the internal limiting membrane (71). Patients with hypertensive retinopathy may not have overt visual

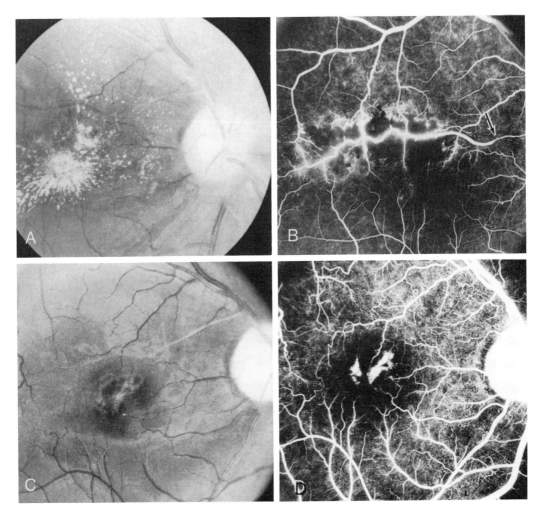

Figure 3.26. Exudative hypertensive retinopathy with vascular occlusion and remodeling in a 28-year-old black man with blood pressure of 240/180 mm Hg. **A.** Acute exudative retinopathy with narrowing of the superior temporal artery and dilation of the distal segment of the artery. **B.** Fluorescein angiogram shows focal narrowing of superotemporal retinal artery (*arrow*) and diffuse dilation and leakage of fluorescein distal to the site of narrowing. Loss of retinal capillaries and dilation and leakage of the adjacent retinal veins are seen. **C.** Photograph of fundus 3 years later with better control of blood pressure. Vascular remodeling is apparent. The artery that was once narrowed is now a fine thread (*arrow*). Irregular pigmentation of the macula is seen. **D.** The narrowed vessel does not perfuse with fluorescein, and the vascular bed has reperfused. The central vision is permanently disrupted.

complaints until complications of the sclerotic phase appear.

Hypertensive Retinopathy after Medical or Surgical Therapy

In recent years, major advances have been made in medical and surgical treatment of systemic hypertension. As a result, the retinal vascular changes in hypertensive patients vary with the efficacy of the therapeutic program. The disease processes in the retina after successful therapy may be evaluated in the following three aspects: (*a*) retinal vascular changes, (*b*) retinal vascular reactivity, and (*c*) exudative changes of the retina.

Retinal Vascular Changes. Retinal vascular changes were studied in patients whose blood pressure had been lowered

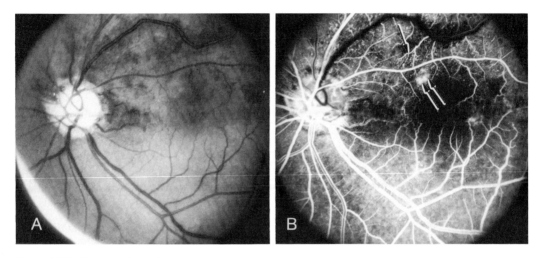

Figure 3.27. Branch retinal vein occlusion as a complication in the sclerotic phase. **A.** Marked engorgement of veins and hemorrhages in the superior hemisphere of the fundus. **B.** Fluorescein angiogram showing little perfusion in the superior temporal vein, while the inferior temporal vein has been completely filled. The retinal capillaries are dilated with numerous microaneurysms (*single arrow*) and focal leakage (*double arrows*) in the perimacular area.

by successful surgical or medical therapy (72). Five of 11 patients with unilateral renal disease, including stenosis of the main renal artery, hydronephrosis, and pyelonephritis, had their blood pressure significantly lowered from preoperative level. All of these patients showed dilation of the smallest retinal arterioles when the mean blood pressure was reduced from 155 to 110 mm Hg. However, the response of the large retinal arteries was variable. Two

additional young patients were treated with guanethidine, and a third had a successful nephrectomy for renal artery stenosis, after which the mean blood pressure was reduced from 138 mm Hg before treatment to 98 mm Hg. These patients showed a general increase in the arterial caliber when the blood pressure was reduced. However, another study of 14 patients with malignant hypertension who had been vigorously treated for 12 months revealed that

Figure 3.28. Retinal arterial macroaneurysm (*arrow*) in a patient with advanced sclerotic phase.

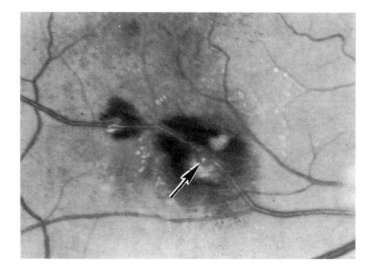

all signs of malignant hypertension had disappeared (68). However, focal and generalized narrowing of the arteries as well as abnormal arteriovenous nicking remained unchanged. It is likely that the promptness with which the blood pressure is lowered, and whether or not permanent damage to the vessels has been sustained, determine whether arteries dilate after treatment.

Retinal Vascular Reactivity. The retinal vascular responses to breathing 100% oxygen at a pressure of 1 atmosphere, to postural changes, or to sympathetic blockage were compared in normal subjects and hypertensive patients (72). Thirteen hypertensive patients ranging in age from 15 to 63 years, whose mean blood pressure ranged between 147 and 173 mm Hg, exhibited less arterial vasoconstriction produced by breathing 100% oxygen at a pressure of 1 atmosphere than did age-matched normal subjects. In addition, the authors examined five hypertensive patients whose mean pretreatment blood pressure was 157 mm Hg. The vasoconstrictive response of the arteries to oxygen was increased after systemic blood pressure was successfully lowered. It should be pointed out that vascular responsiveness to oxygen and other stimuli varies with age and that blood vessels in older individuals or in patients with chronic hypertension may show less reactive constriction than do the arteries of a young patient with acute hypertension. Severe arterial constriction of rapid onset may be reversible when the blood pressure is lowered. It is interesting to note that focal retinal arterial constrictions in rats in early stages of malignant hypertension were observed to be reversed by reducing the blood pressure by deepening the level of anesthesia (73).

Retinal Exudative Changes. Retinal hemorrhages, cotton-wool spots, waxy exudates, and papilledema disappear within 6 to 12 months after blood pressure is controlled. Inadequate control of elevated blood pressure delays the regression of the retinopathy. Papilledema, cotton-wool spots, and hemorrhages usually disappear first.

The waxy exudates disappear more slowly. It has been emphasized that the exudative retinopathy improved even if the blood pressure was lowered but not necessarily normalized and that the exudative retinopathy did not necessarily reappear if the blood pressure was subsequently mildly elevated again after a period of adequate control (68). This observation is analogous to the hypothesis that, when blood pressure is reduced below the limit of autoregulation of cerebral vessels, fibrinoid necrosis of the vascular wall may heal and the autoregulatory mechanism may be restored (76, 77). The same process may also take place in the retina.

Pathophysiological Mechanisms of Hypertensive Retinopathy

In the vasoconstrictive phase of hypertensive retinopathy, a sharp rise in systemic blood pressure stimulates the vascular tone of muscular arteries of the retina by way of a myogenic autoregulatory mechanism. If the elevated blood pressure is controlled by medications or by surgery, the retinal blood vessels may dilate and return to their normal state, inflicting no permanent pathological changes.

If the blood pressure remains highly elevated, the vascular tone further increases, and a reduction in the lumen of the precapillary arterioles results. Disruption of the blood-retinal barrier occurs, and the exudative phase of retinopathy ensues. It has also been hypothesized that degeneration of vascular smooth muscle leads to focal disruption of the vascular endothelium (10, 76) and that endothelial necrosis is essential for leakage to occur. However, by horseradish peroxidase tracer technique, leakage of the tracer has been observed to occur without necrosis of the retinal capillary endothelium (Fig. 3.29) (30). It is possible that either necrosis of the endothelium or disruption of cell junctions between endothelial cells, or both processes taking place simultaneously, may occur in exudative retinopathy. Plasma and red blood cells leak into the vessel wall and infiltrate around the degenerated per-

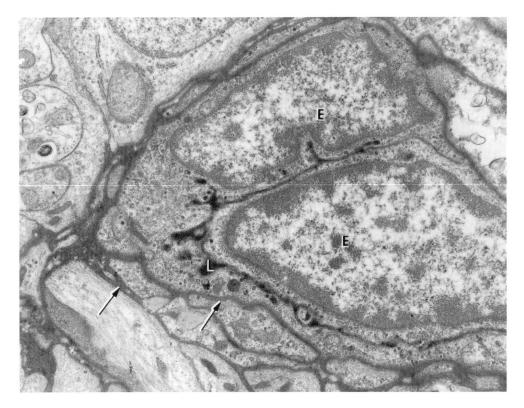

Figure 3.29. Electron micrograph of retinal capillary in a baboon with severe systemic hypertension. Severe narrowing of the vascular lumen (*L*) and early disruption of the blood-retinal barrier with leakage of horseradish peroxidase tracer are seen. Leakage causes a granular staining of the basement membrane (*arrows*) and extracellular space of the retina. *E* indicates endothelium (× 11200).

icytes and muscle cells. The process has been called plasmatic vasculosis. In very severe hypertension, fibrinoid necrosis of the vessel wall occurs; the vascular tone is lost as autoregulation fails, and the blood vessel dilates (Fig. 3.30). The capillary bed is exposed to high intraluminal pressure, which leads to disruption of the blood-retinal barrier and to leakage. In experimental hypertension using a horseradish peroxidase tracer technique, disruption of both the outer blood-retinal barrier at the retinal pigment epithelium and the inner blood-retinal barrier at the retinal vasculature has been found (30).

With damage to the vessel wall, reduction in blood flow occurs, and ischemia develops. One of the signs of retinal ischemia is the appearance of cotton-wool spots. Leakage of fluorescein from the retinal arteries has been observed before the

development of cotton-wool spots (77, 78). Cotton-wool spots are an accumulation of axoplasmic components in the nerve fiber layer, consisting of mitochondria, lamellated dense bodies, and axoplasmic ground substance in the proximal or distal ends of axons in the ischemic area. Disturbance of both retrograde and orthograde axoplasmic transport occurs.

When the blood pressure is mildly elevated, moderate hyperplasia of the tunica media of the retinal artery takes place (Fig. 3.31). If hypertension persists for a period of time, hyaline degeneration of the retinal vessels occurs, accompanied by the loss of muscle cells in the vessel wall (Fig. 3.32). These hyalinized retinal vessels will show diminished autoregulation.

In patients with damaged vessel walls, thrombosis may occur, accelerating the ischemic process. In the chronic reparative

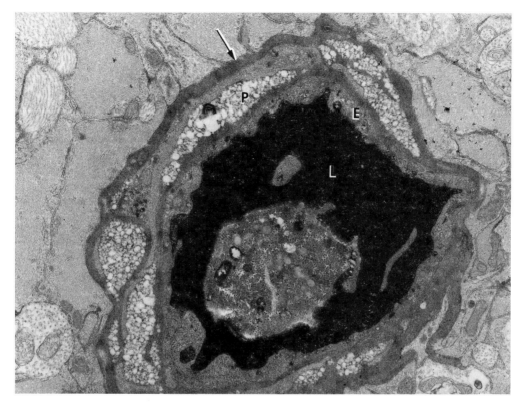

Figure 3.30. Electron micrograph of retinal capillary in a hypertensive baboon showing degeneration of pericytes (*P*). *E* indicates endothelium; *L*, lumen; *arrow*, horseradish peroxidase staining of basement membrane of pericyte (×5667).

phase, vascular remodeling takes place. When nonperfused arteries become recanalized, capillaries may reopen, and a smooth muscle coat may develop around capillaries as they form collaterals. Unfortunately, despite this vascular remodeling, visual function does not usually return to the previously infarcted retina.

Hypertensive Optic Neuropathy

Clinical Findings

Hypertension may cause a variety of changes in the optic nerve head. In patients with accelerated hypertension, optic disc edema may be seen. The optic nerve head exhibits a blurred margin, filling of the optic cup, and congestion of the retinal veins (Fig. 3.33). Exudative changes may be seen in the macula (Fig. 3.34). Hyper-

tensive encephalopathy may or may not be present.

A second group of patients with hypertensive retinopathy may present with a generalized or altitudinal pallor and atrophy of the optic disc. These patients may have had previous central or branch retinal artery or vein occlusions. They usually have severe visual loss, accompanied by varying degrees of visual field defects.

A third group of patients may present with the acute onset of blurring of vision. Ophthalmoscopically, the optic disc is mildly swollen. Two or three flame-shaped or linear hemorrhages are present at the margin of the optic nerve head. Altitudinal or arcuate nerve fiber bundle defects may be observed. Fluorescein angiography may demonstrate sectorial leakage in the optic nerve head. Optic atrophy with retinal arterial narrowing soon develops. Besides

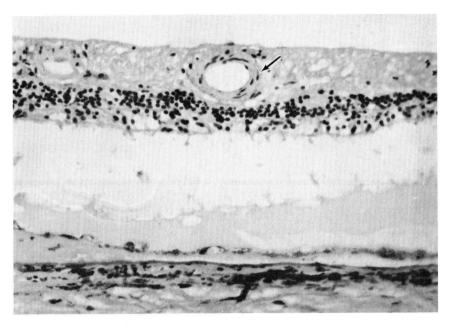

Figure 3.31. Retinal vessels in sclerotic phase of hypertensive retinopathy showing moderate hyperplasia of the tunica media (*arrow*) (hematoxylin-eosin: ×320).

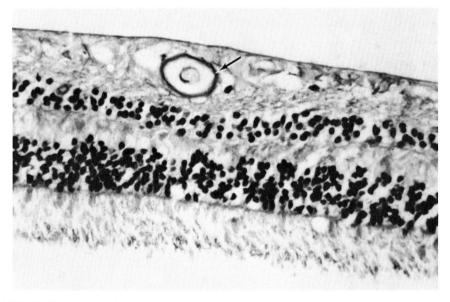

Figure 3.32. Hyaline degeneration of a retinal vessel in a patient with hypertensive retinopathy, showing loss of muscle cells in the vessel wall (*arrow*) (hematoxylin-eosin: ×320).

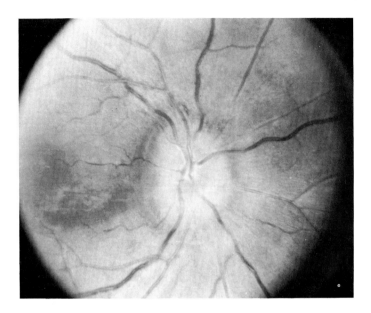

Figure 3.33. Photograph of the retina of a 26-year-old black female patient with hypertensive optic disc edema. Note that extensive hypertensive retinopathy is absent.

hypertension, a history of diabetes is frequently obtained. Giant cell arteritis, embolic diseases, and hematological disorders must be ruled out; however, some ophthalmologists believe that some cases of this form of ischemic optic neuropathy may represent hypertensive optic nerve infarction (79). Others note a statistically significant association between systemic hypertension and anterior ischemic optic neuropathy in patients under 65 years of age (80).

Pathophysiological Mechanisms of Hypertensive Optic Neuropathy

The pathogenetic mechanisms responsible for such varied presentations of optic neuropathy in systemic hypertension depend upon the structure and the pathophysiological control of blood vessels of the optic nerve head. The optic nerve head has a complex blood supply (81). It is supplied anteriorly by branches of the central retinal artery and posteriorly by pial vessels and branches of the short posterior ciliary arteries passing through the choroid and border tissue of Elschnig. The branches of the central retinal artery supplying the optic nerve head anterior to the lamina cribrosa are devoid of sympathetic

innervation; the central retinal artery and vein in the optic nerve head posterior to the lamina cribrosa are regulated by sympathetic tone (20). A portion of the optic nerve head in the region of the lamina choroidalis is partially supplied by a branch of the short posterior ciliary arteries that passes through the choroid (81). This branch is also controlled by the sympathetic nervous system. Angiotensin II, a powerful vasoconstrictor, may leak through the choriocapillaries, permeate the optic nerve head through the border tissue of Elschnig (82), and produce marked vasoconstriction in the region of the lamina choroidalis (83). The pathological processes of hypertensive optic neuropathy have not been fully defined (84–86). In a recent study of experimental hypertension in monkeys, three phases in the pathological process were observed (85): (*a*) an acute ischemic phase, (*b*) a resolution phase, and (*c*) an atrophic phase. In each of these phases, the blood vessels in the anterior optic nerve head showed different pathological changes when compared with those of the optic nerve head behind the lamina cribrosa.

In the acute ischemic phase, the blood vessels in the lamina retinalis (the portion of the optic nerve head anterior to the lam-

Figure 3.34. Photograph of the retina of a patient with hypertensive optic neuropathy showing exudative phase of hypertensive retinopathy with hard exudate, perivascular macular star, marked swelling of the optic disc (*arrows*), and filling of the optic cup.

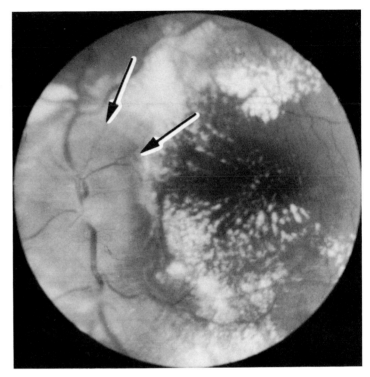

ina cribrosa) showed mild constriction, intact endothelial cells, but degenerated pericytes (Fig. 3.35). However, the blood vessels that supplied the posterior part of the optic nerve head, particularly the pial blood vessels, exhibited severe constriction and swelling of the endothelial cells and degeneration of pericytes, which resulted in the obliteration of the vessel lumina. The pial arterial system, which supplies the retrolaminar portion of the optic nerve, appeared to react much more intensely (Fig. 3.36) than the retinal vessels to the accelerated hypertension of the animal model.

In the resolution phase (Figs. 3.37, 3.38), the blood vessels in the lamina retinalis were less constricted and showed no leakage of tracer, but the endothelial cells and pericytes of the pial blood vessels showed extensive hydropic degeneration and extensive leakage into the perivascular tissue.

In the atrophic phase, the differences between the lamina retinalis and the myelinated optic nerve were dramatic. In spite of the constriction of the retinal arterioles in the lamina retinalis in the acute ischemic phase, some of the blood vessels remained patent in the atrophic phase. In contrast, the pial vessels were necrotic. The ischemia appeared much more severe in the myelinated optic nerve supplied by the pial arteries and the retrolaminar segment of the central retinal artery than it did in the lamina retinalis, which is supplied by branches of retinal arteries. The posterior vessels, probably under sympathetic control, show much more severe ischemic changes in accelerated hypertension than the anterior vessels.

Experimental studies on disc edema secondary to systemic hypertension (30) showed delay in axoplasmic transport and an accumulation of axoplasmic components in the region of the lamina retinalis and the lamina choroidalis anterior to the lamina scleralis (Fig. 3.39). This condition resulted in swelling of the axons at the optic nerve head, which led to optic disc edema. The pathogenetic mechanism of axoplasmic stasis is possibly multifacto-

Figure 3.35. Electron micrographs. **A.** Lamina retinalis in acute phase of hypertensive optic neuropathy. Blood vessel shows slit-like lumen (*arrows*), suggesting vasoconstriction. Pericytes (*P*) exhibit spectrum of degenerative changes, ranging from hydropic swelling to densification of cytoplasm. Some axons (*a*) show hydropic swelling; others (*A*) exhibit disruption of axolemma and loss of axoplasm. Perivascular glial cells (*G*) are swollen (original magnification ×4000). **B.** Lamina choroidalis in acute phase of hypertensive optic neuropathy. Lumen (*arrow*) of blood vessel is occluded. Pericyte (*P*) shows mild hydropic swelling. Some axons (*a*) have watery axoplasm with disrupted axolemma (*arrowheads*) (×4600).

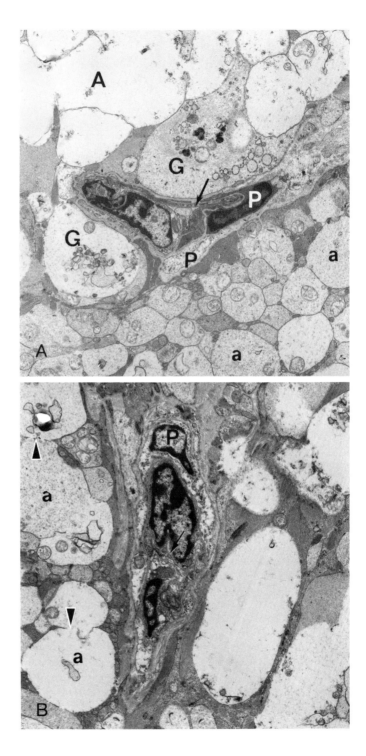

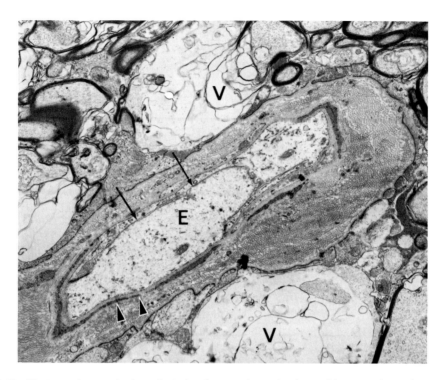

Figure 3.36. Electron micrograph of myelinated optic nerve in acute phase of hypertensive optic neuropathy. Pial blood vessel shows severe swelling of endothelial cell (*E*) and degeneration of pericytes (*arrowheads*). Lumen (*arrows*) is obliterated. Interlamellar spaces of myelin sheath of axons are enlarged, forming vacuoles (*V*) (×6750).

rial. Ischemia of the optic nerve head may produce axoplasmic stasis. The optic nerve head is under the influence of intraocular pressure anteriorly, and intracranial pressure in the subarachnoid space posteriorly. Alteration of the cerebrospinal fluid pressure, intraocular pressure, or interstitial pressure may affect the axoplasmic transport in the optic nerve head. Furthermore, the vascular constriction and subsequent ischemia in the retrolaminar optic nerve may also contribute to the delay in axoplasmic transport.

Systemic Hypertension and Ocular Diseases

Systemic hypertension may influence the course of other diseases of the retina, choroid, or optic nerve. Hypertensive ocular disease can occur simultaneously with another ocular diseases and accentuate the manifestations of these diseases. In dis-

eases affecting the retinal vasculature, such as diabetes or systemic lupus erythematosus, systemic hypertension intensifies and accelerates the retinal exudative process. In diseases affecting the choroid, the additional presence of systemic hypertension may be a major factor in the development of neurosensory retinal detachment following breakdown of the posterior blood-ocular barrier. Following microsphere occlusion of the choriocapillaris of monkeys, neurosensory retinal detachment occurred only following induction of systemic hypertension (87).

In a population-based study of diabetic retinopathy in southern Wisconsin, it was found that a higher prevalence of systemic hypertension existed among diabetic patients than was indicated in previous studies involving nondiabetic patients whose age was similar to those in the Wisconsin study (88). Hypertension was present in 21.9% of Wisconsin diabetic patients whose

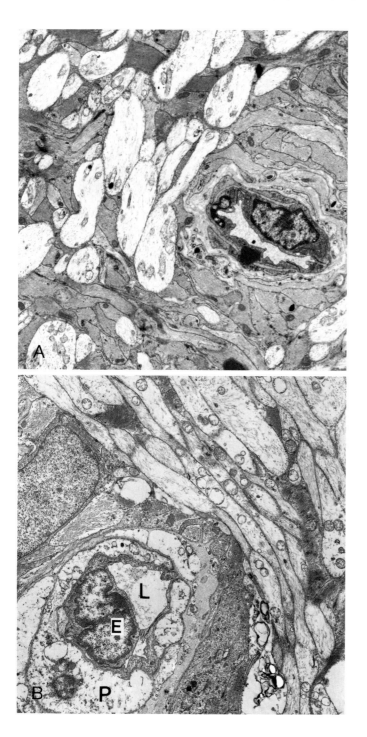

Figure 3.37. Electron micrographs. **A.** Lamina retinalis in resolution phase of hypertensive optic neuropathy. Blood vessel is less constricted. Axons are less swollen (×5550). **B.** Lamina scleralis in reparative phase. Blood vessel shows severe degeneration of pericytes (P). Axons display mild swelling. L, lumen of blood vessel; E, endothelial cell (×4100).

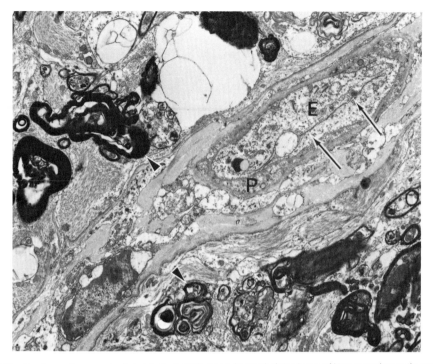

Figure 3.38. Electron micrograph of myelinated optic nerve in resolution phase of hypertensive optic neuropathy. Endothelial cell (*E*) and pericytes (*P*) of a pial blood vessel show extensive hydropic degeneration. Lumen (*arrows*) is mostly occluded. Note fragments of collapsed myelin sheath without axons (*arrowheads*) (×5100).

onset occurred at less than 30 years of age and in 58% of diabetic patients whose onset occurred at 30 years of age or older. Advanced age at the time of examination, presence of proteinuria, increased body mass, gender, and longer duration of diabetes were associated with higher systolic blood pressure.

Previous studies have not clearly shown a relationship between progression of background or proliferative diabetic retinopathy and levels of systemic systolic and diastolic blood pressure. There has been recent evidence of a relationship between elevated diastolic blood pressure and progression of diabetic retinopathy in diabetic patients with onset of disease before 30 years of age but not in diabetic patients with onset of disease at 30 years of age or older (89). It remains unclear whether hypertension is a primary event or the result of advancing diabetic nephropathy. Therefore, there is difficulty in determining if the hypertension and/or nephropathy were

causal events or simply associated events in patients with severe, generalized microvascular disease.

Patients whose diabetic retinopathy has progressed should have their blood pressure evaluated. Normalization of elevated blood pressure might improve the retinopathy and help prevent progressive nephropathy and other complications (90, 93).

Systemic hypertension may play a role in the development and progression of ocular disease associated with rheumatic diseases. Connective tissue diseases, particularly systemic lupus erythematosus (SLE) (see Chapter 1), may cause posterior segment disease regardless of the presence of hypertension. Hypertension that often coexists with connective tissue disorders may worsen the ocular manifestations. Cotton-wool spots with or without retinal hemorrhages are seen in the microangiopathy of SLE (94) (see Chapter 1). In these cases, vaso occlusion may be widespread (95). Histopathologically, there is immune

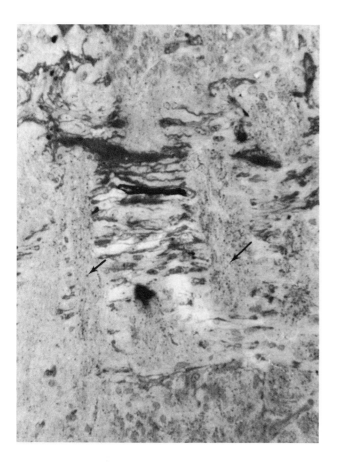

Figure 3.39. An autoradiograph of the optic nerve head of a hypertensive baboon with mild papilledema. Note the accumulation of silver grains (*arrows*) in the region of lamina retinalis and choroidalis, anterior to lamina scleralis (toluidine blue: ×320).

complex deposition within the vessel walls, which may be responsible for the microangiopathy (96). Systemic hypertension may accelerate the microangiopathy and cause the retinal exudative process to progress.

A less common ocular manifestation of SLE is lupus choroidopathy (94–97). Histopathological studies have revealed mononuclear inflammatory cells in the choroid of patients with untreated SLE. Lupus choroidopathy may exhibit multiple leaks in the retinal pigment epithelium and neurosensory retinal detachment. Systemic hypertension is often present and may be partially responsible for the development of the neurosensory retinal detachment.

Hypertension is often found to be associated with systemic vasculitides such as polyarteritis nodosa (see Chapter 1). Retinal or choroidal vasculitis may be present, and associated severe hypertensive ocular disease may also exist.

Hypertension may influence the ocular presentation of thrombotic thrombocytopenic purpura (TTP) and other vasculopathies (98, 99) (see Chapter 2). In TTP, idiopathic thrombocytopenic purpura (ITP), and disseminated intravascular coagulation (DIC), the choriocapillaries are obstructed by platelet and fibrin microthrombi. Though hypertension is not a prerequisite, systemic hypertension may increase the probability of associated neurosensory retinal detachment (96).

Preeclampsia and eclampsia are forms of pregnancy-induced hypertension (61–63, 100) (see Chapter 10). Ocular findings secondary to the hypertension are common and are indistinguishable from those of other forms of accelerated hypertension.

Systemic hypertension may be a risk factor in development of age-related macular degeneration. Analysis of data on 1828 subjects in the Framingham heart and eye study demonstrates a small and consistent association between age-related maculopathy and systemic hypertension (101). The association was found using blood pressure and medical history data collected both 25 years before the eye examination and at a time concurrent with the eye examination. The prevalence of age-related maculopathy (most commonly the dry form of the disease) progressively increased with increasing duration of systemic hypertension. The association was greatest for moderate to severe categories of age-related macular degeneration, which are represented by the following manifestations: obvious or severe pigmentary disturbance; small macular drusen greater than 10 in number; large macular drusen; or serous, hemorrhagic, or proliferative elevation of macular pigmented or neurosensory epithelium. Elevated blood pressure was defined as systolic blood pressure 160 mm Hg or greater, or diastolic blood pressure 95 mm Hg or greater, or use of medication to lower the blood pressure. It is doubtful if the changes in the choroid or choriocapillaris in age-related macular degeneration are a direct result of hypertension. The role of hypertension in age-related macular degeneration is unclear, but the association may be a risk factor.

ACKNOWLEDGMENTS

Supported in part by Grant EY1903 and Core Grant IP30 EY 1792 from the National Institutes of Health (Dr. Tso) and unrestricted grants from Research to Prevent Blindness, Inc. (Dr. Abrams and Dr. Jampol). Dr. Tso is the recipient of a Senior Scientific Investigator Award from Research to Prevent Blindness, Inc. Sandra Brown assisted with the preparation of the classification system demonstrated in Figures 3.18–3.21.

This chapter was modified, with permission, from Chapter 31, Hypertensive Retinopathy, Choroidopathy and Optic Neuropathy of Hypertensive Disease, by MOM Tso and Lee M Jampol, in Hypertension: Pathophysiology, Diagnosis, and Management (JH Laragh, BM Brenner, eds). NY: Raven Press, 1990, pp 433–465.

Figures 3.8–3.11, 3.23, 3.25, 3.26, 3.28–3.33, 3.39 are published courtesy of Ophthalmology (1982;89:1132–1145) with permission of the American Academy of Ophthalmology. Figures 3.1 and 3.34 were reprinted with permission of WB Saunders Co., Philadelphia. Figure 3.5 is reprinted with permission from XXIII Concilium Ophthalmologicum Kyoto, 1978, pp 239–241 (Elsevier Science Publishers). Figures 3.3, 3.4, 3.6, and 3.7 are reprinted from Arch Ophthalmol 1987;105:681, with permission of the American Medical Association. Figures 3.12–3.17 are reprinted from Arch Ophthalmol 1985;103:1189, and Figures 3.35–3.38 from Arch Ophthalmol 1985;103:1198, with permission of the American Medical Association.

References

1. Kaplan NM. Clinical hypertension. 4th ed. Baltimore: Williams & Wilkins, 1986.
2. Joint National Committee on Detection, Evaluation, and Treatment of High Blood Pressure. The 1984 Report of the Joint National Committee on the Detection, Evaluation, and Treatment of High Blood Pressure. Arch Intern Med 1984;144:1045–1057.
3. Fine BS, Yanoff M. Ocular histology; a text and atlas. New York: Harper & Row, 1972:273.
4. Weiter JJ, Schachar RA, Ernest JT. Control of intraocular blood flow. I. Intraocular pressure. Invest Ophthalmol 1973;12:327–331.
5. Gunn M. On ophthalmoscopic evidence of general arterial disease. Trans Ophthalmol Soc UK 1898;18:356–381.
6. Keith NM, Wagener HP, Barker NW. Some different types of essential hypertension: their course and prognosis. Am J Med Sci 1939; 197:332–343.
7. Wagener HP, Clay GE, Gipner JF. Classification of retinal lesions in the presence of vascular hypertension. Trans Am Ophthalmol Soc 1947;45:57–73.
8. Scheie HG. Evaluation of ophthalmoscopic changes of hypertension and arteriolar sclerosis. Arch Ophthalmol 1953;49:117–138.
9. Leishman R. The eye in general vascular disease; hypertension and arteriosclerosis. Br J Ophthalmol 1957;41:641–701.
10. Garner A, Ashton N, Tripathi R, et al. Pathogenesis of hypertensive retinopathy; an exper-

imental study in the monkey. Br J Ophthalmol 1975;59:3–44.

11. Seitz R. The retinal vessels: comparative ophthalmoscopic and histologic studies on healthy and diseased eyes. Translated by F.C. Blodi. St. Louis: CV Mosby, 1964:67–74.

12. Kagan A, Aurell E, Dobree J, et al. A note on signs in the fundus oculi and arterial hypertension: conventional assessment and significance. Bull WHO 1966;34:955–960.

13. Dollery CT, Ramalho PS, Patterson JW. Retinal vascular alterations in hypertension. In: Gross F, ed. Antihypertensive therapy; principles and practice, an international symposium. New York: Springer, 1966:152.

14. Wise GN, Dollery CT, Henkind P. The retinal circulation. New York: Harper & Row, 1971:325.

15. Breslin DJ, Gifford RW Jr, Fairbairn JF II. Essential hypertension; a twenty year follow-up study. Circulation 1966;33:87–97.

16. Breslin DJ, Gifford RW Jr, Fairbairn JF II, Kearns TP. Prognostic importance of ophthalmoscopic findings in essential hypertension. JAMA 1966;195:335–338.

17. Stokoe NL. Fundus changes in hypertension—a long-term clinical study. In: Cant JS, ed. William Mackenzie Centenary Symposium on the Ocular Circulation in Health and Disease. London: Kimpton, 1969:117–135.

18. Stokoe NL. Clinical assessment of the hypertensive fundus. Trans Ophthalmol Soc UK 1975;95:463–471.

19. Walsh JB. Hypertensive retinopathy. Description, classification, and prognosis. Ophthalmology 1982;89:1127–1131.

20. Laties AM. Central retinal artery innervation; absence of adrenergic innervation to the intraocular branches. Arch Ophthalmol 1967;77:405–409.

21. Hogan MJ, Alvarado JA, Weddell JE. Histology of the human eye; an atlas and textbook. Philadelphia: WB Saunders, 1971:508–513.

22. Tso MOM, Fine BS. Electron microscopic study of human papilledema. Am J Ophthalmol 1976;82:424–434.

23. Michaelson IC. Retinal circulation in man and animals. Springfield, IL: Thomas, 1954.

24. Michaelson IC, Steedman HF. Injection of the retinal vascular system in enucleated eyes. Br J Ophthalmol 1949;33:376–379.

25. Toussaint D, Kuwabara T, Cogan DG. Retinal vascular patterns. Part II. Human retinal vessels studied in three dimensions. Arch Ophthalmol 1961;65:575–581.

26. Shimizu K, Ujiie K. Structure of ocular vessels. Tokyo: Igaku-Shoin, 1978:9.

27. Tso MOM. Pathology of the blood-retinal barrier. In: Cunha-Vaz JG. The blood-retinal barriers. New York: Plenum Press, 1980:235–250.

28. Deem CW, Futterman S, Kalina RE. Induction of endothelial cell proliferation in rat retinal venules by chemical and indirect physical trauma. Invest Ophthalmol 1974;13:580–585.

29. Wallow IH, Engerman RL. Permeability and patency of retinal blood vessels in experimental diabetes. Invest Ophthalmol Vis Sci 1977;16:447–461.

30. Tso MOM, Jampol LM. Pathophysiology of hypertensive retinopathy. Ophthalmology 1982;89:1132–1145.

31. Ernest JT. Regulatory mechanisms of the choroidal vasculature in health and disease. In: Tso MOM, ed. Retinal diseases; biomedical foundations and clinical management. Philadelphia: JB Lippincott, 1988:125–130.

32. Bill A, Sperber G, Ujiie K. Physiology of the choroidal vascular bed. Int Ophthalmol 1983;6:101–107.

33. Alm A, Bill A. Ocular and optic nerve blood flow at normal and increased intraocular pressure in monkeys (*Macaca irus*): a study of radioactively labeled microspheres including flow determinations in brain and some other tissues. Exp Eye Res 1973;15:15–29.

34. Russell RW. Evidence for autoregulation in human retinal circulation. Lancet 1973;2:1048–1050.

35. Ffytche TJ, Bulpitt CJ, Kohner EM, et al. Effect of changes in intraocular pressure on the retinal microcirculation. Br J Ophthalmol 1974;58:514–522.

36. Riva CE, Sinclair SH, Grunwald JE. Autoregulation of retinal circulation in response to decrease of perfusion pressure. Invest Ophthalmol Vis Sci 1981;21:34–38.

37. Riva CE, Grunwald JE, Petrig BL, Sinclair SH. Effect of breathing pure oxygen on human retinal blood flow measured by laser doppler velocimetry. ARVO Abstracts. Invest Ophthalmol Vis Sci 1982;22(suppl):194.

38. Frayser R, Hickam JB. Retinal vascular response to breathing increased carbon dioxide and oxygen concentrations. Invest Ophthalmol 1964;3:427–431.

39. Deutsch TA, Read JS, Ernest JT, Goldstick TK. Effects of oxygen and carbon dioxide on the retinal vasculature in humans. Arch Ophthalmol 1983;101:1278–1280.

40. Sinclair SH, Grunwald JE, Riva CE, et al. Retinal vascular autoregulation in diabetes mellitus. Ophthalmology 1982;89:748–750.

41. Sieker HO, Hickam JB. Normal and impaired retinal vascular reactivity. Circulation 1953;7:79–83.

42. Kohner EM, Hamilton AM, Saunders SJ, et al. The retinal blood flow in diabetes. Diabetologica 1975;11:27–33.

43. Goldstick TK, Ernest JT, Engerman RL. Imparied retinal vascular reactivity in diabetic dogs. ARVO Abstracts. Invest Ophthalmol Vis Sci 1981;20(suppl):92.

44. Yoneya S, Tso MOM. Angioarchitecture of the human choroid. Arch Ophthalmol 1987;105:681–687.

45. Torczynski E, Tso MOM. The architecture of the choriocapillaris at the posterior pole. Am J Ophthalmol 1976;81:428–440.

46. Hayreh SS. The choriocapillaris. Albrecht von Graefes Arch Klin Exp Ophthalmol 1974; 192:165–179.

47. Goldbaum MH, Galinos SO, Apple D, et al. Acute choroidal ischemia as a complication of photocoagulation. Arch Ophthalmol 1976;94:1025–1035.

48. Dizon-Moore RV, Jampol LM, Goldberg MF. Chorioretinal and choriovitreal neovascularization; their presence after photocoagulation of proliferative sickle cell retinopathy. Arch Ophthalmol 1981;99:842–849.

49. Parver LM, Auker C, Carpenter DO. Choroidal blood flow as a heat dissipating mechanism in the macula. Am J Ophthalmol 1980;89:641 646.

50. Parver LM, Auker CR, Carpenter DO, Doyle T. Choroidal blood flow. II. Reflexive control in the monkey. Arch Ophthalmol 1982;100:1327–1330.

51. Ernest JT. The effect of systolic hypertension on rhesus monkey eyes after ocular sympathectomy. Am J Ophthalmol 1977;84:341–344.

52. Kishi S, Tso MOM, Hayreh SS. Fundus lesions in malignant hypertension. I. A pathologic study of experimental hypertensive choroidopathy. Arch Ophthalmol 1985;103:1189–1197.

53. Bill A. Intraocular pressure and blood flow through the uvea. Arch Ophthalmol 1962; 67:336–348.

54. Weiter JJ, Schachar RA, Ernest JT. Control of intraocular blood flow. II. Effects of sympathetic tone. Invest Ophthalmol 1973;12:332–334.

55. Friedman E, Smith TR, Kuwabara T, Beyer CK. Choroidal vascular patterns in hypertension. Arch Ophthalmol 1964;71:842–850.

56. Klien BA. Ischemic infarcts of the choroid (Elschnig spots); a cause of retinal separation in hypertensive disease with renal insufficiency; a clinical and histophathologic study. Am J Ophthalmol 1968;66:1069–1074.

57. Morse PH. Elschnig's spots and hypertensive choroidopathy. Am J Ophthalmol 1968;66:844–852.

58. Burian HM. Pigment epithelium changes in arteriosclerotic choroidopathy. Am J Ophthalmol 1969;68:412–416.

59. Uyama M. Histopathological studies on vascular changes, especially on involvements in the choroidal vessels, in hypertensive retinopathy. Acta Soc Ophthalmol Jpn 1975;79:357–370.

60. de Venecia G, Wallow I, Houser D, Wahlstrom M. The eye in accelerated hypertension. I. Elschnig's spots in nonhuman primates. Arch Ophthalmol 1980;98:913–918.

61. de Venecia G, Jampol LM. The eye in accelerated hypertension. II. Localized serous detachments of the retina in patients. Arch Ophthalmol 1984;102:68–73.

62. Fastenberg DM, Fetkenhour CL, Choromokos E, Shoch DE. Choroidal vascular changes in toxemia of pregnancy. Am J Ophthamol 1980;89:362–368.

63. Gitter KA, Houser BP, Sarin LK, Justice J Jr. Toxemia of pregnancy; an angiographic interpretation of fundus changes. Arch Ophthalmol 1968;80:449–454.

64. Kenny GS, Cerasoli JR. Color fluorescein angiography in toxemia of pregnancy. Arch Ophthalmol 1972;87:383–388.

65. Skalina MEL, Annable WL, Kliegman RM, Fanaroff AA. Hypertensive retinopathy in the newborn infant. J Pediatr 1983;103:781–786.

66. Svärdsudd K, Wedel H, Aurell E, Tibblin G. Hypertensive eye growth changes; prevalence, relation to blood pressure, and prognostic importance. The study of men born in 1913. Acta Med Scand 1978,204.159–167.

67. Kagan A, Aurell E, Tibblin G. Signs in the fundus oculi and arterial hypertension; unconventional assessment and significance. Bull WHO 1967;36:2231–241.

68. Bock KD. Regression of retinal vascular changes by antihypertensive therapy. Hypertension 1984;6(6 pt 2): III158–162.

69. Orlin C, Lee K, Jampol LM, Farber M. Retinal arteriolar changes in patients with hyperlipidemias. Retina 1988;8:6–9.

70. Jampol LM, White S, Cunha-Vaz J. Vitreous fluorophotometry in patients with hypertension. Arch Ophthalmol 1983;101:888–890.

71. Jampol LM. Arteriolar occlusive diseases of the macula. Ophthalmology 1983;90:534–539.

72. Ramalho PS, Dollery CT. Hypertensive retinopathy. Caliber changes in retinal blood vessels following blood-pressure reduction and inhalation of oxygen. Circulation 1968;37:580–588.

73. Byrom FB. Vascular crisis in hypertension. In: Gross F, ed. Antihypertensive therapy; principles and practice, an international symposium. New York: Springer, 1966:125.

74. Lassen NA, Agnoli A. The upper limit of autoregulation of cerebral blood flow—on the pathogenesis of hypertensive encephalopathy. Scand J Clin Lab Invest 1972;30:113–116.

75. Strandgaard S, Olesen J, Skinhoj E, Lassen NA. Autoregulation of brain circulation in severe arterial hypertension. Br Med J 1973;1:507–510.

76. Ashton N. The eye in malignant hypertension. Trans Am Acad Ophthalmol Otolaryngol 1972;76:17–40.

77. Hodge JV, Dollery CT. Retinal soft exudates. A clinical study by colour and fluorescence photography. Quart J Med 1964;33:117–131.

78. Tso MOM, Kurosawa A, Benhamou E, et al. Microangiopathic retinopathy in experimental diabetic monkeys. Trans Am Ophthalmol Soc 1988;86:389–421.

79. Smith JL, Goldhammer Y. Hypertensive optic neuropathy. Trans Am Acad Ophthalmol Otolaryngol 1975;79:OP520–523.

80. Guyer DR, Miller NR, Auer CL, Fine SL. The risk of cerebrovascular and cardiovascular disease in patients with anterior ischemic optic neuropathy. Arch Ophthalmol 1985;103:1136–1142.

81. Hayreh SS. Structure and blood supply of the optic nerve. In: Heilmann K, Richardson KT, eds. Glaucoma; conceptions of a disease, pathology, diagnosis, therapy. Philadelphia: WB Saunders, 1978: 78–96.

82. Tso MOM, Shih CY, McLean IW. Is there a blood-brain barrier at the optic nerve head? Arch Ophthalmol 1975;93:815–825.

83. Kishi S, Tso MOM, Hayreh SS. Fundus lesions in malignant hypertension. II. A pathologic study of experimental hypertensive optic neuropathy. Arch Ophthalmol 1985;103:1198–1206.

84. Paton L, Holmes G. The pathology of papilloedema. A histological study of sixty eyes. Brain 1911;33:389–432.

85. Meadows SP. The swollen optic disc. Trans Ophthalmol Soc UK 1959;79:121–143.

86. Hayreh SS. Optic disc edema in raised intracranial pressure. V. Pathogenesis. Arch Ophthalmol 1977;95:1553–1565.

87. Stern WH, Ernest JT. Microsphere occlusion of the choriocapillaris in rhesus monkeys. Am J Ophthalmol 1974;78:438–448.

88. Klein R, Klein BEK, Moss SE, DeMets DL. Blood pressure and hypertension in diabetes. Am J Epidemiol 1985;122:75–89.

89. Krolewski AS, Canessa M, Warram JH, et al. Predisposition to hypertension and susceptibility to renal disease in insulin-dependent diabetes mellitus. N Engl J Med 1988;318:140–145.

90. Klein R, Klein BEK, Moss S, DeMets DL. Proteinuria in diabetes. Arch Intern Med 1988;148:181–186.

91. Janka HU, Ziegler AG, Valsania P, Warram JH, Krolewski AS. Impact of blood pressure on diabetic retinopathy. Diabete Metab 1989;15(5 Pt 2):333–337.

92. Teuscher A, Egger M, Herman JB. Diabetes and hypertension. Blood pressure in clinical diabetic patients and a control population. Arch Intern Med 1989;149:1942–1945.

93. Perkovich BT, Meyers SM. Systemic factors affecting diabetic macular edema. Am J Ophthalmol 1988;105:211–212.

94. Gold DH, Morris DA, Henkind P. Ocular findings in systemic lupus erythematosus. Br J Ophthalmol 1972;56:800–804.

95. Jabs DA, Fine SL, Hochberg MC, Newman SA, Helner GG, Stevens MB. Severe retinal vasoocclusive disease in systemic lupus erythematosus. Arch Ophthalmol 1986;104:558–563.

96. Karpik AG, Schwartz MM, Dickey LE, et al. Ocular immune reactants in patients dying with systemic lupus erythematosus. Clin Immunol Immunopathol 1985;35:295–312.

97. Jabs DA, Hanneken AM, Schachat AP, Fine SL. Choroidopathy in systemic lupus erythematosus. Arch Ophthalmol 1988;106:230–234.

98. Cogan DG. Ocular involvement in disseminated intravascular coagulopathy. Arch Ophthalmol 1975;93:1–8.

99. Lambert SR, High KA, Cotlier E, Benz EJ Jr. Serous retinal detachments in thrombotic thrombocytopenic purpura. Arch Ophthalmol 1985;103:1172–1174.

100. Ober RR. Pregnancy-induced hypertension (preeclampsia-eclampsia). In: Ryan SJ, ed. Retina, Vol 2. St Louis: Mosby, 1989:441–447.

101. Sperduto RD, Hiller R. Systemic hypertension and age-related maculopathy in the Framingham Study. Arch Ophthalmol 1986;104:216–219.

CHAPTER 4

Ophthalmic Manifestations of Carotid Artery Disease

Gary C. Brown, Gabriel Coscas, Froncie A. Gutman, David H. Orth, and Kurt A. Gitter

INTRODUCTION

Atherosclerotic disease of the carotid artery affects the eye in a number of ways. Fibrin-platelet emboli and cholesterol emboli can arise from the carotids and pass into the retinal arterial system, causing amaurosis fugax and branch or central retinal artery obstruction. Additionally, a severe carotid stenosis may cause the ocular ischemic syndrome, which is the subject of this chapter.

Alternatively known as venous stasis retinopathy (1), ischemic ocular inflammation (2), or ischemic oculopathy (3), the ocular ischemic syndrome (OIS) is characterized by ocular symptoms and signs that occur secondary to severe atherosclerotic carotid artery obstruction (4). When the disease was first described in 1963 (1), it was called "venous-stasis retinopathy." Since the same nomenclature has also been used to describe mild, or nonischemic, central retinal vein obstruction (5), an entity that pathophysiologically and clinically differs from OIS, the name "ocular ischemic syndrome" seems preferable. The term "ischemic ocular inflammation" (2) is probably not optimal because, despite the fact that approximately 20% of eyes present with anterior uveitis (4), signs of inflammation are usually lacking when

histopathological examination of the posterior segment is performed (6).

DEMOGRAPHICS

The ocular ischemic syndrome generally affects persons from 50 to 90 years of age; the mean age is about 65 years (4). Males outnumber females by a ratio of 2:1, but no racial preference has been demonstrated (1–4). One eye does not appear to be affected more than the other. The incidence of bilaterality is close to 20% (4).

No carefully collected data exist to establish the incidence of OIS. The disease was noted (7) in six patients seen over a period of 2 years in a hospital serving a population of 400,000; this figure represents 7.5 cases/million persons/year. Assuming a population of 245 million people in the United States, more than 1800 cases/year would be expected. However, this figure is probably an underestimate; OIS can be confused with other diseases such as central retinal vein obstruction and diabetic retinopathy.

Twenty-two cases of OIS were found among 600 patients with intermittent insufficiency or thrombosis of the carotid arterial system (1). Thus, it appears that nearly 5% of patients with marked carotid obstructive disease also have OIS.

SYMPTOMS

Visual Loss and Pain

Of all individuals in whom OIS is diagnosed, 90% are found to have loss of vision at the time of diagnosis, and, in fact, visual loss is usually the factor that brings them to the ophthalmologist. Most commonly, the decreased vision develops gradually over a period of weeks to months as ischemia to the eye increases. However, abrupt visual loss occurs in about 12% of cases (4). In such instances, a cherry-red spot is usually seen in the fundus. This condition most often develops secondary to closure of the central retinal artery when perfusion pressure in this vessel is exceeded by increased intraocular pressure due to neovascular glaucoma (8, 9). About 10% of patients with OIS have a history of amaurosis fugax (4).

Blurred vision in affected eyes following exposure to bright light has been noted by a number of authors (10–12). Positive after-images have also been described. It is believed that these phenomena occur due to photochemical effects, possibly secondary to choroidal vascular insufficiency leading to a compromise of photoreceptor metabolism (12).

Pain, which occurs in approximately 40% of patients with OIS (4), is most often described as a dull ache affecting the globe or ipsilateral orbital region. In some cases, it is attributable to increased intraocular pressure from neovascular glaucoma, but, among eyes in which the intraocular pressure is normal, the discomfort may result from ischemia to the globe or dura. The term "ocular angina" has been applied to the pain (4).

SIGNS

Visual Acuity

The visual acuity at presentation is quite variable (4). The vision in approximately 35% of eyes ranges from 20/20 to 20/40; the vision in another 30% ranges from 20/50 to 20/400. In the remaining 35%, it var-

ies from count fingers to no light perception. Only in the very advanced stages of the disease, usually in conjunction with neovascular glaucoma, do patients lack the capacity to perceive light.

Anterior Segment

Corneal abnormalities are usually absent until the late stages of the disease. Striae accompanied by wrinkling of Descemet's membrane can be present, and corneal edema can be seen when the intraocular pressure is elevated.

In 1965, the anterior segment inflammation seen in some OIS eyes was described (2). Flare is commonly seen in the anterior chamber in OIS eyes, particularly in those with rubeosis iridis. A cellular response is present in about 20% of eyes (4) but generally does not exceed grade 2 of the Schlaegel classification (13). The cells are most prominent in the anterior chamber but can also be seen in the vitreous cavity (2). Small keratic precipitates are occasionally visible on the corneal endothelium (2, 4). Most often, when an anterior uveitis is present, concomitant posterior segment signs of OIS can also be seen. OIS should be considered in the differential diagnosis of uveitis beginning in an adult over 50 years of age.

The presence of rubeosis iridis and neovascular glaucoma associated with carotid artery obstruction was described in 1962 (14). Ensuing publications have consistently noted rubeosis iridis to be a part of the spectrum of the disease (1–4, 7, 12). At the time of presentation, iris neovascularization is seen in about two-thirds of eyes (Fig. 4.1)(4), although this percentage would theoretically be lower if the disease were diagnosed in an earlier stage. Despite the fact that angle closure often develops, only about 50% of eyes with rubeosis iridis progress to neovascular glaucoma (rubeosis iridis + intraocular pressure >22 mm Hg). The intraocular pressure probably fails to rise substantially in these eyes because of impaired ciliary body perfusion and decreased aqueous production secondary to the carotid stenosis (3, 12). The finding of

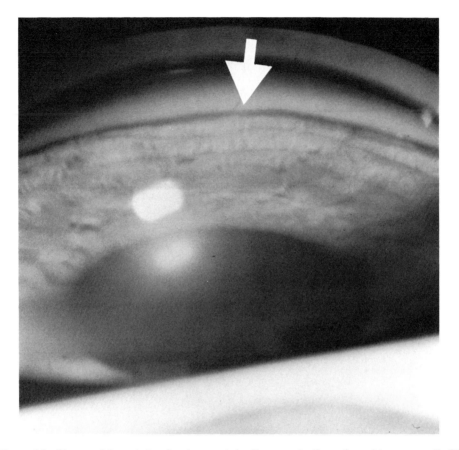

Figure 4.1. Closure of the anterior chamber angle by fibrovascular tissue (*arrow*) in an eye with OIS.

rubeosis iridis in the eye of an older, non-diabetic patient with no obvious predisposing factor, such as a retinal vein obstruction, should arouse suspicion of OIS (15).

Mature cataract can be seen in end-stage disease, probably occurring secondary to the ischemic insult. At the time of initial examination, there appears to be little difference in lens opacities between the affected side and unaffected side in unilateral cases (4).

Posterior Segment

Most eyes with OIS demonstrate narrowing of the retinal arteries. Except for the most extreme cases, in which retinal arteries are threadlike, the observation is subjective. It is difficult to base the diagnosis of OIS solely upon narrowed retinal arteries, since many elderly persons without OIS also have arteries of a reduced caliber.

Twenty-five years ago, it was pointed out (1, 16) that the retinal veins are often irregularly dilated and beaded in OIS (Fig. 4.2). When present, the beading is generally more subtle than that seen with severe preproliferative or proliferative diabetic retinopathy. The fundi of eyes with OIS, an inflow abnormality, generally do not demonstrate venous tortuosity (4), in contrast to central retinal vein obstruction, an outflow abnormality in which the retinal veins are frequently dilated and tortuous. Rarely, arteriovenous communications can be seen (personal communication, Dr. James Bolling, Philadelphia, 1989).

Midperipheral retinal hemorrhages are

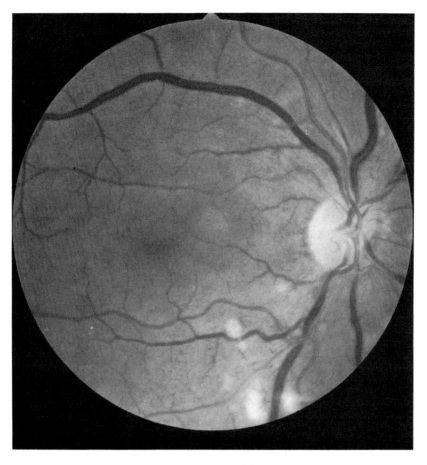

Figure 4.2. Dilated retinal veins in the fundus of an eye with OIS. Some beading is present, although tortuosity is generally absent. The retinal arteries are narrowed, and cotton-wool spots are evident inferiorly.

a recognized feature of OIS (1–4, 7, 8, 12, 16–18). In this region, they are of the dot and blot variety (Fig. 4.3). The hemorrhages can also extend into the posterior pole, where they appear mostly round, although superficial streak hemorrhages also are occasionally observed. Approximately 80% of eyes with OIS have retinal hemorrhages (4).

Microaneurysms are also a commonly encountered sign (Fig. 4.4). Similar to retinal hemorrhages, they predominate in the more peripheral retina but can also be seen in the posterior pole (4, 17–19). Macular telangiectatic changes may be present as well (20).

Neovascularization of the optic disc (NVD) is found in over one-third of persons with OIS (Fig. 4.5); neovascularization of the retina (NVE) is present in about 8% (Fig. 4.6)(4). The neovascularization may be mild, or it may be severe enough to cause traction retinal detachment. On occasion, the neovascularization leads to vitreous hemorrhage. The neovascularization has been observed in association with retinal capillary nonperfusion in cases of OIS, but it is uncertain whether retinal capillary shutdown is a prerequisite for its development (4). As is the case with rubeosis iridis, the occurrence of posterior segment neovascularization in the fundus

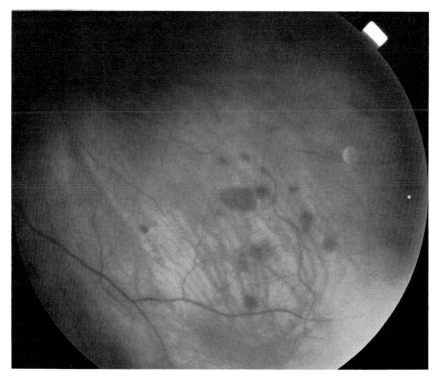

Figure 4.3. Dot and blot retinal hemorrhages occurring secondary to severe carotid artery stenosis.

Figure 4.4. Fluorescein angiogram demonstrating numerous peripheral hyperfluorescent microaneurysms in an eye with OIS.

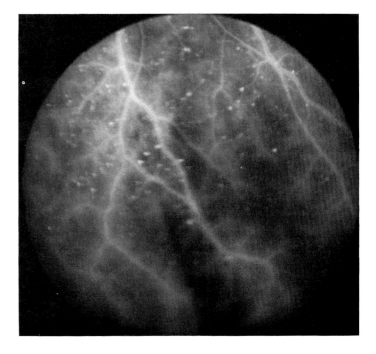

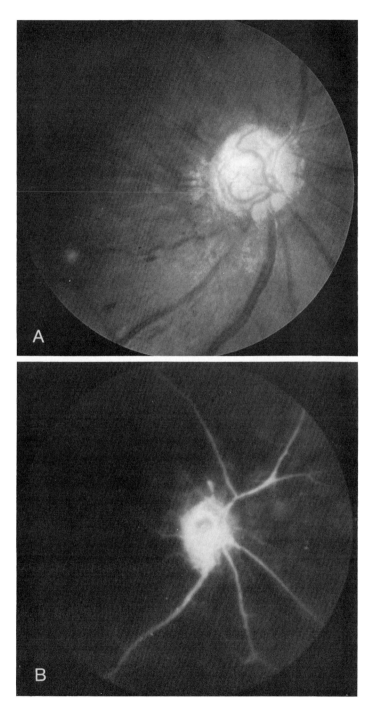

Figure 4.5. A. Neovascularization of the optic disc in an eye with OIS. **B**. Fluorescein angiogram of the same eye reveals marked hyperfluorescence of the optic disc due to leakage of dye from the new vessels. (Reprinted, with permission, from: Brown GC, Magargal LE, Simeone FA, et al. Ophthalmology 1982;89:139–146.)

Figure 4.6. Fluorescein angiogram of an eye with OIS, demonstrating areas of hyperfluorescence secondary to leakage of dye from neovascularization of the retina. Associated regions of retinal capillary nonperfusion (*NP*) can be seen.

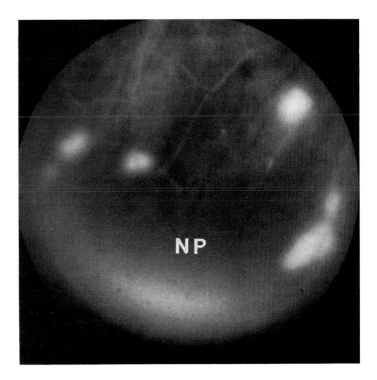

of a nondiabetic, elderly person, without the presence of another predisposing factor such as retinal venous obstruction or sickling hemoglobinopathy, should alert the clinician that OIS may be present.

A cherry-red spot can occur secondary to emboli within the central retinal artery, hemorrhage under an atherosclerotic plaque, or a number of other mechanisms, but that seen in about 12% of eyes presenting with OIS usually develops when increased intraocular pressure from neovascular glaucoma exceeds the central retinal arterial perfusion pressure (8, 9). Abrupt visual loss is usually present, but the cherry-red spot is frequently milder than that seen after acute central retinal artery obstruction in the absence of OIS (Fig. 4.7)(8). When a person with a history of recent, abrupt visual loss presents with concomitant rubeosis iridis and an acute cherry-red spot, the diagnosis of OIS should be strongly suspected.

Central retinal artery obstruction alone, in the absence of carotid obstructive disease, can lead to the development of both rubeosis iridis and posterior segment neovascularization (21). In these cases, the iris neovascularization develops at a mean time of 4 weeks after the central artery obstruction. Thus, whereas neovascularization of the iris in association with central retinal artery obstruction at the time of the acute obstruction suggests the coexistence of carotid artery obstructive disease, the development of rubeosis iridis after central retinal artery obstruction does not necessarily suggest an associated carotid stenosis.

Cotton-wool spots (Fig. 4.2) have been reported in 6% of persons with OIS (4). These small, superficial areas of retinal whitening are found in the posterior pole, where the nerve fiber layer is the thickest. They have been shown to develop secondary to axoplasmic damming within the nerve fiber layer as a result of focal areas of retinal ischemia (22).

Spontaneous retinal arterial pulsations (Fig. 4.8) have been noted in 4% of eyes with OIS. In the absence of cardiac valvular disease associated with a large pulse

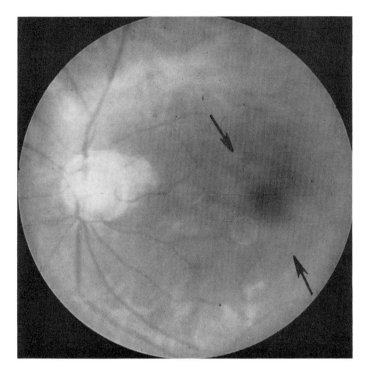

Figure 4.7. Mild cherry-red spot (*arrows*) in an eye with OIS.

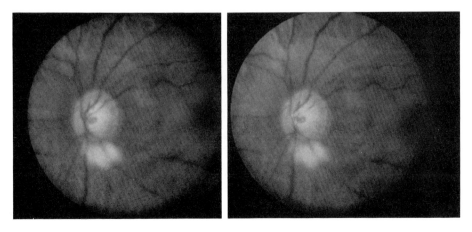

Figure 4.8. Spontaneous retinal arterial pulsations in an eye with OIS. The retinal arterial system on the right is closed at several seconds after the picture on the left was taken. (Reprinted, with permission, from Brown GC, Magargal LE. Int Ophthalmol 1988;11:239–251. Courtesy of Dr. Larry Magargal.)

pressure, the finding of spontaneous retinal arterial pulsations in the eye of an older adult is most suggestive of OIS.

Kearns (23) has emphasized that ophthalmodynamometry is helpful in differentiating OIS from mild central retinal vein obstruction. In unilateral cases of OIS, the readings are invariably lower on the affected side, whereas in central retinal vein obstruction, the measurements of diastolic and systolic pressures are often normal. If

an ophthalmodynamometer is not readily available, light digital palpation upon the globe in OIS eyes generally induces prominent retinal arterial pulsations. These pulsations are best seen on the optic disc and in the peripapillary area.

Anterior ischemic optic neuropathy has been observed in conjunction with OIS (Fig. 4.9), but it is a rare manifestation (24). Hypoperfusion within the short posterior ciliary circulation, probably in part due to

Figure 4.9. A. Anterior ischemic optic neuropathy in an eye with OIS. **B**. Fluorescein angiogram of the same eye reveals hypofluorescence of the optic disc and peripapillary choroid. (From: Brown GC. J Clin Neuro Ophthalmol 1986;6:39–42.)

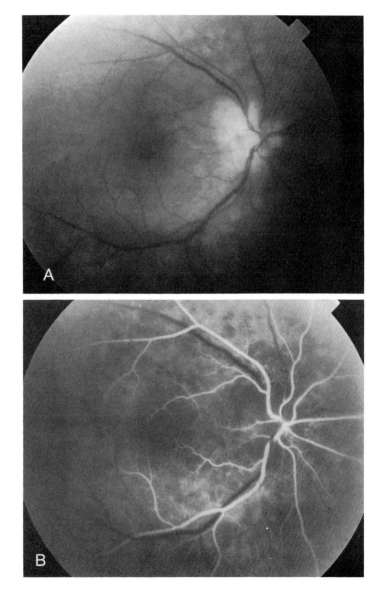

vascular compromise from the carotid stenosis, most likely predisposes to this condition. Emboli can occasionally be seen in the disease (4). Pronounced cobblestone degeneration has also been observed in some eyes with OIS (19, 25).

As noted by Kearns and Hollenhorst (1) in their landmark original treatise, hard exudates are generally not found in the fundi of persons with OIS. The exceptions to this rule are those eyes that have a combination retinopathy secondary to both carotid stenosis and diabetes mellitus.

A summary of the prominent symptoms and signs seen with OIS is shown in Table 4.1.

ANCILLARY STUDIES

Fluorescein Angiography

Fluorescein angiography is helpful to the ophthalmologist in making the diagnosis of OIS. Angiographic signs include (a) delayed arm-to-choroid and arm-to-retina circulation times, (b) slow, patchy choroidal filling, (c) prolonged retinal arteriovenous transit time, (d) late staining of the retinal vessels, (e) microaneurysms, (f) retinal capillary nonperfusion, (g) macular

Table 4.1. Ocular Ischemic Syndrome Features

Symptoms	
Visual loss	90%
Pain	40%
Signs	
Anterior segment	
Anterior uveitis (cells & flare)	20%
Rubeosis iridis	67%
Posterior segment	
Narrowed retinal arteries	Most
Dilated (not tortuous) retinal veins	Most
Retinal hemorrhages	80%
Neovascularization	35%
Cherry-red spot	12%
Cotton-wool spots	6%
Spontaneous retinal arterial pulsations	4%

leakage, and (h) optic disc hyperfluorescence (4, 26).

A delay in arm-to-choroid circulation (normal duration is <20 seconds with antecubital injection) is frequently seen in eyes with OIS (26). It must be kept in mind, however, that this time can be quite variable, depending upon the site of injection, the rate of injection of fluorescein dye, and cardiac status.

Normally, the choroid is completely filled by 5 seconds after the dye first appears within it. Delayed, patchy filling is seen in 60% of eyes with OIS (Fig. 4.10)(4).

The most frequently encountered fluorescein angiographic sign in eyes with OIS is a delayed retinal arteriovenous transit time (time from the first appearance of dye within the retinal arteries until the retinal veins in the temporal arcade are completely filled. Normal transit time is <11 seconds). This abnormality is seen in 95% of eyes (4).

Late staining of the retinal vessels, particularly the large vessels, is a prominent fluorescein angiographic feature, seen in 85% of eyes (Figs. 4.11, 4.12)(4). The arteries tend to stain to a greater degree than do the veins. This leakage of dye through the vessel walls probably occurs due to endothelial damage from the ischemia.

Microaneurysms are seen as hyperfluorescent foci that leak as the study progresses. Although more commonly located outside the posterior pole, they also can be seen in the macular region.

Retinal capillary nonperfusion is most often seen in the midperiphery (Figs. 4.6, 4.13). In general, the transition from a perfused retinal capillary bed to one that is shut down is more subtle than is the transition seen in diabetic retinopathy or in branch retinal vein obstruction. In OIS eyes, loss of endothelial cells and pericytes in the retinal capillaries has been observed, particularly in the more peripheral vessels (6, 19). In some instances, only acellular tubes can be seen; these probably correlate with the areas of retinal capillary shutdown visible on fluorescein angiography.

Macular edema with fluorescein leakage is present in about 17% of eyes (17). The

Figure 4.10. A. Fundus photograph showing retinal arterial narrowing in the ocular ischemic syndrome. Myelinated nerve fibers are seen in the inferior peripapillary region. **B**. Fluorescein angiogram of the same eye at approximately 1 minute after injection discloses patchy choroidal filling and delayed filling of the retinal arteries and veins. A leading edge of dye (*arrow*) is seen within a retinal artery. (Courtesy of Dr. Larry Magargal.)

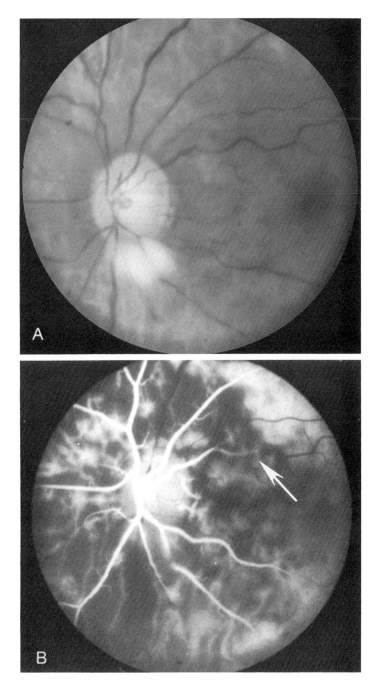

retinal thickening is usually subtle. Although single foveal cysts have been seen, the multiple, prominent intraretinal cystic changes found with diabetic retinopathy or following cataract surgery have not been described. Fluorescein angiography demonstrates intraretinal accumulation of dye, which presumably occurs due to leakage from incompetent retinal vessels (Fig. 4.14). When macular edema is present, the optic

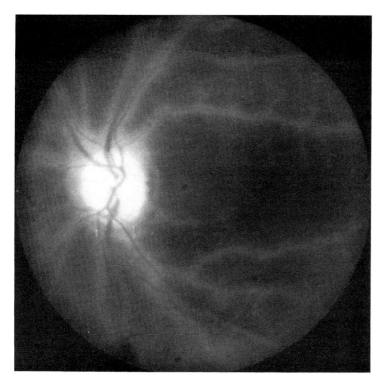

Figure 4.11. Retinal vascular staining, particularly of the arteries, in late-phase fluorescein angiogram of an eye with OIS.

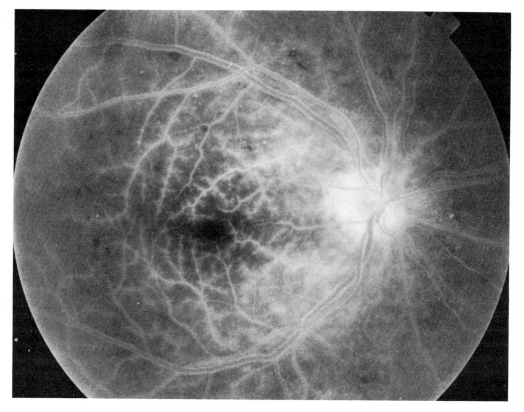

Figure 4.12. Staining of the larger retinal vessels in the posterior pole in OIS.

Figure 4.13. Fluorescein angiogram of midperiphery of an eye with OIS demonstrates areas of retinal capillary nonperfusion (*NP*).

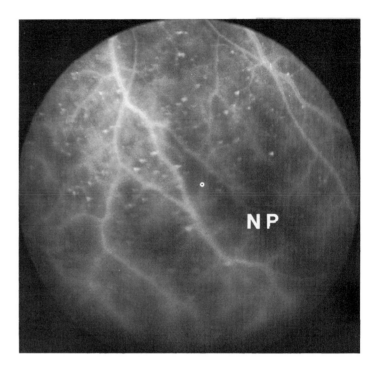

nerve head also is generally hyperfluorescent, despite the absence of clinical disc swelling.

Electroretinography

In cases of central retinal artery obstruction with inner layer retinal vascular compromise and ischemia, the b-wave is often diminished in amplitude (27, 28). When outer layer retinal ischemia due to choroidal vascular compromise is present, in addition, the a-wave is also decreased. Thus, with OIS, both the a- and b-waves are diminished in approximately 80% of eyes (Fig. 4.15)(4).

Carotid Artery Evaluation

Usually, a minimum of 90% or greater stenosis of the ipsilateral internal or common carotid artery is necessary to induce OIS (Fig. 4.16) (4). A 90% stenosis has been demonstrated to be necessary before significant lowering of the retinal arterial pressure occurs (29). In approximately half of the unilateral cases, there is also at least a 50% stenosis in the contralateral carotid system (4). With bilateral cases, the carotid obstruction is also bilateral; in the majority of these instances, at least one of the carotid vessels is 100% occluded (4).

A number of noninvasive tests are available to evaluate the carotid system in persons with suspected OIS (30, 31). Included among these are ultrasonography, Doppler flow studies, and oculoplethysmography, which in combination can detect high-grade carotid stenosis with approximately 90% accuracy (31). Despite improvements in these tests, carotid angiography, whether by conventional or digital subtraction techniques, remains the definitive diagnostic modality. Nevertheless, it should probably be reserved for those cases in which carotid endarterectomy is being considered.

SYSTEMIC ASSOCIATIONS

As might be expected, diseases that predispose to the development of atheroscle-

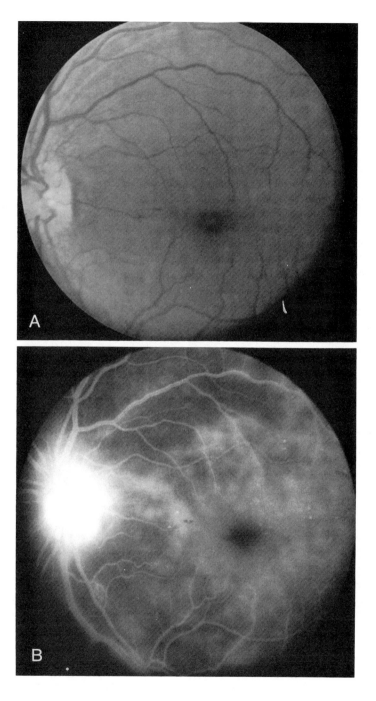

Figure 4.14. **A**. Fundus photograph showing a central macular cyst in an eye with OIS. **B**. Fluorescein angiogram of the same eye discloses macular edema, characterized by intraretinal leakage of dye. (Reprinted, with permission, from: Brown GC. Am J Ophthalmol 1986;102:442–448. Copyright Ophthalmic Publishing Company.)

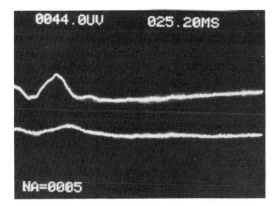

Figure 4.15. Upper electroretinographic tracing corresponds to normal right eye, while lower tracing of left eye with OIS reveals diminished amplitude of both the a- and b-waves.

rosis and those that occur secondary to atherosclerosis are prevalent in patients with OIS. Approximately 55% have a history of systemic arterial hypertension, 45% have diabetes, and 35% have atherosclerotic cardiovascular disease (4). Nearly one-fourth have experienced a previous cerebrovascular accident, either contralateral or ipsilateral to the ischemic eye, prior to their initial examination for OIS by an ophthalmologist (4). The stroke rate after ophthalmic presentation is about 4% per year (32).

The five-year mortality rate in persons with OIS is 40% (32). The majority of deaths

Figure 4.16. A. Carotid arteriogram in a patient with OIS reveals total occlusion of the right common carotid artery. **B.** On the corresponding left side, a marked constriction (*arrow*) of the left internal carotid artery can be seen. (Reprinted, with permission from Brown GC, Magargal LE. Int Ophthalmol 1988;11:239–251.)

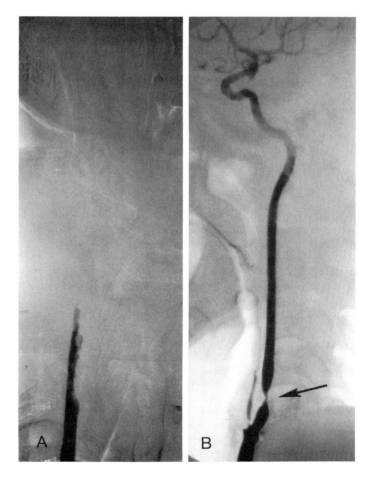

occur secondary to cardiovascular disease, followed in order by stroke and cancer.

DIFFERENTIAL DIAGNOSIS

Carotid artery stenosis most frequently causes OIS, but chronic ophthalmic artery obstruction can produce a similar clinical picture (8, 33, 34). Obstruction of the ophthalmic artery can best be demonstrated with conventional or arterial digital subtraction carotid angiography.

Although giant cell arteritis could theoretically cause OIS, the authors have not seen such cases. The atherosclerosis that produces carotid obstruction in OIS probably occurs more slowly than does vascular obstruction due to giant cell arteritis. The faster time course most likely accounts for the relative absence of the latter entity as a cause.

Magargal and associates (35) reported a case of a 58-year-old man with a fundus appearance characterized by dilated veins, dot and blot retinal hemorrhages, microaneurysms, and retinal capillary nonperfusion due to embolic obstruction of the central retinal artery on the optic disc. Following spontaneous disappearance of the embolus, the retinopathy resolved.

The aortic arch syndrome (obliteration of the large arteries as they arise from the aortic arch) can also cause OIS (25), particularly when the etiology is atherosclerosis. Takayasu's disease, an idiopathic inflammatory disease producing obliteration of the major arteries of the aortic arch, predominantly in young Japanese females, can cause a bilateral fundus picture similar to that of OIS (3). However, the retinal vessels are often tortuous in this disease (Fig. 4.17), in contrast to typical OIS. In addition to Takayasu's disease and atherosclerosis, other causes of the aortic arch syndrome include syphilis and dissecting aneurysm (36).

The entities that are most frequently confused with the appearance of the fundus in OIS are mild central retinal vein obstruction and diabetic retinopathy. Differentiating features are shown in Table 4.2.

TREATMENT

The most effective therapeutic modality has not yet been determined, either for OIS or for carotid artery obstructive disease unassociated with ocular signs (37). Additionally, the natural history of OIS is not totally clear. Nevertheless, when most of the ophthalmic features discussed in this chapter are present, the visual prognosis without treatment is poor.

Reversal of the carotid stenosis is theoretically the most efficacious way to preserve or improve vision. Carotid endarterectomy has been demonstrated to reverse OIS (8, 38), and it is probably most helpful when performed prior to the onset of rubeosis iridis (39). Evaluation for therapy should be relatively prompt, since central retinal artery obstruction has been observed in patients soon after the diagnosis of OIS was made (39). It should be remembered that, in many cases, the visual acuity is good at the time of initial diagnosis.

In general, carotid endarterectomy cannot be successfully performed when a 100% carotid obstruction is present, since a thrombus often propagates retrograde from the site of blockage to the next major vessel. Carotid bypass surgery has been attempted in such cases, but it does not seem to reduce the incidence of ischemic stroke (40). Although bypass surgery has been noted to cause resolution of OIS (41), no long-term beneficial effect on vision can be demonstrated in most instances (39).

When endarterectomy is not a viable alternative, such as in cases of 100% carotid obstruction or general medical debility, local ocular therapeutic measures can be considered. Panretinal photocoagulation for OIS eyes is generally not as effective in causing resolution of rubeosis iridis as it is in cases occurring secondary to diabetic retinopathy, but it will induce regression in some instances (39, 42, 43). Once the anterior chamber angle is closed by fibrovascular tissue in eyes with rubeosis, there is probably little reason to perform panretinal photocoagulation unless a glaucoma filtering procedure is also being con-

Figure 4.17. **A.** Fundus photograph showing tortuous retinal vessels in Takayasu's disease. **B.** Fluorescein angiogram of the same area confirms the tortuosity.

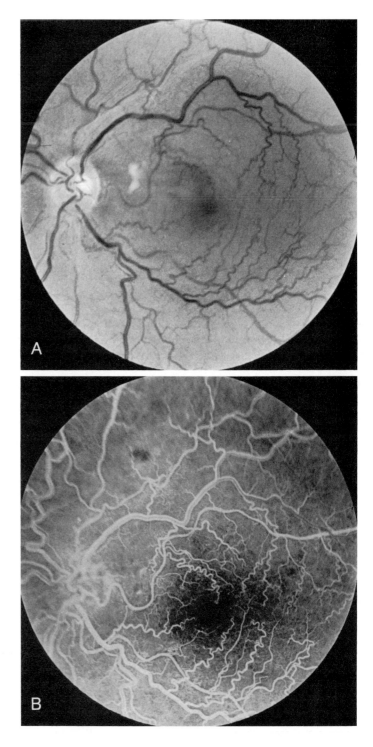

Table 4.2. Differentiating Features of the Ocular Ischemic Syndrome, Mild Central Retinal Vein Obstruction, and Diabetic Retinopathy

	Ocular Ischemic Syndrome	Mild Central Vein Obstruction	Diabetic Retinopathy
Laterality	Unilateral—80%	Unilateral	Bilateral
Ophthalmoscopy			
Optic disc	Normal	Swollen	Normal
Veins	Dilated, beaded	Dilated, tortuous	Dilated, beaded
Microaneurysms	Midperiphery	Variable	Posterior pole
Hard exudate	Absent	Rare	Common
Fluorescein Angiography			
Choroidal filling	Delayed—60%	Normal	Normal
Vessel staining	Arterial & venous	Venous	Generally absent
Perfusion pressure (retinal arterial)	Decreased	Normal	Normal

sidered. In these cases, it is important to decrease iris neovascularization, which could lead to scar tissue formation and closure of the filter. Cyclocryotherapy and cyclodiathermy are also therapeutic options when angle closure is present and the intraocular pressure is increased.

References

1. Kearns TP, Hollenhorst RW. Venous-stasis retinopathy of occlusive disease of the carotid artery. Proc Mayo Clin 1963;38:304–312.
2. Knox DL. Ischemic ocular inflammation. Am J Ophthalmol 1965;60:995–1002.
3. Young LHY, Appen RE. Ischemic oculopathy; a manifestation of carotid artery disease. Arch Neurol 1981;38:358–361.
4. Brown GC, Magargal LE. The ocular ischemic syndrome. Clinical, fluorescein angiographic and carotid angiographic features. Int Ophthalmol 1988;11:239–251.
5. Hayreh SS. So-called "central retinal vein occlusion." II. Venous stasis retinopathy. Ophthalmologica 1976;172:14–37.
6. Kahn M, Green WR, Knox DL, Miller NR. Ocular features of carotid occlusive disease. Retina 1986;6:239–252.
7. Sturrock GD, Mueller HR. Chronic ocular ischaemia. Br J Ophthalmol 1984;68:716–723.
8. Brown GC, Magargal LE, Simeone FA, et al. Arterial obstruction and ocular neovascularization. Ophthalmology 1982;89:139–146.
9. Hayreh SS, Podhajsky P. Ocular neovascularization with retinal vascular occlusion. II. Occurrence in central and branch retinal artery occlusion. Arch Ophthalmol 1982;100:1585–1596.
10. Furlan AJ, Whisnant JP, Kearns TP. Unilateral visual loss in bright light; an unusual symptom of carotid artery occlusive disease. Arch Neurol 1979;36:675–676.
11. Ross-Russell RW, Page NER. Critical perfusion of brain and retina. Brain 1983;106:419–434.
12. Jacobs NA, Ridgway AEA. Syndrome of ischaemic ocular inflammation: six cases and a review. Br J Ophthalmol 1985;69:681–687.
13. Tessler HH. Classification and symptoms and signs of uveitis. In: Duane TD, ed. Clinical ophthalmology. Hagerstown: Harper & Row, 1983; Vol 4, Chap 32.
14. Smith JL. Unilateral glaucoma in carotid occlusive disease. JAMA 1962;182:683–684.
15. Brown GC, Magargal LE, Schachat A, Shah H. Neovascular glaucoma; etiologic considerations. Ophthalmology 1984;91:315–320.
16. Hedges TR Jr. Ophthalmoscopic findings in internal carotid artery occlusion. Am J Ophthalmol 1963;55:1007–1012.
17. Brown GC. Macular edema in association with severe carotid artery obstruction. Am J Ophthalmol 1986;102:442–448.
18. Kearns TP. Ophthalmology and the carotid artery. Am J Ophthalmol 1979;88:714–722.
19. Michelson PE, Knox DL, Green WR. Ischemic ocular inflammation; a clinicopathologic case report. Arch Ophthalmol 1971;86:274–280.
20. Campo RV, Reeser FH. Retinal telangiectasia secondary to bilateral carotid artery occlusion. Arch Ophthalmol 1983;101:1211–1213.
21. Duker JS, Brown GC. Iris neovascularization associated with obstruction of the central retinal artery. Ophthalmology 1988;95:1244–1249.
22. McLeod D, Marshall J, Kohner EM, Bird AC. The role of axoplasmic transport in the pathogenesis of retinal cotton-wool spots. Br J Ophthalmol 1977;61:177–191.
23. Kearns TP. Differential diagnosis of central retinal vein obstruction. Ophthalmology 1983;90:475–480.
24. Brown GC. Anterior ischemic optic neuropathy occurring in association with carotid artery obstruction. J Clin Neuro Ophthalmol 1986;6:39–42.
25. Kahn M, Knox DL, Green WR. Clinicopathologic

studies of a case of aortic arch syndrome. Retina 1986;6:228–233.

26. Ridley ME, Walker PM, Keller A, Chew EY. Ocular perfusion in carotid artery disease. Scientific Poster. Ophthalmology 1986;93(Suppl):125.

27. Henkes HE. Electroretinography in circulatory disturbances of the retina. II. The electroretinogram in cases of occlusion of the central retinal artery or one of its branches. Arch Ophthalmol 1954; 51:42–53.

28. Carr RE, Siegel IM. Electrophysiologic aspects of several retinal diseases. Am J Ophthalmol 1964;58:95–107.

29. Kearns TP, Sickert GR, Sundt TM Jr. The ocular aspects of bypass surgery of the carotid artery. Mayo Clin Proc 1979;54:3–11.

30. Sanborn GE, Miller NR, Langham ME, Kumar AJ. An evaluation of currently available, noninvasive tests of carotid artery disease. Ophthalmology 1980;87:435–439.

31. Bosley TM. The role of carotid noninvasive tests in stroke prevention. Semin Neurol 1986;6:194–203.

32. Sivalingam A, Brown GC, Magargal LE, Menduke H. The ocular ischemic syndrome. II. Mortality and systemic morbidity. Int Ophthalmol 1989;13:187–191.

33. Madsen PH. Venous-stasis retinopathy in insufficiency of the ophthalmic artery. Acta Ophthalmol 1966;44:940–947.

34. Bullock JD, Falter RT, Downing JE, Snyder HE. Ischemic ophthalmia secondary to an ophthalmic artery occlusion. Am J Ophthalmol 1972;74:486–493.

35. Margaral LE, Sanborn GE, Zimmermann A. Venous stasis retinopathy associated with embolic obstruction of the central retinal artery. J Clin Neuro Ophthalmol 1982;2:113–118.

36. Henkind P, Chambers JK. Arterial occlusive disease of the retina. In: Duane TD, ed. Clinical ophthalmology. Hagerstown: Harper & Row, 1983; Vol 3, Chap 14.

37. Becker WL, Burde RM. Carotid artery disease; a therapeutic enigma. Arch Ophthalmol 1988; 106:34–39.

38. Neupert JR, Brubaker RF, Kearns TP, Sundt TM. Rapid resolution of venous stasis retinopathy after carotid endarterectomy. Am J Ophthalmol 1976;81:600–602.

39. Sivalingam A, Brown GC, Magargal LE. Visual prognosis and the effect of treatment in eyes with the ocular ischemic syndrome (submitted for publication).

40. The EC/IC Bypass Study Group. The failure of extracranial-intracranial arterial bypass to reduce the risk of ischemic stroke; results of an international randomized trial. N Engl J Med 1985;313:1191–1200.

41. Kearns TP, Younge BR, Peipgras DG. Resolution of venous stasis retinopathy after carotid artery bypass surgery. Mayo Clin Proc 1980;55:342–346.

42. Eggleston TF, Bohling CA, Eggleston HC, Hershey FB. Photocoagulation for ocular ischemia associated with carotid artery occlusion. Ann Ophthalmol 1980;12:84–87.

43. Carter JE. Panretinal photocoagulation for progressive ocular neovascularization secondary to occlusion of the common carotid artery. Ann Ophthalmol 1984;16:572–576.

CHAPTER 5

Acquired Immune Deficiency Syndrome

Herbert L. Cantrill and Keith Henry

INTRODUCTION

In June 1981, the Centers for Disease Control (CDC) reported an outbreak of *Pneumocystis carinii* pneumonia and Kaposi's sarcoma in previously healthy homosexual males living in New York and California (1, 2). Within one year, over 500 cases of this unique syndrome of opportunistic infection and neoplasia with unexplained, severe immunodeficiency were reported to the CDC (3). The 1983 CDC definition of the disease has been used, with minor modifications, since that time (4, 5). The disease was called acquired immunodeficiency syndrome (AIDS) and was characterized by opportunistic infections or tumors in the presence of underlying cellular immunodeficiency. Within a short time, cases of AIDS were reported in most of the United States, with a predominance of cases in New York and California. By 1986, AIDS had been reported in all 50 states and in at least 16 European countries (6, 7). Cases were also reported in Australia, Canada, Central America, South America, and several countries in Asia and Africa. Since 1981, 133,000 cases of AIDS resulting in 81,000 deaths have been reported in the United States (8) (Fig. 5.1). It is estimated that, by 1992, there will have been 365,000 cases of AIDS and an annual death rate of 66,000, making AIDS one of the 10 leading causes of death in the United States (8) (Fig. 5.2).

VIRAL ETIOLOGY

It was clear from the beginning that cases of AIDS were associated with certain high-risk behaviors (9). The most frequently affected groups were homosexual or bisexual males and intravenous drug abusers. By 1982, clusters of cases were reported in Haitians living in the United States (10), in patients with hemophilia (11), and in people who had received blood transfusions (12). Cases were also reported in female sexual partners of patients with AIDS and in infants born to women with AIDS (13, 14). Because of the clustering of these cases, a blood-borne transmissible agent was suspected.

An intense search for the etiological agent of AIDS ensued. In 1983, investigators at the Pasteur Institute in Paris isolated a viral agent from a patient with generalized lymphadenopathy who was at risk for developing AIDS (15). The virus was called "lymphadenopathy-associated virus" or LAV. In 1984, investigators at the National Institutes of Health in the United States isolated a similar virus from a patient with AIDS (16). They noted the similarity of this virus to retroviruses known to cause T-cell leukemia/lymphoma, and they

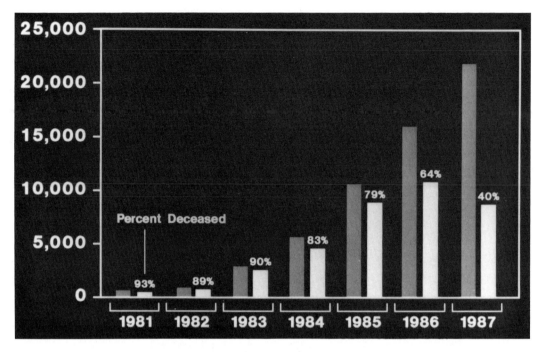

Figure 5.1. Frequency distribution diagram that illustrates the course of the AIDS epidemic since 1981. The number of cases continues to increase, but at a slightly reduced rate. The number of new cases reported each year is designated by the *blue bar*. The percentage of patients who have died is designated by the *white bar*.

named the virus human T-cell leukemia/lymphoma virus (HTLV-3). Retroviruses contain the enzyme reverse transcriptase, which generates DNA from viral RNA within the host cell. Assay for reverse transcriptase has become a marker for the virus, but it is not specific for the AIDS virus (17). The virus was also identified within T lymphocytes by electron microscopy (18). The AIDS virus is now referred to as human immunodeficiency virus (HIV) (19). At least two closely related retroviruses, HIV-1 and HIV-2, can cause AIDS (20). HIV-2 is found almost exclusively in Western Africa (21).

MOLECULAR BIOLOGY

More is probably known about the AIDS virus than about any other piece of biological material known to mankind. The structure of the virus has been precisely determined (Fig. 5.3) (22). The virus contains only 11 genes, compared with 50,000 to 100,000 genes in human cells. These genes code for the enzyme reverse transcriptase, core proteins (p7, p17, and p24), envelope proteins (gp41, gp120, and gp160), and products required to regulate the expression of genes.

The origin of HIV is controversial. At one time, it was believed by some that HIV may have evolved from a simian (monkey) virus, found in the African green monkey. The simian immunodeficiency virus (SIV) does not cause disease in the African green monkey, but in other primates it causes a syndrome similar to AIDS. Homology studies, on the other hand, have found that SIV shares only a 50% homology with HIV (23). Studies of the divergence of HIV strains have suggested than an HIV-like virus has probably existed in some human populations for 40 to 100 years (24). The human virus probably became pathogenic for man by a mutation that has occurred relatively recently. Sporadic cases of unexplained immunodeficiency possibly due to HIV

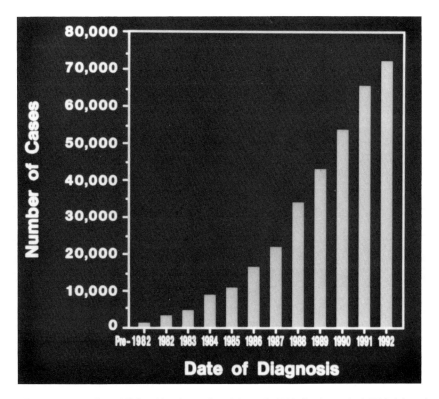

Figure 5.2. Future course of the AIDS epidemic predicted through 1992. By the end of 1992, it is estimated that there will have been 365,000 AIDS cases with an estimated 66,000 deaths in 1992 alone.

have occurred in this country since 1959, long before the recognition of the AIDS epidemic in the early 1980s (25). The route of dissemination of HIV throughout the world is not well understood.

This virus preferentially infects T-helper lymphocytes (26). The receptor for the virus is the CD-4 antigen on the surface. This receptor has also been identified on other cells, including macrophages, monocytes, glial cells, and Langerhans cells. After the virus enters the cell, DNA is generated from viral RNA by reverse transcriptase. The DNA is used as a template to produce viral RNA. Several viral proteins, including envelope proteins and core proteins, are produced later in the course of infection. Antibodies to these proteins are markers for HIV infection (27) and are the basis of most widely used tests for HIV.

Three types of infection may occur (Fig. 5.4). In T lymphocytes, a lytic infection results in the production and release of virus particles. In some cells, the viral genetic material is incorporated into the host genome, where it remains latent. After months or years of latency, HIV may reactivate, leading to progressive destruction of the CD-4 lymphocyte pool. The latency of the virus may be influenced by other factors, such as infection with other viruses (28). Finally, passive infection occurs in macrophages, accounting for the wide dissemination of the virus throughout the body, including the central nervous system.

IMMUNOLOGY

The most important immunological abnormality in patients with AIDS is a profound drop in the number of T-helper/inducer lymphocytes (26). Since the T-helper cell is essential to a variety of im-

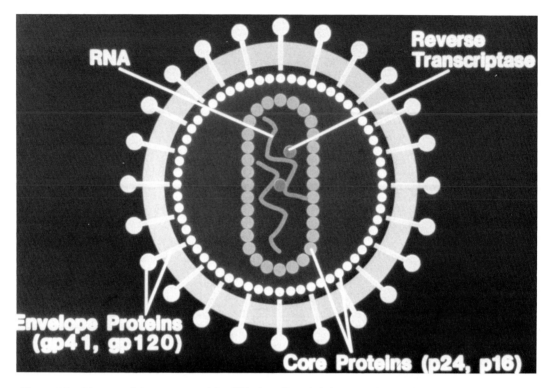

Figure 5.3. Diagram of the structure of the HIV virus. Genetic information is contained in RNA. The reverse transcriptase enzyme complex is responsible for generating viral DNA within the host cell. Core and envelope proteins complete the viral structure.

mune functions, its destruction results in the profound immunodeficiency that characterizes AIDS. All phases of the cellular immune response are impaired (29). These include decreased cytotoxic response (30), cutaneous anergy (31), decreased lymphoproliferative response to mitogens (32), and impaired lymphokine production (interleukin 2 and gamma interferon) (33). There is polyclonal activation of the B-cell system, resulting in an increase in the levels of serum immunoglobulins, beta-2 microglobulin, and circulating immune complexes (34). T-cell abnormalities also prevent normal processing of antigens, thereby impairing the normal antibody response (35). HIV appears to have no effect on polymorphonuclear leukocyte function other than to reduce their number. The complement system is not affected.

EPIDEMIOLOGY

Since 1981, the CDC has monitored the course of the AIDS epidemic in this country (36). Cases are reported to local and state health authorities in all 50 states. This information is passed along anonymously to the CDC. The distribution of cases has been followed according to age, sex, race, ethnic group, and geographical area. By June 1990, 133,000 cases of AIDS resulting in 81,000 deaths (8) had been reported in the United States. These figures are probably under-reported by 10% to 20%.

Virtually all cases have been confined to groups with certain high-risk behavior (36). The distribution of cases has shifted toward a larger fraction related to use of intravenous drugs (Fig. 5.5A). Sixty-three percent of cases are seen in homosexual or bisexual men not known to have abused

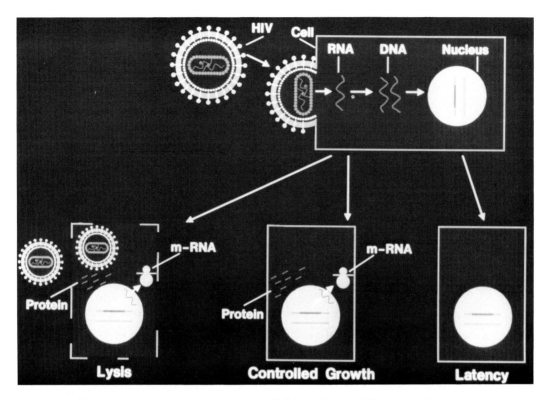

Figure 5.4. Three types of infection may occur in cells infected by the HIV virus. In T-helper lymphocytes, a lytic infection results, with the release of numerous virus particles. In some cells, controlled growth of the virus occurs without major disruption of cellular function. Finally, the viral genome may be incorporated into host genetic material, where it remains latent indefinitely.

IV drugs. Nineteen percent are IV drug abusers. An additional 7% are homosexual or bisexual drug abusers. Four percent have acquired the disease by heterosexual contact, usually as a sexual partner of an IV drug abuser. Three percent of cases have resulted from blood transfusion or the use of contaminated blood products. One percent of cases has occurred in hemophiliacs. Three percent of cases have occurred in patients who have no obvious high-risk factors, although these cases remain under investigation.

AIDS has also been reported among children (36). By July 1990, 2315 cases with a fatality rate of 59% had been reported in children under 13 years of age (8). Seventy-eight percent of the affected children are offspring of parents who have AIDS or are in high-risk groups (Fig. 5.5B). Nine-

teen percent are believed to have acquired the disease by blood transfusion. The etiology is undetermined in 3%.

The distribution of AIDS cases appears to be changing slightly. The incidence in gay men is declining (37). This is probably due to changes in sexual behavior brought about by educational programs. Protection of the blood supply, which occurred in 1985 after the development of accurate antibody tests, will virtually eliminate AIDS in hemophiliacs and other transfusion recipients. On the other hand, AIDS is increasing in other groups, particularly among IV drug abusers (38). This is due in part to the failure of efforts to control the drug abuse problem and to other sociological factors that isolate this group (39). Intravenous cocaine use is considered to present a higher risk for HIV than does heroin

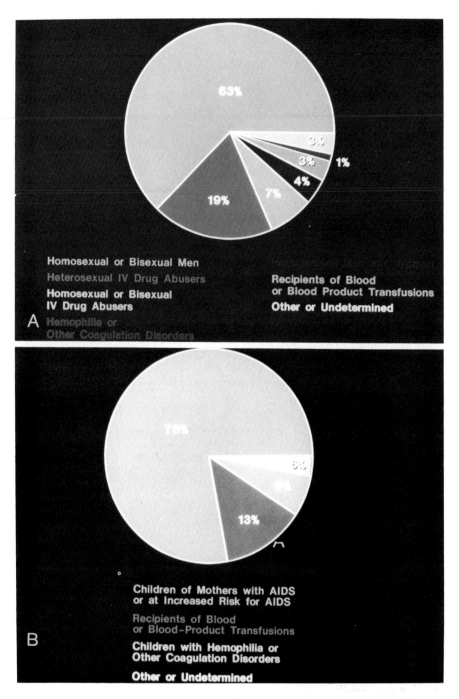

Figure 5.5. A. Diagram illustrating the distribution of AIDS cases among adults. The distribution of cases has remained fairly stable except for increases in cases among heterosexual individuals and IV drug abusers. **B.** Diagram illustrating the distribution of AIDS cases among children under the age of 13. The vast majority of cases are in children of patients with AIDS or of patients at high risk of developing AIDS.

use because of the "drugs for sex" exchange (39).

AIDS has increased in the heterosexual population as well. This has been attributed to the high rate of infection in the sexual partners of IV drug abusers. There does not appear to be an increase in the heterosexual population without high-risk behavior. However, heterosexual spread appears to be the primary means of transmission in Africa (40). Prostitution has played a major role in the heterosexual spread of AIDS in Africa, with urban prostitutes showing a rate of HIV infection of up to 90% (41). Contamination of the blood supply, the use of unsterilized needles and syringes, and ritual practices may also contribute to the spread of AIDS in the African population (42). In the United States, the rate of HIV infection among prostitutes varies widely by location, but generally is much lower than rates in some Central African populations (43). Nevertheless, there remains the possibility that AIDS may enter the heterosexual population as a result of bisexuality, prostitution, or IV drug abuse (44, 45).

The most dramatic increase in the incidence of AIDS has been not in adults but in children. Studies from New York indicate that 1 in 66 infants born in New York City in 1987 was HIV positive (46). The prevalence of HIV infection outside the metropolitan area was 0.18%. The risk of seroconversion from congenital infection is estimated to be 30% to 50% (47, 48).

The distribution of AIDS cases reveals a concentration on the East and West Coasts. In 1986, New York and San Francisco accounted for almost 40% of all AIDS cases (49). AIDS is now the leading cause of death in New York City among men between the ages of 25 and 44 and women between the ages of 25 and 34. By 1991, New York and California will account for only 20% of the cases as the epidemic spreads to other metropolitan areas throughout the country. Ninety percent of patients with AIDS are between 20 and 49 years of age (50). Ninety-two percent are male (50). Cases of AIDS are 2 to 3 times more prevalent in the black

and Hispanic populations, primarily due to the high rate of IV drug abuse in these groups (36). There is concern that the rates of HIV infection are increasing more rapidly among these segments of the population.

The prevalence of HIV infection is highest in those risk groups that account for the majority of AIDS cases (51). The prevalence of HIV infection in homosexual or bisexual men ranges from 20% to 50%, depending upon demographic location. In San Francisco, approximately 50% of the male homosexual population is infected. The prevalence in IV drug abusers also varies with geographical location. Rates are 50% to 60% in major East Coast cities and 5% in other parts of the country. Heterosexual partners of HIV-positive individuals have an infection rate of 10% to 50%, with the highest rates among heterosexual partners of IV drug abusers. HIV prevalence in the general population has been assessed by large-scale screening studies (52). Only 0.04% of the first-time blood donors are HIV-positive. Testing of Job Corps applicants, predominantly inner-city, disadvantaged youths between the ages of 16 and 21, showed a seroprevalence of 0.33%. Screening of military recruits showed an overall prevalence of 0.14%. Probably the most accurate information comes from anonymous HIV antibody testing of hospitalized patients. Based on 18,809 test results, the age-and-sex adjusted prevalence of infection was found to be 0.32%. Based on these figures, it is estimated that between 1 and 1.5 million Americans, or 1 in 225, are HIV-positive.

CLASSIFICATION AND DIAGNOSIS

The CDC has divided infection with HIV into four categories (Table 5.1) (53). Initial infection with HIV may result in acute flu-like illness lasting 4 to 6 weeks (Stage I). Although patients at this stage of the disease are potentially infectious, antibody tests are often negative. After seroconversion occurs, a prolonged period of asymptomatic disease results (Stage II). Patients enter a transition phase with persistent

Table 5.1.   Classification System for Human Immunodeficiency Virus Infection

Stage I.	Acute infection—mononucleosis-like syndrome associated with seroconversion of HIV antibody.
Stage II.	Asymptomatic infection—absence of signs or symptoms of HIV infection.
Stage III.	Persistent generalized lymphadenopathy—palpable lymphadenopathy involving two or more noninguinal sites and persisting for more than 3 months in the absence of concurrent illness.
Stage IV.	Acquired immune deficiency syndrome.
Subgroup A.	Constitutional disease—fever, involuntary weight loss, or diarrhea in the absence of concurrent illness.
Subgroup B.	Neurological disease—dementia, myelopathy, or peripheral neuropathy in the absence of concurrent illness.
Subgroup C.	Opportunistic infections.
Category C-1	Includes *Pneumocystis carinii* pneumonia, cryptosporidiosis, toxoplasmosis, strongyloidiasis, isosporiasis, candidiasis, cryptococcosis, histoplasmosis, mycobacterial infection with *M. avium intracellulare* or *M. kansasii*, cytomegalovirus, chronic mucocutaneous or disseminated herpes simplex, or progressive multifocal leukoencephalopathy.
Category C-2	Includes oral hairy leukoplakia, multidermatomal herpes zoster, recurrent *Salmonella* bacteremia, nocardiosis, tuberculosis, or oral candidiasis.
Subgroup D.	Secondary cancers including Kaposi's sarcoma, non-Hodgkin's lymphomas, or primary lymphoma of the brain.
Subgroup E.	Miscellaneous conditions.

lymphadenopathy and evidence of mild immune dysfunction with decreased numbers of CD-4 cells and a decrease in the CD-4/CD-8 ratio (Stage III). With progressive immune dysfunction, systemic symptoms of HIV infection, opportunistic infection, or neoplasia may develop (Stage IV). The virus can readily be detected in the blood, and levels of antibody may decline. The clinical stages of HIV infection together with levels of detectable virus and antibody are illustrated in Fig. 5.6.

The CDC further subdivided Stage IV into five categories. Stage IVa is characterized by constitutional symptoms, including fever, night sweats, chronic diarrhea, and weight loss of over 10% of body weight. This stage was previously called AIDS-related complex or ARC. Stage IVb includes patients with neurological symptoms, including dementia, peripheral neuropathy, and aseptic meningitis. Stage IVc is characterized by opportunistic infections, and Stage IVd is characterized by tumors such as Kaposi's sarcoma and non-Hodgkin's lymphoma. Stage IVe is a miscellaneous category including complications such as myocarditis, nephritis, and thrombocytopenia.

The diagnosis of HIV infection depends on the demonstration of antibody to viral protein, the detection of HIV antigen in serum, or the culture of HIV from body fluid or tissue (54). Beginning in 1984, reliable antibody tests based on enzyme immunoassay were developed (26). Other tests include immunoprecipitation, immunofluorescence, and Western blotting. These tests are highly sensitive and specific. Tests for HIV antigen detect the amount of virus present in serum, plasma, or other body fluids. The tests are based on the neutralization of viral antigens by antibodies present on polystyrene beads. The recovery of HIV antigen increases with the stage of disease and the deterioration of the patient's clinical condition (55). Serum antigen is present in only 19% of patients with Stage II disease but increases to 46% with Stage III and 64% in Stage IV. Culture of HIV depends upon the cocultivation of blood or infected tissue with transformed lymphocytes from HIV antibody–negative donors (56). The culture technique is tedious and time-consuming and includes the risk of laboratory-acquired infection. Combining the culture technique with the antigen assay has resulted in the most sen-

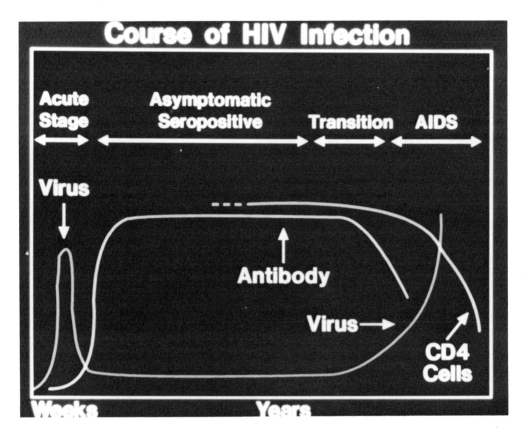

Figure 5.6. The course of HIV infection begins with an acute phase of viremia lasting 4 to 6 weeks. Antibodies can be detected as the virus is cleared from the blood. A prolonged asymptomatic phase then results. During the transition phase, levels of antibody typically decline as the virus again can be cultured. Signs of impaired immune function, such as a decrease in the number of T-helper lymphocytes, precede the onset of progressive immune dysfunction.

sitive test for the presence of HIV. Refinements in these techniques have resulted in detection of HIV in virtually all HIV antibody–positive individuals (57).

COURSE OF SYSTEMIC HIV INFECTION

Estimates have also been made concerning the rate of progression of HIV infection (58). Cohort studies of gay men living in San Francisco have examined serum samples obtained in the late 1970s and the early 1980s. Clinical disease rarely occurs during the first 2 years after infection occurs. After 8.5 years, more than 40% of the HIV-infected group will have developed AIDS, and a similar proportion of those infected will have symptoms of HIV infection. Based on this cohort, it is predicted that, in the absence of treatment, close to 100% of HIV-infected persons will have developed AIDS or ARC within 13 years. Data from patients with infection acquired by transfusion suggest that the rate of progress increases with age with the exception of neonatally acquired AIDS, which has the highest rate of progression. Of all patients with AIDS, over 50% have died (50). Of those diagnosed before 1984, 71% have died (50). There are no reports of spontaneous recovery of immune function in patients with AIDS. It is assumed that nearly all HIV antibody–positive individuals will ultimately develop AIDS and die from its infectious or neoplastic complications. Once opportunistic infection or malignancy occurs, most patients begin a progressive downhill course. Patients with opportunistic infection have a particularly poor prognosis, with a median survival in the absence of any treatment or prophylactic therapy of only 8 months (59). Patients with Kaposi's sarcoma have a more favorable prognosis, with median survival of 14 months (59).

TRANSMISSIBILITY

It is clear from the epidemiology of AIDS that it is spread by a transmissible agent through parenteral or sexual contact. It does not appear that AIDS is spread by casual contact such as droplet infection, insect vectors, fecal-oral contamination, or kissing. Studies of family members of AIDS patients have failed to show a single case of transmission, except to sexual partners of an infected person and to children born to infected mothers. The risk of transmitting the disease in schools and offices is presumably even lower. The risk to health-care workers has been investigated, and worldwide there are 30 well-documented cases of seroconversion following exposure to blood or body fluid of infected patients (60). Included in these were 3 cases of nonparenteral exposure, all with gross, unprotected contact with blood or body secretions. In a series of 489 accidental parenteral exposures (most of which were accidental needle sticks), only 3 seroconversions were documented (61). Two additional cases of laboratory-acquired infection have been reported.

It is useful to compare the risk associated with exposure to HIV with the risk of hepatitis B (62). In 1986, 18,000 health-care workers acquired hepatitis B, with an estimated 200 deaths in the U.S. alone. It is estimated that there is a 25% to 30% risk of infection following parenteral exposure to hepatitis B. The risk of infection after significant exposure to HIV is 0.4%.

Nevertheless, HIV has been isolated from several body fluids, including saliva (63), breast milk (64), pulmonary secretions (65), cerebral spinal fluid (66), and tears (67). The risk of transmitting the virus from these sources is theoretically possible but has not been proven. HIV has also been recovered from tissue, including lymph nodes (68), bone marrow (68), peripheral nerve (66), brain (66), conjunctiva (69), and corneal epithelium (70). AIDS has also been transmitted through organ transplantation (71). Although corneal transplants have been performed with inadvertent use of tissue from HIV-positive individuals, seroconversion has not yet been documented (72).

Because of concern about transmission of infectious agents to health-care workers, the CDC has recommended a policy of universal blood and body fluid precautions (73). All blood and body fluid should be considered potentially infectious, regardless of its source. Universal precautions apply not only to HIV but also to hepatitis B virus (HBV) and other blood-borne pathogens. Universal precautions apply to all blood and body fluid containing visible blood. Universal precautions also apply to semen, vaginal secretions, and cerebral spinal fluid. Universal precautions do not apply to nasal secretions, sputum, sweat, tears, urine, feces, or vomitus unless they contain visible blood. There is a risk of exposure to saliva and breast milk, particularly with regard to the transmission of hepatitis B. Protective barriers are recommended to reduce the risk of exposure of skin or mucous membranes to all potentially infected material. This protection would include the use of masks, gowns, gloves, and protective eyewear.

Because HIV has been recovered from tears, there is a risk of transmitting the virus as a result of routine office procedures such as tonometry (74). The virus has an envelope and can be easily destroyed by brief contact with 70% isopropyl alcohol, 3% hydrogen peroxide, or 1:10 bleach (0.525% sodium hypochlorite). On contact lenses, the virus can be inactivated with commercial hydrogen peroxide sterilizing solution or heat (75).

EFFICIENCY OF TRANSMISSION

Although the primary means of HIV transmission are well known, the ease with which HIV can be transmitted by any particular means is not as clear (76). Probably the most efficient means of acquiring AIDS is via blood transfusion. Over 90% of individuals exposed to HIV-infected blood by transfusion will seroconvert within 23 months (77). The risk of perinatal infection is about 25% to 50% (47, 48). Perinatal transmission can occur during pregnancy, at birth, or shortly after birth. Since HIV antibodies cross the placenta, it is hard to determine whether the infant is infected with HIV or has received HIV antibody passively. Due to the illicit nature of drug trafficking, it is difficult to estimate the risk associated with sharing contaminated needles. HIV infection clearly spreads rapidly when introduced into the drug-using community (38). Homosexual transmission appears to depend upon the number of contacts and the nature of sexual practices. The risk is greatest for receptive anal intercourse (78). The risk of heterosexual transmission can be estimated from the rates of seroconversion of sexual partners of infected individuals. In long-term female partners of male IV drug abusers, the risk is about 25% to 50% (79). Sexual partners of hemophiliacs and of people infected via blood transfusion have a rate of HIV infection averaging 10% (80). Rates in spouses of bisexual men are similar. The risk of male-to-female transmission appears to be higher than that of female-to-male transmission (81).

OCULAR MANIFESTATIONS OF AIDS

Clinical and autopsy studies show that up to 75% of patients with AIDS will have ocular findings (82–84). All parts of the visual system can be affected by AIDS. Ocular involvement can also be the presenting sign of AIDS (85). Because of the high frequency of ocular involvement, it is appropriate for ophthalmologists to be knowledgeable concerning this condition.

AIDS RETINOPATHY

The most common ocular manifestation of AIDS is a form of retinopathy consisting of cotton-wool spots, hemorrhages, and capillary abnormalities (Fig. 5.7) (86). This retinopathy is seen in up to 71% of patients with AIDS (87). AIDS retinopathy is usually asymptomatic. The etiology of the cotton-wool spots is the subject of controversy (88). It was initially thought that these microvascular changes were the result of associated hematological abnormalities. An alternative theory proposed that cotton-wool spots were an early manifestation of cytomegalovirus (CMV) retinitis. Culture and histopathological study of these lesions, however, has been negative for opportunistic pathogens, such as CMV, although the lesions are frequently associated with systemic CMV infection (89). It has been suggested that AIDS retinopathy is the result of endothelial damage by circulating immune complexes (87). Immunofluorescent studies have shown deposition of immunoglobulins, but other components of the immune-complex reaction, such as neutrophilic infiltration and complement, were not seen (87).

The exact role of HIV in AIDS retinopathy has also been investigated. Sophisticated testing for HIV using in situ hybridization techniques has failed to identify HIV genomes in the retina (90). Viral particles compatible with HIV have been seen, however, by electron microscopy (91). HIV has been recovered from the retina by culture from patients with AIDS, and, in one case, HIV was localized within the retinal vascular endothelium by immunofluorescent techniques (92, 93). Therefore, it is possible that the microvascular changes of AIDS retinopathy are the direct result of HIV infection.

CMV RETINITIS

CMV retinitis is the most common ocular opportunistic infection in patients with AIDS. It presents as a necrotizing retinitis with associated retinal hemorrhages and vasculitis (Fig. 5.8A). A typical lesion is a

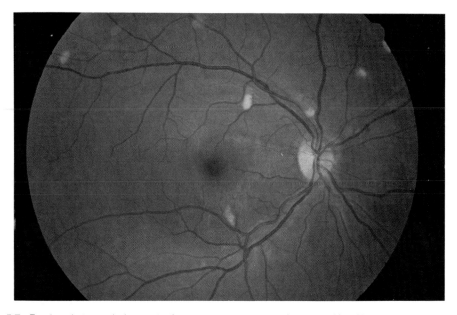

Figure 5.7. Fundus photograph demonstrating numerous cotton-wool spots and focal hemorrhages characteristic of AIDS retinopathy. These lesions are usually asymptomatic and may indicate infection of the retina by HIV itself.

zone of white retinal infiltration with translucent, slightly irregular margins. Multicentric origin and bilateral disease are frequently seen. As the lesions mature, they become more granular and ultimately become transparent (Fig. 5.8B). Faint pigment stippling is seen at the level of the retinal pigment epithelium. Focal deposits of lipid, calcium, and glial tissue may be seen within inactive lesions. The retinal vessels become markedly attenuated, and secondary optic atrophy develops. A zone of active necrotizing retinitis remains at the margin of inactive lesions (Fig. 5.8C).

Histopathology shows total destruction of the retina in areas of involvement (Fig. 5.9A). There is glial proliferation and prominent pigment phagocytosis by macrophages. A mild infiltration of the vitreous with mononuclear cells is also seen. The retinal architecture is preserved in areas that are uninvolved. Intranuclear and intracytoplasmic inclusions are associated with infection (Fig. 5.9B).

The reason for the high incidence of CMV retinitis in the AIDS population is unclear. Clinical and autopsy series indicate a

prevalence of 17% to 34% (83, 87). Other immunocompromised patients, such as the organ transplant population, have a much lower prevalence of CMV retinitis, although the rate of CMV viremia and viruria is quite high (94). Some geographical differences exist; the incidence of CMV retinitis is lower in the African population with AIDS (95).

One possible explanation of the high prevalence of CMV retinitis in the AIDS population is interaction with other viruses, particularly HIV. Experimental studies demonstrate transactivation of HIV by CMV in vitro (96). In the retina, HIV appears to infect the retinal vascular endothelium and is likely the cause of AIDS retinopathy (90, 91). CMV, on the other hand, is a neurotropic virus and is less likely to infect retinal vascular endothelium. In the presence of both viruses, HIV may cause endothelial damage, allowing CMV access to retinal tissue. It is not known whether viral transactivation may occur locally within retinal tissue.

There are several mechanisms for visual loss in CMV retinitis. Absolute scotomata

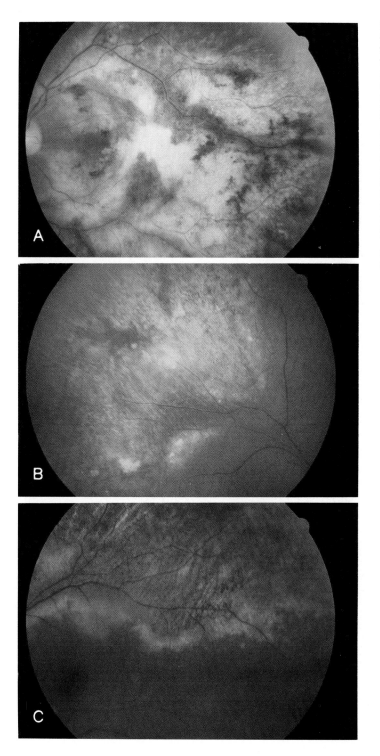

Figure 5.8. A. Fundus photograph showing necrotizing retinitis, hemorrhage, and retinal vasculitis characteristic of CMV retinitis. **B.** Fundus photograph showing a zone of inactive CMV retinitis. Within the lesion there is pigment stippling and atrophy. The retinal vessels are attenuated. Clumps of lipid material and calcific deposits indicate extensive degeneration of the retina. **C.** Fundus photograph showing active necrotizing retinitis along the border of an inactive CMV lesion. The surrounding retina is edematous, and there is some overlying vitreous debris. The inactive lesion is characterized by pigment stippling and atrophy.

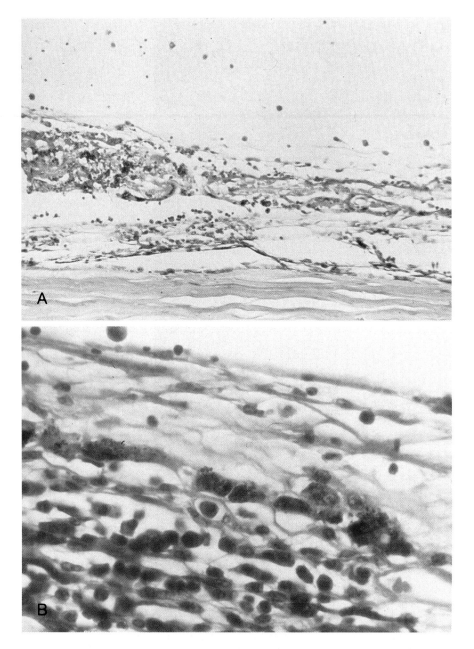

Figure 5.9. A. Photomicrograph showing a zone of inactive CMV retinitis. The sensory retina shows total disorganization. There is extensive replacement by glial cells. Numerous pigment-laden macrophages are present. There is a moderate infiltration of mononuclear cells in the overlying vitreous (hematoxylin and eosin: ×10). **B.** High-power photomicrograph showing both nuclear and cytoplasmic inclusions. The characteristic owl's eye cell has an enlarged nucleus with a clear rim of surrounding nucleoplasm (hematoxylin and eosin: ×160).

correspond to zones of inactive retinitis. Ischemia and edema adjacent to active zones may lead to visual loss, particularly in the macula. CMV may affect the optic nerve, causing a loss of vision either by direct infection or by secondary ischemic damage. Finally, CMV retinitis may result in retinal detachment in up to 29% of cases (97). Retinal holes typically occur near the posterior border of inactive zones of necrotizing retinitis. A significant number of patients develop proliferative vitreoretinopathy. Repair of these detachments frequently requires vitrectomy techniques, and the results of surgery are poor.

Without treatment, CMV retinitis is relentlessly progressive, leading to loss of vision from involvement of the optic nerve and macula or from retinal detachment. In the immunosuppressed population, withdrawal of immunosuppression may lead to resolution, but in the AIDS population, immunosuppression is irreversible. CMV retinitis typically progresses over a period of months, with expansion of old lesions and the development of new ones. Rarely, it may progress rapidly.

Before 1984, treatment of CMV retinitis was usually ineffective. Investigators had attempted specific antiviral therapy with such agents as idoxuridine (98), vidarabine (99), trifluoridine (100), acyclovir (101), and alpha interferon (102). None of these agents proved to be effective. In 1983, ganciclovir, a derivative of acyclovir, became available (Fig. 5.10A). Against CMV, ganciclovir has in vitro activity 10 to 100 times as great as that of acyclovir (103). CMV lacks the viral thymidine kinase required to convert acyclovir to acyclovir triphosphate, the active form of the drug (Fig. 5.10B). Ganciclovir is selectively phosphorylated in CMV-infected cells by cellular enzymes. Ganciclovir triphosphate competitively inhibits viral DNA polymerase, preventing viral replication. There is overwhelming clinical evidence that ganciclovir is effective in the management of CMV retinitis and other significant systemic CMV infections (Figs. 5.11A, 5.11B) (104–108). Unfortunately, the drug is virostatic and must be taken indefinitely,

unlike acyclovir. Furthermore, ganciclovir has significant systemic toxicity. Maintenance treatment with ganciclovir is complicated by significant myelosuppression requiring discontinuation of the drug in 30% to 50% of patients (105–108). Intravitreal treatment with ganciclovir has been reported and appears to be an effective alternative in those patients who cannot be treated systemically (109–110).

Foscarnet is another antiviral agent that is effective against CMV, with a slightly different spectrum of toxicity (111). Foscarnet inhibits viral DNA polymerase by a mechanism different from that of ganciclovir. Nephrotoxicity is the most significant adverse effect of foscarnet. Because of the different toxic effects of the two drugs, they may be used sequentially to control CMV retinitis. We have much less clinical experience with foscarnet in this country.

OTHER OPPORTUNISTIC INFECTIONS

Opportunistic infections other than CMV are much less common. Other viruses of the herpes group, including both herpes simplex and herpes zoster, may cause necrotizing retinitis (112, 113). Culture of these viruses from extraocular sites may be helpful in establishing the diagnosis. Protozoan infections with either *Pneumocystis carinii* or *Toxoplasma gondii* are also seen in the AIDS population. Toxoplasmosis may present with a particularly fulminant retinochoroiditis resembling endophthalmitis (114). *Pneumocystis* has been associated with cotton-wool spots, but until recently, it was uncertain whether *Pneumocystis* was a cause of retinal infection (115). It is now known that disseminated *Pneumocystis* may cause a multifocal choroiditis that may remain asymptomatic for long periods of time (116). The characteristic changes in the fundus are large, yellow, placoid lesions located in the choroid, without overlying retinal or vitreous involvement (Fig. 5.12). The choroiditis will respond to specific systemic treatment. The incidence of *Pneumocystis* choroiditis may increase as more patients are prophylactically treated with aerosolized pentami-

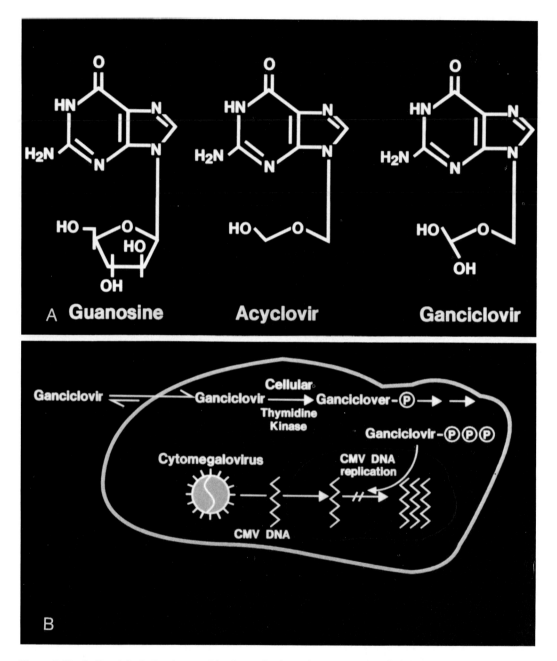

Figure 5.10. A. Ganciclovir closely resembles the purine base deoxyguanosine. Ganciclovir differs from acyclovir by the addition of a single hydroxyl group to the side chain. **B.** The antiviral activity of ganciclovir depends upon its phosphorylation by enzymes within the host cell. Ganciclovir triphosphate is a potent inhibitor of viral DNA polymerase, and it is also incorporated into viral DNA, causing chain termination.

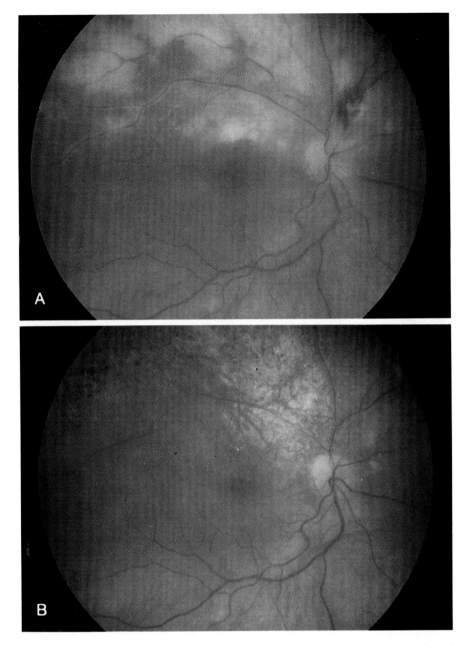

Figure 5.11. A. Fundus photograph showing active CMV retinitis extending into the posterior pole and partially surrounding the optic nerve head. **B.** After 3 months of induction and maintenance treatment with ganciclovir, the area of CMV retinitis is entirely inactive. There is segmental optic atrophy corresponding to the large area of inactive CMV retinitis. An absolute scotoma corresponds to the lesion, but the visual acuity remains 20/25.

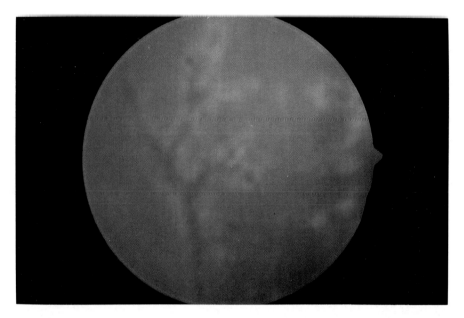

Figure 5.12. Fundus photograph showing multiple, yellowish placoid lesions at the level of the choroid. The lesions have slightly irregular margins and no overlying retinal or vitreous involvement.

dine. Such treatment does not prevent dissemination of the organism. Mycobacterial infection as a complication of systemic *M. avium intracellulare* has also been reported (82, 84, 87). Fungal infections with *Candida*, *Histoplasma*, and *Cryptococcus* have also been reported (83, 87, 117). *Cryptococcus* is a common opportunistic pathogen in the central nervous system. Ocular involvement usually occurs secondary to meningeal infection extending along the optic nerve sheath. Syphilis is usually a rare cause of ocular disease, but, in the AIDS population, syphilis is not infrequently seen, and retinochoroiditis has been reported (118).

NEURO-OPHTHALMIC SIGNS AND SYMPTOMS

Probably the most common neurological manifestation of AIDS is dementia, but the visual system is also affected as a result of CNS involvement (87, 89, 119). Eye movement disorders, disconnection syndromes, visual field defects, and pupillary abnormalities have also been reported.

Neuro-ophthalmic signs and symptoms are also associated with various opportunistic infections of the central nervous system.

NEOPLASMS

Kaposi's sarcoma is the most common neoplastic disease in patients with AIDS (120). Kaposi's sarcoma classically involves the lower extremities and visceral organs, but, in patients with AIDS, the disease is much more aggressive, causing lesions on the face and ocular surface, lid dysfunction, and orbital pain (Fig. 5.13) (82). The lesions usually require no treatment, but they can be locally excised or treated with radiation or chemotherapy. Non-Hodgkin's lymphoma is the second most common neoplasm (121).

In Africa, Burkitt's lymphoma is frequently associated with AIDS and may involve the orbit in up to 50% of cases (122). The association of Burkitt's lymphoma with the Epstein-Barr virus (EBV) raises the possibility of viral interaction of EBV and HIV, which may explain the disseminated

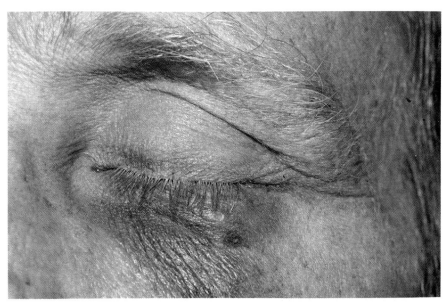

Figure 5.13. Clinical photograph of the areas of purplish induration characteristic of Kaposi's sarcoma. Lesions may be seen in the lid and conjunctiva and in the orbit. The lesions are locally invasive but usually do not impair visual function.

nature of the disease in the AIDS population.

Viral interaction may also be involved in the pathogenesis of Kaposi's sarcoma. It is possible that interaction of HIV with other viruses (such as the newly identified herpes virus type 6) may be important in the development of Kaposi's sarcoma (123). Recently, HIV-infected T lymphocytes have been found to produce a potent growth factor, which may explain the endothelial proliferation that is characteristic of Kaposi's sarcoma (124).

OTHER OCULAR MANIFESTATIONS

Other miscellaneous ocular manifestations have been reported that are questionably related to HIV infection. Acute glaucoma, for example, has been reported in three patients (125). The glaucoma resulted from ciliary body swelling and secondary angle closure. Two cases responded to cycloplegic therapy, and the third improved after drainage of suprachoroidal fluid.

Mild anterior uveitis is infrequently reported in patients with AIDS. This has usually been associated with CMV retinitis. Unlike other forms of viral retinitis, the uveitis associated with CMV retinitis is mild. Fine, filamentous keratic precipitates, similar to those seen in Fuch's heterochromic cyclitis, have been associated with CMV retinitis (126). Although HIV has been recovered from the cornea, iris, and ciliary body, it has not been associated with specific clinical findings (92).

Other nonspecific forms of ocular involvement may be seen, including conjunctivitis, keratoconjunctivitis sicca, peripheral corneal thinning, and orbital pseudotumor (82, 127). These changes are not associated with a particular opportunistic infection and may be a result of hematological changes or circulating immune complexes.

HIV TREATMENT

Chemotherapy directed against HIV has progressed slowly. Drugs have been developed that may affect viral replication by interfering with many of the steps of virus synthesis. These include cellular binding, viral uncoating, inhibition of reverse transcriptase, viral protein synthesis, viral assembly, and budding (Fig. 5.14). The only drug that has proved to be effective against HIV is zidovudine (ZDV). Like acyclovir and ganciclovir, ZDV is a prodrug and must be converted to the active triphosphate form by cellular enzymes (Fig. 5.15A). ZDV is an inhibitor of reverse transcriptase and acts as a terminator of chain synthesis when incorporated into viral DNA (Fig. 5.15B). ZDV has been evaluated in controlled clinical trials and has been shown to decrease the amount of HIV antigen present in serum and to prolong survival in AIDS patients (128). ZDV modestly improves immunological response by increasing the number of CD-4 lymphocytes. It improves skin-test reactivity in patients with Stage III disease (129). ZDV may also have a beneficial effect on AIDS-related neurological disease (130). The primary toxic effect of ZDV is bone marrow suppression. Approximately 40% to 50% of AIDS patients receiving full-dose ZDV (1200 mg to 1500 mg/day) require either a blood transfusion or discontinuation of the drug (131). Several recent, unpublished studies demonstrate that lower doses of ZDV (500 mg to 600 mg/day) have clinical benefits equal to those of the higher doses, with lower toxicity. In addition, persons that have anemia due to ZDV can be treated with human recombinant erythropoietin (132). Because the toxicity of ZDV is similar to that of ganciclovir, patients treated with ZDV generally cannot tolerate simultaneous treatment with ganciclovir. Other thymidine analogs have been developed and are undergoing evaluation. Dideoxycytidine was found to have intolerable neurological side effects in the initial Phase I clinical trial and is now being studied at a lower dose in combination with zidovudine (133).

Currently, the dideoxynucleoside that is receiving the most attention is dideoxyinosine (DDI). It appears to have clinical efficacy similar to that of ZDV with a different toxicity (peripheral neuropathy, pancreatitis, and hyperuricemia). At the present time, the drug is available through compassionate use programs and through three federal drug trials (134).

Attempts to restore immunological function have been largely unsuccessful. Early experience with agents such as interleukin 2 (135) or isoprinosine (136) in patients with Stage IV disease showed little effect on immune dysfunction. These agents may be of some benefit at early stages of the disease. Other agents have been identified that have activity against retroviruses. Agents such as suramin show activity against HIV in peripheral blood lymphocytes, but systemic side effects have limited their usefulness (137).

Ribavirin is a guanosine analog that inhibits HIV replication at a later stage in viral synthesis. It has undergone Phase I clinical trials in Stage III and Stage IV disease (138). In clinical trials, the drug failed to show significant effects at low doses, but it may be more effective in higher doses. Minimum toxicity was demonstrated. It is possible that treatment with higher doses would be effective, but enthusiasm currently is limited.

Ampligen is another agent with in vitro activity against HIV. Ampligen is a mismatched, double-stranded RNA preparation (Poly I:Poly C) that inhibits HIV replication at a posttranscriptional step. Studies have shown a reduction in serum HIV antigen concentration and clinical improvement, as well as some improvement in tests of immune function (139). Again, greater clinical effects were noted in patients with less advanced disease. In initial studies, ampligen was well tolerated and had minimal toxicity. Preliminary data suggested ampligen may be clinically beneficial, but a more recent study found no evidence of clinical efficacy, prompting the sponsoring pharmaceutical company to withdraw funding (140).

Other unique approaches to anti-HIV therapy are being evaluated. Several manufacturers have mass-produced the CD-4 protein, which is the major target of HIV on the outer surface of T-helper lymphocytes. The CD-4 protein appears to protect

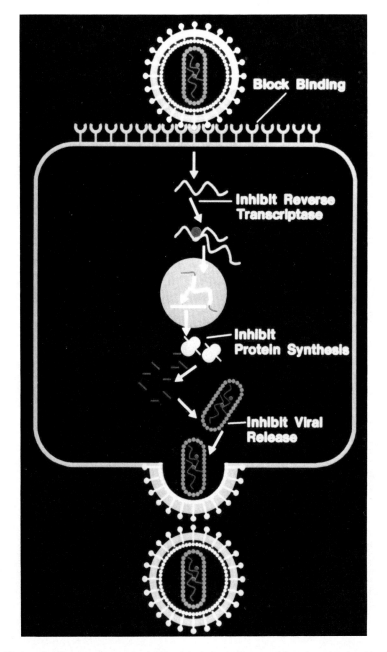

Figure 5.14. Viral replication may be prevented by interfering with any of the steps involved in viral synthesis. Cellular binding of HIV to the CD-4 receptor may be blocked, for example, by an antibody. RNA-dependent DNA polymerase is inhibited by drugs such as zidovudine. Other drugs, such as ampligen, may interfere with the synthesis and assembly of viral proteins. Release of virus from the cell might be another point of chemotherapeutic intervention.

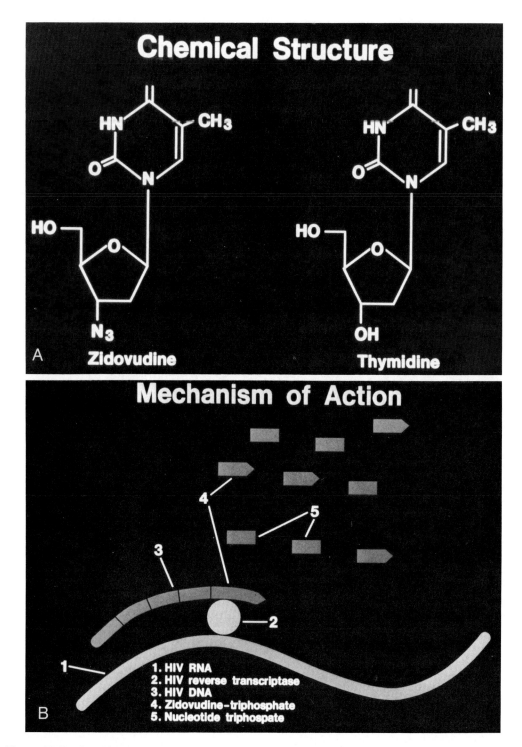

Figure 15.15. A. Azidothymidine (zidovudine) is a thymidine analog that differs by a substitution at a single carbon atom. **B.** Zidovudine prevents HIV replication by inhibiting reverse transcriptase. Like acyclovir and ganciclovir, zidovudine must be phosphorylated by cellular enzymes to its active form, the triphosphate. Zidovudine also causes chain termination when incorporated into the viral genome.

T-helper cells from HIV in cell culture, and initial clinical trials involving CD-4 protein have begun to measure clinical benefit and toxicity (141, 142). Investigators have also noted that several highly sulfated polysaccharides (for example, heparin, dextran sulfate) can inhibit syncytia formation and HIV entry into T-helper lymphocytes in vivo (143). Dextran sulfate has become a popular drug among AIDS patients because of its availability from mail-order houses and alternative clinics. A Phase I/II clinical trial evaluating the toxicity and efficacy of dextran sulfate is underway. Recently, reports of severe bloody diarrhea due to dextran sulfate as well as a concern about its oral absorption have lessened the enthusiasm for its use (144).

Combination therapy with a variety of agents may allow continuous treatment while reducing toxicity. A true synergistic effect may be possible because the agents appear to affect different steps in viral replication. Such synergistic effects have already been demonstrated with acyclovir and ZDV (145). Other drugs that counteract specific toxic effects may be used. For example, ZDV might be combined with either erythropoietin or granulocyte-macrophage colony stimulating factor (GM-CSF) to counteract the myelosuppressive effects (146). Combination therapy with immunomodulator agents and antivirals is also underway.

Vaccine development has also progressed slowly (147). Until recently, no primate animal model of the disease was available for testing. Early in the course of infection, the virus is incorporated into the host genome, where it remains latent for many years. A vaccine would not be expected to be effective against latent virus. The large population of latently infected individuals would, therefore, probably not benefit. The virus shows a high rate of mutation in its envelope protein, making the development of a vaccine difficult. Preliminary results show that vaccines may induce antibodies against HIV but do not consistently confer immunity (148). As of 1990, there is some renewed hope that vaccine development might result in large clinical trials by later in the decade (149).

SOCIOECONOMIC ISSUES

AIDS, in many ways, is a unique disease in the history of epidemic infections. The disease is uniformly fatal. There is no apparent cure, and a long, asymptomatic latent period exists between exposure and onset of the disease. In addition, it strikes individuals in the prime of life, and it has significant social and moral dimensions. Because AIDS occurs in already stigmatized groups—homosexual or bisexual males, IV drug abusers, and prostitutes—response to the problem is complicated by moralistic attitudes and assignment of blame. The persistent fear of casual transmission remains, despite mounting scientific evidence to the contrary. In this atmosphere, discrimination and prejudice may impair our ability to identify and control the disease.

Probably the most effective means of dealing with the disease is through modification of behavior—sexual practices and IV drug abuse. Educational programs based upon knowledge of the spread of the disease have already been effective. The rate of HIV infection has been reduced in a cohort of homosexual males in San Francisco (150). Annual HIV seroconversion rates have declined 88%, from 6% at the beginning of 1985 to 0.7% at the end of 1987. There was a parallel decrease in the incidence of other sexually transmitted diseases. Modification of sexual behavior, avoidance of high-risk practices, use of condoms, and voluntary abstinence of individuals known to be HIV-infected could greatly reduce the risk of sexual transmission. More effective management of the drug abuse problem in general, with adequate facilities for treatment, a reduction in the supply and demand for drugs, or perhaps the distribution of needles and syringes to selected groups, are other possible approaches to the problem. Public health measures, such as case identification, contact tracing, and the elimination of sites where the disease is spread, could ultimately control the spread of disease (151). The disease is suited to control by these public health measures because the risk is concentrated among high-risk groups and patterns of behavior.

TESTING FOR HIV

Accurate tests for HIV infection became available in 1985 (27). Mandatory testing of blood, tissue, and organ donors has virtually eliminated the risk of infection via this route. A few cases have been acquired during the silent phase of early infection when antibody tests are still negative. Mandatory testing in other situations remains controversial. The major issues are confidentiality and discrimination (152, 153). Recent data from a major national trial suggest that early use of ZDV, even in asymptomatic HIV-infected individuals, may confer clinical benefit (154). Therefore, it is more important than ever for an individual to know his or her HIV status. By discouraging voluntary testing, the disease may be driven underground, preventing effective public health measures and clinical benefit (152–155). Routine testing of patients entering hospitals is not cost-effective in most areas of the United States. The institution of universal blood precautions should greatly decrease the risk to health-care workers, not only from HIV infection but from other blood-borne infections, in particular hepatitis B. Likewise, premarital testing seems to be less effective than educational programs. Voluntary testing and aggressive education in high-risk groups remain the most important public health measures we have.

MEDICAL-LEGAL IMPLICATIONS

Health-care professionals have a moral obligation to treat patients with all forms of illness, including HIV infection and AIDS (156). They also have a right to know the occupational risk and to take reasonable precautions. Likewise, in social situations or in the work place, there should not be discrimination against or fear of patients with HIV infection, given our knowledge of the way the infection is spread. This principle has already been tested in the courts, which have upheld laws prohibiting discrimination in housing, education, and employment (156).

There also are issues of consent and confidentiality (157–159). Present law does not restrict testing in the setting of a communicable disease, although informed consent is strongly recommended. Some states have required specific consent for HIV antibody testing. Since the results of this test have such major implications concerning a patient's socioeconomic status and the medical prognosis, the HIV antibody test cannot be considered as other routine laboratory tests. Testing should be done only in a setting where counseling is also available. States have become increasingly protective of the contents of both hospital and private physician records. The necessity to maintain confidentiality must be balanced against the legitimate requests of health-care workers concerning an individual's HIV antibody status. Confidentiality of test results is a major factor in promoting voluntary testing, a key part of the program to prevent the spread of infection.

Exceptions to the preservation of confidentiality exist when a third party is at risk. In almost all states, physicians are protected from liability in warning third parties. The AMA has offered guidelines that apply specifically to the spread of AIDS (156). Physicians should (a) attempt to persuade the infected individual to change his behavior; (b) report the individual to public health authorities, if persuasion fails; and (c) notify the third party if authorities take no action. Clearly, great sensitivity is needed since voluntary contact notification is another powerful weapon in preventing the spread of infection.

In rare instances, it may be necessary to restrict personal freedom of infected individuals. Intentional or reckless attempts to transmit HIV through sexual conduct, blood donation, spitting, and biting have resulted in criminal prosecution. Isolation of infected individuals may be necessary in rare cases.

ECONOMIC IMPACT

The economic costs of AIDS involve both monetary and nonmonetary issues (160–162). Direct costs include the costs of medical care, as well as the costs for education, testing, and research. Indirect costs include the foregone earnings of AIDS patients. Nonmonetary costs include the value of individuals to their families and society. Unlike many other diseases, AIDS strikes individuals in the prime of life, greatly increasing the indirect and nonmonetary burden of the disease.

The lifetime direct cost of AIDS care has been estimated to be $80,000 per patient, which is comparable to that of other serious illnesses such as heart disease or cancer (160). The indirect costs, however, are 6 to 8 times higher. To place the cost of AIDS in perspective, estimates can be made comparing the cost of AIDS with that of other infectious diseases and illnesses (160). In 1986, direct cost of AIDS accounted for 0.5% of all illnesses and 24% of the costs of infectious diseases. By 1991, AIDS will exceed the cost of all other infectious diseases but will account for only 2% of all medical costs. The costs of AIDS will have only a modest effect on the total cost of health care in the United States.

Unfortunately, a disproportionate share of the cost has fallen on certain geographical areas where the incidence of the disease is high (160). While hospital occupancy rates for AIDS nationally were only 0.4% in 1986, the rates for New York City and San Francisco were 3% and 2.7%, respectively. In 1991, the rates in these cities will be 12.4% and 8.1%, respectively. Hospitalization alone will cost residents of these cities between 100 and 350 dollars per person per year. Financial resources for patients with AIDS are also unique. Medicare, for example, pays for less than 2% of AIDS-related health care costs. Private insurance covers only 17% of the cost. 27% of AIDS patients have no insurance. In most cases, Medicaid assumes financial responsibility after personal resources have been exhuasted.

CONCLUSION

Until the recognition of AIDS in 1981, most infectious diseases were not thought to pose a great threat to mankind and society. The AIDS pandemic has altered this perception and dramatically changed the course of medicine and society. The disease is insidious, caused by a relatively frail virus that slowly incorporates itself into its host and gradually undermines its immune system. The mysterious origin of AIDS and the rapid spread of the epidemic has created great fear and uncertainty among health-care professionals and the public in general. Through its association with homosexuality and IV drug abuse and its concentration in certain socioeconomic groups, AIDS has elicited prejudices that have interfered with a rational approach to the epidemic. Despite the mobilization of impressive technological resources, the disease remains incurable. Instead, we have been challenged to deal with the epidemic through modifications of behavior rather than through specific medical measures.

The world has been changed because of AIDS, and the way in which we confront the epidemic will have a major impact on all aspects of society. Despite these challenges, involvement in the care of HIV patients can be intellectually exciting and personally rewarding and is an endeavor that needs wide support throughout the medical profession.

ACKNOWLEDGMENTS

Supported in part by the Minnesota Lions Eye Bank and a grant from Research to Prevent Blindness.

References

1. Gottlieb MS, Schroff R, Schanker HM, et al. *Pneumocystis carinii* pneumonia and mucosal candidiasis in previously healthy homosexual men: evidence of a new acquired cellular immunodeficiency. N Engl J Med 1981;305:1425–1431.

2. Masur H, Micholic MA, Croono JB, et al. An outbreak of community-acquired *Pneumocystis carinii* pneumonia: initial manifestation of cellular immune dysfunction. N Engl J Med 1981;305:1431–1438.

3. Update on Kaposi's sarcoma and opportunistic infections in previously healthy persons—United States. MMWR 1982;31:294, 300–301.

4. Update: Acquired immunodeficiency syndrome (AIDS)—United States. MMWR 1983;32:389–391.

5. Update: Acquired immunodeficiency syndrome (AIDS)—United States. MMWR 1983;32:465–467.

6. Cases of specified notifiable disease, United States, weeks ending August 2, 1986 and August 3, 1985 (31st week). MMWR 1986;35:497.

7. Update: Acquired immunodeficiency syndrome · Europe. MMWR 1986;35:35–38, 43–46.

8. Centers for Disease Control. HIV/AIDS Surveillance Report. June 1990;1–18.

9. Update on acquired immune deficiency syndrome (AIDS)—United States. MMWR 1982;31:507–508, 513–514.

10. Opportunistic infections and Kaposi's sarcoma among Haitians in the United States. MMWR 1982;31:353–354, 360–361.

11. Evatt BL, Chorba TL. Acquired immunodeficiency syndrome (AIDS) in hemophilia. Clin Lab Med 1984;4:333–344.

12. Curran JW, Lawrence DN, Jaffe H, et al. Acquired immunodeficiency syndrome (AIDS) associated with transfusions. N Engl J Med 1984;310:69–75.

13. Harris C, Butkus-Small C, Klein RS, et al. Immunodeficiency in female sexual partners of men with the acquired immunodeficiency syndrome. N Engl J Med 1983;308:1181–1184.

14. Unexplained immunodeficiency and opportunistic infections in infants—New York, New Jersey, California. MMWR 1982;31:665–667.

15. Barre-Sinoussi F, Chermann JC, Rey F, et al. Isolation of a T-lymphotropic retrovirus from a patient at risk for acquired immune deficiency syndrome (AIDS). Science 1983;220:868–871.

16. Popovic M, Sarngadharan MG, Read E, Gallo RC. Detection, isolation, and continuous production of cytopathic retroviruses (HTLV-III) from patients with AIDS and pre-AIDS. Science 1984;224:497–500.

17. Poiesz BJ, Ruscetti FW, Gazdar AF, et al. Detection and isolation of type C retrovirus particles from fresh and cultured lymphocytes of a patient with cutaneous T-cell lymphoma. Proc Natl Acad Sci USA 1980;77:7415–7419.

18. Gallo RC, Salahuddin SZ, Popovic M, et al. Frequent detection and isolation of cytopathic retroviruses (HTLV-III) from patients with AIDS and at risk for AIDS. Science 1984;224:500–503.

19. Curran JW, Evatt BL, Lawrence DN. Acquired immune deficiency syndrome: the past as prologue. Ann Intern Med 1983;98:401–403.

20. Clavel F. HIV-2, the West African AIDS virus. AIDS 1987;1:135–140.

21. Update: HIV-2 infection—United States. MMWR 1989;38:572–574, 579–580.

22. Haseltine WA, Wong-Staal F. The molecular biology of the AIDS virus. Sci Am 1988;259:52–62.

23. Essex M, Kanki PJ. The origins of the AIDS virus. Sci Am 1988;259:64–71.

24. Smith TF, Srinivasan A, Schochetman G, et al. The phylogenetic history of immunodeficiency viruses. Nature 1988;333:573–575.

25. Garry RF, Witte MH, Gottlieb AA, et al. Documentation of an AIDS virus infection in the United States in 1968. JAMA 1988;260:2085–2087.

26. Klatzmann D, Barre-Sinoussi F, Nugeyre MT, et al. Selective tropism of lymphadenopathy associated virus (LAV) for helper-inducer T lymphocytes. Science 1984;225:59–63.

27. Veronese FD, Sarngadharan MG, Rahman R, et al. Monoclonal antibodies specific for p24, the major core protein of human T-cell leukemia virus type III. Proc Natl Acad Sci USA 1985;82:5199–5202.

28. Rando RF, Pellett PE, Luciw PA, et al. Transactivation of human immunodeficiency virus by herpesviruses. Oncogene 1987;1:13–18.

29. Fauci AS, Macher AM, Longo DL, et al. Acquired immunodeficiency syndrome: epidemiologic, clinical, immunologic and therapeutic considerations. Ann Intern Med 1984;100:92–106.

30. Shearer GM, Salahuddin SZ, Markham PD, et al. Prospective study of cytotoxic T lymphocyte responses to influenza and antibodies to human T lymphotropic virus-III in homosexual men. J Clin Invest 1985;76:1699–1704.

31. Schroff RW, Gottlieb MS, Prince HE, et al. Immunological studies of homosexual men with immunodeficiency and Kaposi's sarcoma. Clin Immunol Immunopathol 1983;27:300–314.

32. Seligmann M, Chess L, Fahey JL, Roberts RB. AIDS—an immunologic reevaluation. N Engl J Med 1984;311:1286–1292.

33. Murray HW, Rubin BY, Masur H, Roberts RB. Imparied production of lymphokines and immune (gamma) interferon in the acquired immunodeficiency syndrome. N Engl J Med 1984;310:883–889.

34. Ammann AJ, Schiffman G, Abrams D, et al. B-cell immunodeficiency in acquired immune deficiency syndrome. JAMA 1984;251:1447–1449.

35. Lane HC, Masur H, Edgar LC, et al. Abnormalities of B-cell activation and immunoregulation

in patients with the acquired immunodeficiency syndrome. N Engl J Med 1983;309:453–458.

36. Heyward WL, Curran JW. The epidemiology of AIDS in the U.S. Sci Am 1988;259(4):72–81.

37. Human immunodeficiency virus infection in the United States: a review of current knowledge. MMWR 1987;36(suppl 6):1–48; erratum: MMWR 1988;37;479,

38. Des Jarlais DC, Friedman SR, Stoneburner RL. HIV infection and intravenous drug use: critical issues in transmission dynamics, infection outcomes, and prevention. Rev Infect Dis 1988;10:151–158.

39. Chaisson RE, Bacchetti P, Osmond D, et al. Cocaine use and HIV infection in intravenous drug users in San Francisco. JAMA 1989;261:561–565.

40. AIDS in sub-saharan Africa. Lancet 1988;1:1260–1261.

41. Kreiss JK, Koech D, Plummer FA, et al. AIDS virus infection in Nairobi prostitutes. Spread of the epidemic to East Africa. N Engl J Med 1986;314:414–418.

42. Hrdy DB. Cultural practices contributing to the transmission of human immunodeficiency virus in Africa. Rev Infect Dis 1987;9:1109–1119.

43. Rosenberg MJ, Weiner JM. Prostitutes and AIDS: a health department priority? Am J Public Health 1988;78:418–423.

44. Holmberg SD, Horsburgh CR Jr, Ward JW, Jaffe HW. AIDS commentary: biologic factors in the sexual transmission of human immunodeficiency virus. J Infect Dis 1989;160:116–125.

45. Handsfield HH. Heterosexual transmission of human immunodeficiency virus. JAMA 1988;260:1943–1944.

46. Novick LF, Berns D, Stricof R, et al. HIV seroprevalence in newborns in New York State. JAMA 1989;261:1745–1750.

47. Blanche S, Rouzioux C, Moscato MLG, et al. A prospective study of infants born to women seropositive for human immunodeficiency virus type 1. HIV Infection in Newborns French Collaborative Study Group. N Engl J Med 1989;320:1643–1648.

48. Katz SL, Wilfert CM. Human immunodeficiency virus infection of newborns. N Engl J Med 1989;320:1687–1689.

49. Morgan WM, Curran JW. Acquired immunodeficiency syndrome: current and future trends. Public Health Rep 1986;101:459–465.

50. Update: Acquired immunodeficiency syndrome—United States. MMWR 1986;35:17–21.

51. Institute of Medicine. Confronting AIDS: Update 1988: HIV prevalence in groups at recognized risk. Washington, DC: National Academy Press, 1988:46–47.

52. Institute of Medicine. Confronting AIDS: Update 1988: HIV prevalence among selected segments of the general population. Washington, DC: National Academy Press, 1988:47–48.

53. Classification system for human T-lympho-
tropic virus type III/lymphadenopathy-associated virus infections. MMWR 1986;35:334–339.

54. Jackson JB, Balfour HH Jr. Practical diagnostic testing for human immunodeficiency virus. Clin Microbiol Rev 1988;1:124–138.

55. Paul DA, Falk LA, Kessler HA, et al. Correlation of serum HIV antigen and antibody with clinical status in HIV-infected patients. J Med Virol 1987;22:357 363.

56. Levy JA, Shimabukuro J. Recovery of AIDS-associated retroviruses from patients with AIDS or AIDS-related conditions and from clinically healthy individuals. J Infect Dis 1985;152:734–738.

57. Jackson JB, Coombs RW, Sannerud K, et al. Rapid and sensitive viral culture method for human immunodeficiency virus type 1. J Clin Microbiol 1988;26:1416–1418.

58. Institute of Medicine Confronting AIDS: Update 1988: Proportion of infected individuals who will develop AIDS. Washington, DC: National Academy Press, 1988;35–36.

59. Bacchetti P, Osmond D, Chaisson RE, et al. Survival with AIDS in New York. N Engl J Med 1988;318:1464–1465.

60. Update: Acquired immunodeficiency syndrome and human immunodeficiency virus infection among health-care workers. MMWR 1988;37:229–234, 239.

61. Henderson DK, Saah AJ, Zak BJ, et al. Risk of nosocomial infection with human T-cell lymphotropic virus type III/lymphadenopathy-associated virus in a large cohort of intensively exposed health care workers. Ann Intern Med 1986;104:644–647.

62. Gerberding JL, Bryant-LeBlanc CE, Nelson K, et al. Risk of transmitting the human immunodeficiency virus, cytomegalovirus, and hepatitis B virus to health care workers exposed to patients with AIDS and AIDS-related conditions. J Infect Dis 1987;156:1–8.

63. Groopman JE, Salahuddin SZ, Sarngadharan MG, et al. HTLV-III in saliva of people with AIDS-related complex and healthy homosexual men at risk for AIDS. Science 1984;226:447–449.

64. Thiry L, Sprecher-Goldberger S, Jonckheer T, et al. Isolation of AIDS virus from cell-free breast milk of three healthy virus carriers. Lancet 1985;2:891–892.

65. Ziza JM, Brun-Vezinet F, Venet A, et al. Lymphadenopathy-associated virus isolated from bronchoalveolar lavage fluid in AIDS-related complex with lymphoid interstitial pneumonitis. N Engl J Med 1985;313:183.

66. Ho DD, Rota TR, Schooley RT, et al. Isolation of HTLV-III from cerebrospinal fluid and neural tissues of patients with neurologic syndromes related to the acquired immunodeficiency syndrome. N Engl J Med 1985;313:1493–1497.

67. Fujikawa LS, Salahuddin SZ, Ablashi D, et al. HTLV-III in the tears of AIDS patients. Ophthalmology 1986;93:1479–1481.

68. Salahuddin SZ, Markham PD, Popovic M, et al.

Isolation of infectious human T-cell leukemia/lymphotropic virus type III (HTLV-III) from patients with acquired immunodeficiency syndrome (AIDS) or AIDS-related complex (ARC) and from healthy carriers: a study of risk groups and tissue sources. Proc Natl Acad Sci USA 1985;82:5530–5534.

69. Fujikawa LS, Salahuddin SZ, Ablashi D, et al. Human T-cell leukemia/lymphotropic virus type III in the conjunctival epithelium of a patient with AIDS. Am J Ophthalmol 1985;100:507–509.

70. Salahuddin SZ, Palestine AG, Heck E, et al. Isolation of the human T-cell leukemia/lymphotropic virus type III from the cornea. Am J Ophthalmol 1986;101:149–152.

71. Prompt CA, Reis MM, Grillo FM, et al. Transmission of AIDS virus at renal transplantation. Lancet 1985;2:672.

72. Pepose JS, MacRae S, Quinn TC, Holland GN. The impact of the AIDS epidemic on corneal transplantation. Am J Ophthalmol 1985;100:610–613.

73. Guidelines for prevention of transmission of human immunodeficiency virus and hepatitis B virus to health-care and public-safety workers. MMWR 1989;38(suppl 6):1–37.

74. Recommendations for preventing possible transmission of human T-lymphotropic virus type III/lymphadenopathy-associated virus from tears. MMWR 1985;34:533–534.

75. Vogt MW, Ho DD, Bakar SR, et al. Safe disinfection of contact lenses after contamination with HTLV-III. Ophthalmology 1986;93:771–774.

76. Institute of Medicine. Confronting AIDS: Update 1986: Efficiencies of transmission. Washington, DC: National Academy Press, 1988:42–43.

77. Ward JW, Deppe DA, Samson S, et al. Risk of human immunodeficiency virus infection from blood donors who later developed the acquired immunodeficiency syndrome. Ann Intern Med 1987;106:61–62.

78. Winkelstein W, Lyman DM, Padian N, et al. Sexual practices and risk of infection by the human immunodeficiency virus. The San Francisco Men's Health Study. JAMA 1987;257:321–325.

79. Curran JW, Jaffe HW, Hardy AM, et al. Epidemiology of HIV infection and AIDS in the United States. Science 1988;239:610–616.

80. Padian N, Marquis L, Francis DP, et al. Male-to-female transmission of human immunodeficiency virus. JAMA 1987;258:788–790.

81. Padian NS. Heterosexual transmission of acquired immunodeficiency syndrome: international perspectives and national projections. Rev Infect Dis 1987;9:947–960.

82. Holland GN, Pepose JS, Pettit TH, et al. Acquired immune deficiency syndrome; ocular manifestations. Ophthalmology 1983;90:859–873.

83. Freeman WR, Lerner CW, Mines JA, et al. A prospective study of the ophthalmologic findings in the acquired immune deficiency syndrome. Am J Ophthalmol 1984;97:133–142.

84. Friedman AH. The retinal lesions of the acquired immune deficiency syndrome. Trans Am Ophthalmol Soc 1984;82:447–491.

85. Henderly DE, Freeman WR, Smith RE, et al. Cytomegalovirus retinitis as the initial manifestation of the acquired immune deficiency syndrome. Am J Ophthalmol 1987;103:316–320.

86. Newsome DA, Green WR, Miller ED, et al. Microvascular aspects of acquired immune deficiency syndrome retinopathy. Am J Ophthalmol 1984;98:590–601.

87. Pepose JS, Holland GN, Nestor MS, et al. Acquired immune deficiency syndrome; pathogenic mechanisms of ocular disease. Ophthalmology 1985;92:472–484.

88. Pepose JS, Nestor MS, Holland GN, et al. An analysis of retinal cotton-wool spots and cytomegalovirus retinitis in the acquired immunodeficiency syndrome. Am J Ophthalmol 1983;95:118–120.

89. Palestine AG, Rodrigues MM, Macher AM, et al. Ophthalmic involvement in acquired immunodeficiency syndrome. Ophthalmology 1984;91:1092–1099.

90. Kennedy PGE, Newsome DA, Hess J, et al. Cytomegalovirus but not human lymphotropic virus type III/lymphadenopathy associated virus detected by in situ hybridisation in retinal lesions in patients with the acquired immunodeficiency syndrome. Br Med J 1986;293:162–164.

91. Schuman JS, Orellana J, Friedman AH, Teich SA. Acquired immunodeficiency syndrome (AIDS). Surv Ophthalmol 1987;31:384–410.

92. Pomerantz RJ, Kuritzkes DR, de la Monte SM, et al. Infection of the retina by human immunodeficiency virus type I. N Engl J Med 1987;317:1643–1647.

93. Cantrill HL, Henry K, Jackson B, et al. Recovery of human immunodeficiency virus from ocular tissues in patients with acquired immune deficiency syndrome. Ophthalmology 1988;95:1458–1462.

94. Fiala M, Payne JE, Berne TV, et al. Epidemiology of cytomegalovirus infection after transplantation and immunosuppression. J Infect Dis 1975;132:421–433.

95. Kestelyn P, Van de Perre P, Rouvroy D, et al. A prospective study of the ophthalmologic findings in the acquired immune deficiency syndrome in Africa. Am J Ophthalmol 1985;100:230–238.

96. Skolnik PR, Kosloff BR, Hirsch MS. Bidirectional interactions between human immunodeficiency virus type I and cytomegalovirus. J Infect Dis 1988;157:508–514.

97. Freeman WR, Henderly DE, Wan WL, et al. Prevalence, pathophysiology, and treatment of rhegmatogenous retinal detachment in treated cytomegalovirus retinitis. Am J Ophthalmol 1987;103:527–536.

98. Conchie AF, Barton BW, Tobin JO. Congenital cytomegalovirus infections treated with idoxuridine. Br Med J 1968;4:162–163.

99. Pollard RB, Egbert PR, Gallagher JC, Merigan TC. Cytomegalovirus retinitis in immunosuppressed hosts. I. Natural history and effects of treatment with adenine arabinoside. Ann Intern Med 1980;93:655–663.

100. Spector SA, Tyndall M, Kelley F. Inhibition of human cytomegalovirus by trifluorothymidine. Antimicrob Agents Chemother 1983;23:113–118.

101. Balfour HH Jr, Bean B, Mitchell CD, et al. Acyclovir in immunocompromised patients with cytomegalovirus disease: a controlled trial at one institution. Am J Med 1982;73(1A):241–248.

102. Chou SW, Dylewski JS, Gaynon MW, et al. Alpha-interferon administration in cytomegalovirus retinitis. Antimicrob Agents Chemother 1984;25:25–28.

103. Mar E-C, Cheng Y-C, Huang E-S, Effect of 9-(1,3-dihydroxy-2-propoxymethyl) guanine on human cytomegalovirus replication in vitro. Antimicrob Agents Chemother 1983;24:518–521.

104. Collaborative DHPG Treatment Study Group. Treatment of serious cytomegalovirus infections with 9-(1,3-dihydroxy-2-propoxymethyl) guanine in patients with AIDS and other immunodeficiencies. N Engl J Med 1986;314:801–805.

105. Holland GN, Sidikaro Y, Kreiger AE, et al. Treatment of cytomegalovirus retinopathy with ganciclovir. Ophthalmology 1987;94:815–823.

106. Jabs DA, Newman C, de Bustros S, Polk BF. Treatment of cytomegalovirus retinitis with ganciclovir. Ophthalmology 1987;94:824–830.

107. Orellana J, Teich SA, Friedman AH, et al. Combined short- and long-term therapy for the treatment of cytomegalovirus retinitis using ganciclovir (BW B759U). Ophthalmology 1987;94:831–838.

108. Henderly DE, Freeman WR, Causey DM, Rao NA. Cytomegalovirus retinitis and response to therapy with ganciclovir. Ophthalmology 1987;94:425–434.

109. Henry K, Cantrill H, Fletcher C, et al. Use of intravitreal ganciclovir (dihydroxy propoxymethyl guanine) for cytomegalovirus retinitis in a patient with AIDS. Am J Ophthalmol 1987;103:17–23.

110. Ussery FM III, Gibson SR, Conklin RH, et al. Intravitreal ganciclovir in the treatment of AIDS-associated cytomegalovirus retinitis. Ophthalmology 1988;95:640–648.

111. Walmsley SL, Chew E, Read SE, et al. Treatment of cytomegalovirus retinitis with trisodium phosphonoformate hexahydrate (Foscarnet). J Infect Dis 1988;157:569–572.

112. Pepose JS, Kreiger AE, Tomiyasu U, et al. Immunocytologic localization of herpes simplex type I viral antigens in herpetic retinitis and encephalitis in an adult. Ophthalmology 1985;92:160–166.

113. Cole EL, Meisler DM, Calabrese LH, et al. Herpes zoster ophthalmicus and acquired immune deficiency syndrome. Arch Ophthalmol 1984;102:1027–1029.

114. Parke DW II, Font RL. Diffuse toxoplasmic retinochoroiditis in a patient with AIDS. Arch Ophthalmol 1986;104:571–575.

115. Schuman JS, Friedman AH. Retinal manifestations of the acquired immune deficiency syndrome (AIDS): cytomegalovirus, *Candida albicans*, *Cryptococcus*, toxoplasmosis and *Pneumocystis carinii*. Trans Ophthalmol Soc UK 1983;103:177–190.

116. Rao NA, Zimmerman PL, Boyer D, et al. A clinical, histopathologic, and electron microscopic study of *Pneumocystis carinii* choroiditis. Am J Ophthalmol 1989;107:218–228.

117. Macher A, Rodrigues MM, Kaplan W, et al. Disseminated bilateral chorioretinitis due to *Histoplasma capsulatum* in a patient with the acquired immunodeficiency syndrome. Ophthalmology 1985;92:1159–1164.

118. Stoumbos VD, Klein ML. Syphilitic retinitis in a patient with acquired immunodeficiency syndrome-related complex. Am J Ophthalmol 1987;103:103–104.

119. Holland GN. Ocular manifestations of the acquired immune deficiency syndrome. Int Ophthalmol Clin 1985;25(2):179–187.

120. Haverkos HW, Drotman DP, Morgan M. Prevalence of Kaposi's sarcoma among patients with AIDS. N Engl J Med 1985;312:1518.

121. Ziegler JL, Beckstead JA, Volberding PA, et al. Non-Hodgkin's lymphoma in 90 homosexual men; relation to generalized lymphadenopathy and the acquired immunodeficiency syndrome. N Engl J Med 1984;311:565–570.

122. Centers for Disease Control Task Force on Kaposi's Sarcoma and Opportunistic Infections. Special report. Epidemiologic aspects of the current outbreak of Kaposi's sarcoma and opportunistic infection. N Engl J Med 1982; 306:248–252.

123. Nakamura S, Salahuddin SZ, Biberfeld P, et al. Kaposi's sarcoma cells: long-term culture with growth factor from retrovirus-infected CD4 + T cells. Science 1988;242:426–430.

124. Lopez C, Pellett P, Stewart J, et al. Characteristics of human herpesvirus-6. J Infect Dis 1988;157:1271–1273.

125. Ullman S, Wilson RP, Schwartz LS. Bilateral angle-closure glaucoma in association with the acquired immune deficiency syndrome. Am J Ophthalmol 1986;101:419–424.

126. Cantrill HL, Novak A, Cameron JD, Skelnik DL. Corneal changes in CMV ocular infection. Ophthalmology 1986;94(suppl):124.

127. Benson WH, Linberg JV, Weinstein GW. Orbital pseudotumor in a patient with AIDS. Am J Ophthalmol 1988;105:697–698.

128. Fischl MA, Richman DD, Grieco MH, et al. The efficacy of azidothymidine (AZT) in the treatment of patients with AIDS and AIDS-related

complex; a double-blind, placebo-controlled trial. N Engl J Med 1987;317:185–191.

129. Yarchoan R, Klecker RW, Weinhold KJ, Markham PD, Lyerly HK, Durack DT. Administration of 3'-azido-3'-deoxythymidine, an inhibitor of HTLV-III/LAV replication, to patients with AIDS or AIDs-related complex. Lancet 1986;1:575–580.

130. Yarchoan R, Berg G, Brouwers P, et al. Response of human-immunodeficiency-virus-associated neurological disease to 3'-azido-3'-deoxythymidine. Lancet 1987;1:132–135.

131. Richman DD, Fischl MA, Grieco MH, et al. The toxicity of azidothymidine (AZT) in the treatment of patients with AIDS and AIDS-related complex; a double-blind, placebo-controlled trial. N Engl J Med 1987;317:192–197.

132. Fischl M, Galpin JE, Levine JD, Groopman JE, Henry DH, Kennedy P, Miles S, Robbins W, Starrett B, Zalusky R, et al. Recombinant human erythropoietin for patients with AIDS treated with zidovudine. N Engl J Med 1990;322:1488–1493.

133. Yarchoan R, Thomas RV, Allain JP, et al. Phase 1 studies of 2',3'-dideoxycytidine in severe human immunodeficiency virus infection as a single agent and alternating with zidovudine (AZT). Lancet 1988;1:76–81.

134. Yarchoan R, Mitsuya H, Thomas RV, et al. In vivo activity against HIV and favorable toxicity profile of 2',3'-dideoxyinosine. Science 1989;245:412–415.

135. Rook AH, Masur H, Lane HC, et al. Interleukin-2 enhances the depressed natural killer and cytomegalovirus-specific cytotoxic activities of lymphocytes from patients with the acquired immune deficiency syndrome. J Clin Invest 1983;72:398–403.

136. Grieco MH, Reddy MM, Manvar D, et al. In-vivo immunomodulation by isoprinosine in patients with the acquired immunodeficiency syndrome and related complexes. Ann Intern Med 1984;101:206–207.

137. Kaplan LD, Wolfe PR, Volberding PA, et al. Lack of response to suramin in patients with AIDS and AIDS-related complex. Am J Med 1987;82:615–620.

138. Crumpacker C, Heagy W, Bubley G, et al. Ribavirin treatment of the acquired immunodeficiency syndrome (AIDS) and the acquired-immunodeficiency-syndrome-related complex (ARC); a phase 1 study shows transient clinical improvement associated with suppression of the human immunodeficiency virus and enhanced lymphocyte proliferation. Ann Intern Med 1987;107:664–674.

139. Carter WA, Strayer DR, Brodsky I, et al. Clinical, immunological and virological effects of ampligen, a mismatched double-stranded RNA, in patients with AIDS or AIDS-related complex. Lancet 1987;1:1286–1292.

140. Kolata G. Poor results bring end to anti-AIDS drug study. New York Times 1988 Oct 14:A17, column 1.

141. Smith DH, Byrn RA, Marsters SA, Gregory T. Groopman JE, Capon DJ. Blocking of HIV-1 infectivity by a soluble, secreted form of the CD4 antigen. Science 1987;238:1704–1707.

142. Lifson JD, Hwang KM, Nara PL, et al. Synthetic CD4 peptide derivatives that inhibit HIV infection and cytopathicity. Science 1988;241:712–716.

143. Mitsuya H, Looney DJ, Kuno S, et al. Dextran sulfate suppression of viruses in the HIV family: inhibition of virion binding to CD4 + cells. Science 1988;240:646–649.

144. Abrams D, Pettinelli C, Power M, et al. A phase I–II dose ranging trial of oral dextran sulfate in HIV P24 antigen positive individuals (ACTG 060): results of a safety and efficacy trial. In: Morisset RA, ed. V International Conference of AIDS; the Scientific and Social Challenge. Montreal, Quebec, 1989. Ottawa: Intl Development Research Centre, 1989;404.

145. Surbone A, Yarchoan R, McAtee N, et al. Treatment of the acquired immunodeficiency syndrome (AIDS) and AIDS-related complex with a regimen of 3'-azido-2',3'-dideoxythymidine (azidothymidine or zidovudine) and acyclovir; a pilot study. Ann Intern Med 1988;108:534–540.

146. Hammer SM, Gillis JM. Synergistic activity of granulocyte-macrophage colony-stimulating factor and 3'-acido-3'-deoxythymidine against human immunodeficiency virus in vitro. Antimicrob Agents Chemother 1987;31:1046–1050.

147. Matthews TJ, Bolognesi DP. AIDS vaccines. Sci Am 1988;259:120–127.

148. Koff WC, Hoth DF. Development and testing of AIDS vaccines. Science 1988;241:426–432.

149. Bolognesi DP. Progress in vaccine development against SIV and HIV. J Acquir Immune Defic Syndr 1990;3:390–394.

150. Winkelstein W Jr, Wiley JA, Padian NS, et al. The San Francisco Men's Health Study: continued decline in HIV seroconversion rates among homosexual/bisexual men. Am J Public Health 1988;78:1472–1474.

151. Rutherford GW, Woo JM. Contact tracing and the control of human immunodeficiency virus infection. JAMA 1988;259:3609–3610.

152. Bayer R, Levine C, Wolf SM. HIV antibody screening; an ethical framework for evaluating proposed programs. JAMA 1986;256:1768–1774.

153. Rhame FS, Maki DG. The case for wider use of testing for HIV infection. N Engl J Med 1989;320:1248–1254.

154. Volberding PA, Lagakos SW, Koch MA, Pettinelli C, Myers MW, Booth DK, Balfour HH JR, Reichman RC, Bartlett JA, Wirsch MS, et al. Zidovudine in asymptomatic human immunodeficiency virus infection. A controlled trial in persons with fewer than 500 CD4-positive cells per cubic milliliter. The AIDS Clinical Trials Group of the National Institute of Allergy and Infectious Diseases. Engl J Med 1990;322:941–949.

155. Cotton DJ. The impact of AIDS on the medical care system. JAMA 1988;260:519–523.

156. Walters L. Ethical issues in the prevention and treatment of HIV infection and AIDS. Science 1988;239:597–603.

157. Dickens BM. Legal limits of AIDS confidentiality. JAMA 1988;259:3449–3451.

158. Henry K, Maki M, Crossley K. Analysis of the use of HIV antibody testing in a Minnesota hospital. JAMA 1988;259:229–232.

159. Bloom DE, Carliner G. The economic impact of AIDS in the United States. Science 1988;239:604–610.

160. Arno PS. The economic impact of AIDS. JAMA 1987;258:1376–1377.

161. Iglehart JK. Financing the struggle against AIDS. N Engl J Med 1987;317:180–184.

162. Andrulis DP, Beers VS, Bentley JD, Gage LS. The provision and financing of medical care for AIDS patients in US public and private teaching hospitals. JAMA 1987;258:1343–1346.

CHAPTER 6

Viral Diseases Affecting the Retina and Choroid

Mary Lou Lewis, Jean-Jacques De Laey,
James S. Tiedeman, and Robert C. Watzke

INFECTIOUS DISEASES AFFECTING THE RETINA AND CHOROID

Almost all infectious diseases of the retina and choroid are of systemic origin even if symptoms appear only in the eye. Although this chapter will discuss viral diseases, an outline follows listing the various organisms that can cause infection. For a further discussion, see References 1–7.

A. Bacteria
  1. Bacterial emboli
     a) Cardiac
     b) Dental
     c) Skin
     d) Other organs with focal abscesses
  2. Tuberculosis
  3. Nocardia
  4. Spirochetes
     a) Syphilis
     b) Lyme disease
B. Rickettsia
  1. Rocky Mountain spotted fever
  2. Typhus
C. Fungi
  1. *Candida albicans*
  2. Coccidioidomycosis
  3. Histoplasmosis
  4. Mucormycosis
  5. Aspergillosis
  6. Blastomycosis
  7. Cryptococcosis
  8. Sporotrichosis
  9. Trichosporosis

D. Parasites
  1. Toxoplasmosis
  2. Nematodes
     a) Diffuse unilateral subacute neuroretinitis (DUSN) (due to at least two as yet unidentified nematodes)
     b) Toxocariasis (canis and cati)
     c) Onchocerciasis
     d) Gnathostomiasis
  3. Ophthalmomyiasis
  4. Cysticercosis
E. Viruses
  1. Herpes Simplex type 1 (HSV-1)
  2. Herpes Simplex type 2 (HSV-2)
  3. Varicella Zoster Virus (VZV)
  4. Rubella
  5. Rubeola
  6. Epstein-Barr Virus (EBV)
  7. Cytomegalovirus (CMV)—see Chapter 5, Acquired Immune Deficiency Syndrome (AIDS)
  8. Rift Valley fever
  9. Mumps
  10. Nonspecific reaction to viruses—postviral syndrome

INTRODUCTION

DNA (herpes viruses) and RNA (rubella, measles) group viruses have a cytolytic effect on the retina. Viruses are obligatory intracellular parasites that cause necrosis and proliferation on a cell-to-cell basis; therefore, viral infections result in severe, often irreversible damage to tissues (8). In addition, the strong antigenicity of viruses may stimulate the immune system, causing immune complex deposition that results in vasculitis and increased vascular permeability leading to retinal ischemia (8). Immunocompromised individuals, tissue transplant recipients and/or those who have been treated with immunosuppressant drugs, patients with immune-mediated diseases or diseases of lymphocyte dysfunction such as acquired immunodeficiency syndrome (AIDS), renal dialysis patients, or burn victims are all more susceptible than are healthy individuals to viral infections of the retina (8).

RUBEOLA

The rubeola virus contains RNA and belongs to the myxovirus group. It is transmitted by direct contact and affects primarily children. The acute illness (measles) is usually mild with fever and rash. One of the most devastating consequences of this infection is the late occurrence of subacute sclerosing panencephalitis (SSPE). Immunization programs have been the only means of decreasing the incidence of SSPE.

Acute Rubeola

Acute rubeola (measles) is highly contagious and usually acquired in childhood. A nonspecific conjunctivitis is common, with conjunctival injection, tearing, and photophobia, which resolve spontaneously without sequelae. Within a week of the onset of the rash, 0.1% to 0.2% of patients develop acute encephalitis manifested by fever, drowsiness, irritability, meningismus, vomiting, and headache. Convulsions and coma, as well as optic neuritis, occur frequently with encephalitis. Rarely, rubeola may cause a severe bilateral neuroretinitis. The onset of neuroretinitis usually occurs 1 to 2 weeks after the initial rash appears. At this time, there is diffuse optic disc and macular edema with venous dilation and often a star figure in the macula. Visual loss is often dramatic (9, 10). The edema subsides, and usually some improvement in

vision follows, but secondary optic atrophy, vascular attenuation, and pigmentary degeneration ensue in weeks to months. The electroretinogram (ERG) is abnormal; visual fields are constricted; and central vision is usually severely decreased. Visual loss resulting from the optic neuritis and pigmentary degeneration may progress over many years. One well-documented case exists in which the degeneration had progressed so completely that the fundus developed an appearance similar to that of pigmented paravenous retinochoroidal atrophy, with sharply outlined zones of atrophy of the retinal pigment epithelium (RPE) that follow the course of the major retinal veins and bilateral, symmetrical migration of pigment into the retina surrounding the retinal veins. However, in pigmented paravenous retinochoroidal atrophy, the optic nerve, retinal vessels, electrophysiological tests, and visual acuity are normal, and many patients are asymptomatic (11). Measles retinopathy may also resemble retinitis pigmentosa, with scattered bone spicule pigmentation in the peripheral retina, optic atrophy, and attenuated vessels.

There is no specific treatment available for the retinopathy. The visual deficit may be managed by utilization of visual aids and training.

Measles may also affect the fetus if the mother is infected during the first trimester of pregnancy. Cardiopathy, cataracts, and retinopathy may occur. The newborn may have a pigmentary retinopathy resembling the salt-and-pepper or stippled pigmentary changes seen in congenital rubella retinopathy. As in rubella, the vision is good, and electrophysiologic tests are normal (12).

Subacute Sclerosing Panencephalitis

Introduction

Subacute sclerosing panencephalitis (SSPE) is a degenerative disease of the central nervous system occuring in children and adolescents. It was first described by Dawson (13) in 1933, then by van Bogaert

Table 6.1. Stages of Rubeola Retinopathy

6 to 12 days after rash:
Acute retinopathy: neuroretinitis, disc edema, dilated vessels, macular star, and occasional retinal hemorrhages.

2 to 8 weeks:

Vision improves; chorioretinal pigmentation—salt-and-pepper or heavy, clumped branching pigmentation in the periphery, attenuated vessels, disc pallor.

2+ months:

Late retinopathy: fundus lesions may progress to resemble retinitis pigmentosa, optic atrophy, and attenuated vessels or pigmented paravenous retinochoroidal atrophy. The ERG is often depressed.

and De Busscher (14), and later by Pette and Doring (15). Histopathologically, inclusion bodies indicate viral infection of the cells involved. When Dawson (13) observed inclusion bodies in the nerve cells and neuroglial cells in a 16-year-old patient who died from SSPE, a viral origin of the disease was considered. Its possible relationship with measles was first suspected by Bouteille et al. (16), who used electron microscopy to demonstrate the presence of the nucleocapsid of a virus similar to the measles virus in the brains of SSPE patients. Connolly et al. (17) noted high measles antibody titers in blood and cerebrospinal fluid (CSF) of SSPE patients and, using immunofluorescence, found measles antigens in the brain. A virus closely related to the measles virus was isolated from brain tissue samples by Horta-Barbosa et al. (18) and Payne et al. (19). However, some studies suggest antigenic differences between the slow virus causing SSPE and the virus causing measles (20).

Epidemiology

Measles virus plays an important role in the pathogenesis of SSPE. Epidemiological studies indicate a positive measles history in 93% of confirmed SSPE patients, almost half of whom contracted measles before their second birthday (21, 22). In industrialized countries, measles is rare in this age group.

About 85% of the patients present the first neurological signs between 5 and 15 years of age (23). The disease is 2 to 4 times more frequent in boys than in girls, but the male-to-female ratio decreases with increasing age at onset (22). Another remarkable feature of SSPE is that its incidence is almost 6 times higher in rural areas, particularly in farming communities, than it is in large cities. A number of studies underline the fact that most SSPE patients come from large families and that they have contracted measles at home from siblings. Usually, it is the youngest child that develops SSPE. From these different facts, Aaby et al. (21) suggested that SSPE results from intensive exposure to measles.

Systemic Manifestations (24)

According to Jabbour et al. (25), the clinical course of SSPE can be divided into four stages (Table 6.2).

The first stage is quite insidious. The parents observe a decrease in school performance, some mental regression, and an increased irritability. In the first stage,

Table 6.2. Stages of SSPE[a]

Stage 1: Cerebral signs (mental-behavioral): irritability, affectionate displays, lethargy, forgetfulness, indifference, withdrawal, drooling, regressive speech, slurred speech.
Stage 2: Convulsion, motor signs: myoclonus of head, limbs, trunk; incoordination of trunk and limbs; dyskinesia-choreoathetoid postures, movements, tremors.
Stage 3: Coma, opisthotonos: no responsiveness to any stimulus; extensor hypertonus; decerebrate rigidity; irregular, stertorous respiration.
Stage 4: Mutism, loss of function of cerebral cortex, myoclonus: pathological laughter, crying, wandering of eyes, flexion of upper and lower limbs, hypotonia, turning of head to one side, occasional limb myoclonus, startling by noise.

[a]Adapted from Jabbour JT, Garcia JH, Lemmi H, et al. Subacute sclerosing panencephalitis; a multidisciplinary study of eight cases. JAMA 1969; 207:2248–2254.

neurological signs, such as intention tremor or involuntary movements, may appear; however, ocular symptoms, such as decreased vision from maculopathy, may be the initial reason patients seek medical advice.

After a few weeks to several months, stage 2 begins. This stage is mainly characterized by myoclonic jerks, consisting of a rapid flexion movement followed by a slow relaxing component. The clinical diagnosis in stage 2 is confirmed by the presence of paroxysmal bursts of high voltage discharge on the EEG, occurring simultaneously with the myoclonus. The mental deterioration progresses, although remissions may sometimes be observed.

Stage 3 is characterized by an increase in spasticity, with decerebrate rigidity and coma following. Sometimes the body temperature increases, probably as a consequence of the dysregulation of autonomic functions.

In Stage 4, the severe hypertonia may diminish, and myoclonus becomes less frequent. This often gives rise to false hopes of recovery; however, all central functions are eventually lost. The disease is fatal, with most patients dying within 5 to 12 months of the onset.

The clinical diagnosis is confirmed by the typical EEG changes, the finding of increased gammaglobulins in the CSF, and high titers of measles antibodies in serum and CSF. Brain biopsy reveals perivascular lymphoblastic infiltrative involvement of neurons and glial cells.

Ocular Manifestations

Ocular symptoms or signs are found in almost 50% of SSPE patients at some time during the disease (26). These symptoms may be divided into three groups (27):

1. Disturbance of higher visual functions, such as visual hallucinations or cortical blindness (28);
2. Motility problems: ocular muscle palsies, supranuclear palsies, ptosis, nystagmus;
3. Ocular fundus changes: papilledema, optic neuritis, optic atrophy, (macular) retinitis.

In exceptional cases, exophthalmos has been decribed in the course of SSPE (29); it may be related to bilateral cavernous sinus thrombosis. The involvement of the optic disc is related to the cerebral manifestations of the disease. Papilledema is an essential sign of the pseudotumor cerebri form of the disease (30). Intranuclear inclusions may be found in the optic nerve by histopathology, explaining the occurrence of optic neuritis (31).

The most striking ocular manifestation is the necrotizing retinitis that was first described by Otradovec in 1963 (32). The lesion is characterized by edema, retinal folds, sometimes superficial hemorrhages, and the absence of inflammatory signs in the vitreous (Fig. 6.1). The lesion usually is solitary, but both eyes may be affected, and more widespread involvement outside the posterior pole is also possible (33). The retinitis may be associated with a localized serous detachment of the neuroepithelium or of the retinal pigment epithelium. Fluorescein angiography performed in the acute stage of the retinitis may reveal some staining of the lesion. More widespread diffusion on fluorescein angiography has been described, mimicking that seen in Harada's disease (33). In the cicatricial stage, the fundus lesions are more or less atrophic and exhibit irregular pigmentation (Fig. 6.2). Modifications of the macular reflexes are sometimes especially striking. Preretinal membranes have been described, as well as macular holes. Because the manifestations in the fundus may precede the neurological signs by several months, these cases are often misdiagnosed. In cases with bilateral involvement, they may be diagnosed as juvenile macular degeneration. The lesion is sometimes mistaken for toxoplasmic chorioretinitis (34).

On histopathology, the internal nuclear layer and the ganglion cells appear more severely affected than the outer retinal layers (35). Disorganization of the RPE and even fragmentation of Bruch's membrane

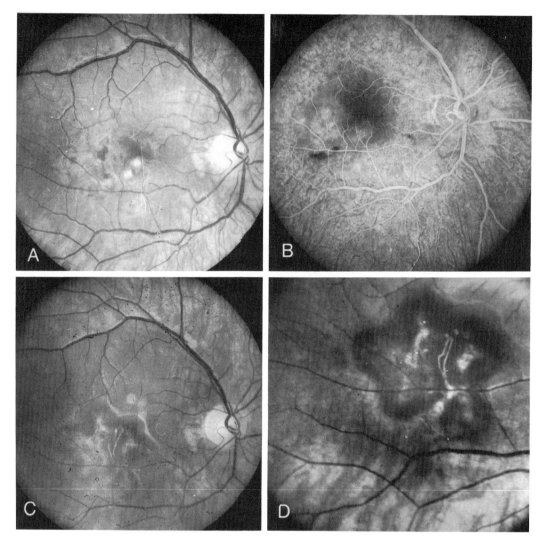

Figure 6.1. **A** and **B**. Ophthalmoscopic and fluorescein angiographic findings at presentation (June 1980). Note the retinal infiltrates. (With permission Doc Ophthalmol.) **C**. Same patient (Sept. 1980). Note the vertical split in the macular region (rupture of the internal limiting membrane). **D**. (Feb. 1981) Note irregular light reflexes. (Reprinted, with permission, from: De Laey JJ, Hanssens M, Colette P, et al. Doc Ophthalmol 1983;56:11–21.)

may occur. Retinal folds and detachment of the inner limiting membrane are observed (Fig. 6.3) (36). The affected retina may be modified into fibroglial scar tissue. The scarcity of inflammatory cells is striking, although, depending on the intensity of the response, marked infiltrates of macrophages are sometimes seen in the retina and choroid (33). Inclusion bodies may be found in the retina (37). Electron microscopy of the retina has demonstrated the

presence of tubular filaments of a paramyxovirus (38), indicating that the fundus lesions due to SSPE are a direct consequence of the viral infection.

Prevention and Treatment

Although SSPE has been described in children who were vaccinated against measles, the incidence of SSPE has dramatically dropped in populations where

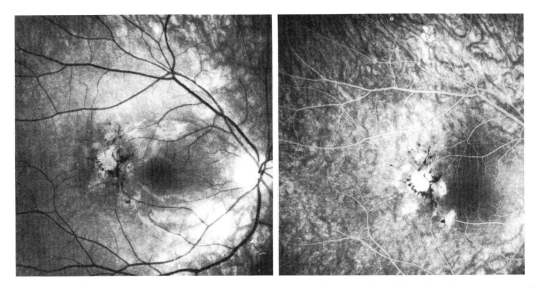

Figure 6.2. Appearance of the fundus and fluorescein angiogram of late pigmentary changes.

mass measles vaccination has been introduced (39). The occurrence of SSPE in vaccinated children can be explained either by incomplete efficacy of the vaccine or by exposure to measles prior to vaccination; this occurs more frequently when children are vaccinated at an older age.

Most antiviral agents have little beneficial effect on the course of SSPE (23).

Amantadine hydrochloride, an anti-DNA agent that blocks the penetration of virus into host cells, has proved to be of limited value in treating SSPE. Isoprinosine (Inosiplex) has variable antiviral activity but also has a possible immunomodulating effect (40). Isoprinosine was found to improve or stabilize SSPE patients. The recommended dosage is 100 mg/kg/day in

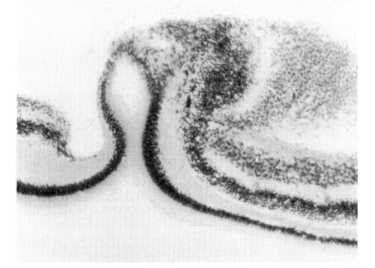

Figure 6.3. Retinal folds in macular region. (Reprinted, with permission, from: De Laey JJ, Hanssens M, Colette P, et al. Doc Ophthalmol 1983;56:11–21.)

divided doses. Treatment should be initiated as early as possible. Because recurrences have been reported in patients in remission whose treatment was ceased, isoprinosine therapy should be continued after apparent remission (23). Panitch et al. (41) recently reported the beneficial effect of repeated intraventricular injections of interferon.

RUBELLA

The rubella virus is common and highly contagious and usually causes a mild infection in children and adults. However, the infection of the fetus in the first trimester is often severe and can have devastating consequences. Fortunately, as a result of immunization programs in the United States, congenital rubella is rare. However, since 20% of the women of child-bearing age in the United States continue to be susceptible to rubella (42), the danger still exists that, if we become complacent, this damaging disease may return. Other countries, particularly the Caribbean Islands, have a much higher incidence of congenital rubella, and with the increasing mobility of the world population, these cases may be seen in any country.

Transmission

Transmission is by direct contact. The clinical signs and symptoms are unreliable for the diagnosis of the disease, and serological confirmation is essential for proof of infection. If symptoms occur, they are usually mild, with fever, lymphadenopathy, and rash. In the fetus, however, the infection results in a serious illness, especially in the first trimester.

Congenital Rubella

Transmission

The maternal infection is often clinically insignificant, with no signs of illness. Viremia occurs within 10 to 12 days of the maternal infection, and the virus crosses the placental barrier and infects the fetus

(43). Reinfection may occur in women who acquired antibodies by infection with live rubella virus vaccines and, years later, became reinfected, but the risk of damage to the fetus in these patients is small (42, 44). Of fetuses infected during the first trimester of pregnancy, 81% will develop one or more of the stigmata of congenital rubella (42). It is a chronic infection beginning in fetal life and continuing into infancy. The virus is excreted for long periods after birth (43). A significant number of the children who have this infection are normal at birth but develop signs of the syndrome later in life (42, 45).

Systemic Manifestations

Hearing loss may be the most common manifestation, but it is difficult to diagnose and is underreported. Heart disease occurs in 67% to 69% of patients with congenital rubella (46). These children may have acute thrombocytopenia at birth, low birth weight, and feeding difficulties. Psychomotor retardation, mental retardation, and/or microcephaly may occur. In 20% to 50% of these children, delayed manifestations occur, including endocrinopathies, deafness, ocular disease (see below), vascular effects, and progressive rubella panencephalitis (42, 45). Most of these children's mothers had rubella in the second or third trimester of the pregnancy. Mechanisms to explain delayed manifestations include continued growth of the virus in tissues, autoimmune responses, genetic susceptibility, vascular damage by the viral infection, and reactive hypervascularization (45).

Ocular Manifestations (47–49)

Ocular involvement occurs in 43% of children with clinical evidence of congenital rubella (43). Cataract and pigmentary retinopathy are the most common ocular manifestations.

Rubella retinopathy consists of a salt-and-pepper pigmentary change or a mottled, blotchy, irregular pigmentation, usually with the greatest density in the macula (Fig. 6.4). The foveal reflex is absent. Pigmentary changes may be found only in the macula or only in the periphery. Monocular involvement may occur, or only one or two quadrants may be involved. The peripheral pigmentary changes are more likely to appear stippled or dust-like. The pigment is usually at a uniform depth under the retinal vessels. The optic nerve may be pale; the retinal vessels are normal. There is minimal to no effect on retinal function. Visual acuity and visual fields are normal and usually do not change with time. Observation of this typical pigmentary retinopathy should raise the question of a congenital rubella infection. The mother may have had no symptoms, but antibody titers may help to establish the diagnosis (49). Development and progression of the pigmentary retinopathy after birth has been reported in cases of congenital rubella (50). It is possible that, after birth, the virus may proliferate in the retinal pigment epithelium as it does in other tissues (50). Fluorescein angiography shows window defects and blocked fluorescence corresponding to the pigmentary changes in the fundus. The formation of a choroidal neovascular membrane in the macula occurs rarely as a late complication and is probably a manifestation of the damage to the RPE due to the rubella infection (Fig. 6.5) (51, 52); this may result in significant reduction in visual acuity.

Other ocular manifestations include glaucoma with optic atrophy and decreased vision, transient corneal clouding (53, 54), microphthalmus, nystagmus, high refractive error, strabismus, and iris hypoplasia. Cataract with microphthalmus has been noted to have a particularly poor prognosis (43, 46).

Differential Diagnosis

The differential diagnosis of pigmentary retinopathy includes rubella retinopathy, tapetoretinal degeneration, choroideremia, ocular albinism, syphilis, and rarely, other viral retinopathies (55). Tapetoretinal degeneration can usually be identified by the severely abnormal or absent electroretinogram. Family history will help rule out choroideremia (51). The retinopathy of syphilis may resemble that of ru-

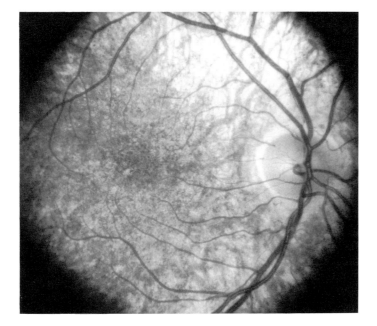

Figure 6.4. Typical rubella retinopathy in a patient with excellent central vision.

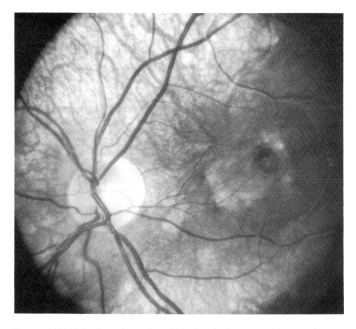

Figure 6.5. Rubella retinopathy with subretinal neovascular membrane.

bella retinopathy. The ERG is usually normal, but the retinal vessels are attenuated, and there may be optic atrophy in severe cases. The serology is most important in this diagnosis. Other viral infections, such as morbilli, varicella, and influenza, are only rarely transmitted transplacentally (55, 56). Exposure to radiation in the first trimester of pregnancy may result in a pigmentary retinopathy, cataract, and/or microphthalmia (55). Congenital toxoplasmosis can usually be recognized by the characteristic chorioretinal scars, with heavy pigmentation at the edges, occurring often in the macula. Grouped pigmentation or "bear tracks" is a form of developmental change in the RPE and is usually easily recognized by pigment groups in one sector that have a pattern like foot prints. Various viruses, including rubella, may rarely result in a pigmentary retinopathy similar to that of congenital rubella when the infection occurs in childhood.

Treatment

Prevention is the most effective form of treatment, and immunization programs have been highly effective, almost eliminating the congenital rubella syndrome in the United States. However, it is estimated that 20% of women of child-bearing age are susceptible to rubella, so congenital infection is still possible (42).

Rubella retinopathy does not require treatment. The choroidal neovascular membranes, which rarely occur, do so later in life. They usually involve the center of the foveal avascular zone or have already formed scars, and most are not amenable to laser treatment (51, 52).

MUMPS VIRUS

Transmission

The mumps virus is a myxovirus transmitted via the airborne route from the saliva of the infected person to the respiratory tract of the new host (57).

Ocular Manifestations

These include follicular conjunctivitis, keratitis, iritis, scleritis, episcleritis, uveitis, glaucoma, extraocular muscle paresis, lacrimal gland inflammation, optic neuritis, choroiditis, and, rarely, central retinal vein occlusion (58–73).

Meningitis and encephalitis may occur within 2 weeks of the onset of the infection, and recovery is usual. Optic neuritis is the most common ocular complication associated with meningitis and encephalitis and is usually bilateral and rarely retrobulbar. The disc is hyperemic, and there is surrounding edema of the retina with visual loss and visual field defects. Although some cases are left with permanent visual deficit, fortunately most cases experience recovery of vision (62, 63, 74). Rare cases of uveitis and chorioretinitis have been reported (75, 76). Generally, the ocular changes are not serious.

Maternal infection with the mumps virus has been reported to result in fetal damage, including congenital cataracts, nystagmus, optic atrophy, and retinal lesions (74, 77).

EPSTEIN-BARR VIRUS

The Epstein-Barr virus has been implicated in the etiology of multifocal choroiditis associated with panuveitis, but Koch's law has not been met as yet. Koch's law states that, to establish the specificity of a pathogenic microorganism, it must be present in all cases of the disease; inoculations of its pure culture must produce the same disease in animals; and from these, it must be again obtained and propagated in pure cultures. The Epstein-Barr virus is a ubiquitous virus, and most adults have been infected with it (78), whether or not they have had a clinically recognized episode of infectious mononucleosis, the prototypical illness caused by the virus (79, 80). The relationship of the Epstein-Barr virus to ocular disease has thus far been demonstrated through observing the occurrence of specific patterns of viral antibodies in patients with syndromes of clinically recognized chorioretinitis.

Typically, a virus is confirmed serologically to be the cause of a clinical disease when a rise in the antibody titer to the virus has been demonstrated during the time of illness (acute and convalescent titers). In the case of the Epstein-Barr virus, specific classes of antibodies are produced that can give evidence as to the status of viral replication within the host without the clinician necessarily having to rely on the finding of changing antibody titers (81, 82). Upon primary infection with Epstein-Barr virus, the first host immunological response is the production of IgG and IgM class antibodies against the structural viral capsid antigens (VCA). Both IgG and IgM antibody titers rise rapidly following primary infection. Although the IgG antibodies persist throughout life, the IgM antibodies return to undetectable levels after the clinical illness has resolved.

Another class of antibodies occurring in Epstein-Barr infection is directed against the so-called early antigens (EA). These protein antigens are coded by the viral DNA and produced in the host cell. The appearance of EA antibodies occurs early in the course of Epstein-Barr infection and subsequently falls to undetectable levels after the acute infection has passed.

A final class of antibodies is those against the Epstein-Barr nuclear antigens (EBNA). Once infected, the host always retains a small fraction of infected B lymphocytes. Over a lifetime, these cells may be targeted and lysed by activated T lymphocytes, thereby releasing EBNA. Thus EBNA antibodies continue to remain in a host that has been infected at any time in the past.

A person who has had an infection with the Epstein-Barr virus in the past, which has now resolved, is then expected to have VCA-IgG antibodies and EBNA antibodies but not VCA-IgM or EA antibodies. The presence of EBNA antibodies is strong evidence that the infection has not been recently acquired, since they take months to develop. EA and VCA-IgM antibodies are evidence of a productive, lytic infection, although there are some apparently healthy adults who have persistently detectable but low EA titers. The simultaneous presence of EBNA along with either VCA-IgM or EA antibodies suggests that infection was acquired in the relatively distant past but that active viral replication is currently taking place.

Against this background, there have been three published reports of chorioretinal disease associated with the Epstein-Barr virus. In the first, Tiedeman (83) reported 10 patients with a multifocal choroiditis and mild panuveitis who all showed elevated EA and/or VCA-IgM titers. These patients had many findings similar to those that exist in the presumed ocular histoplasmosis syndrome (POHS), including multiple, small chorioretinal scars, peripapillary pigmentary changes, macular and peripapillary choroidal neovascularization, and disciform scarring (Fig. 6.6A and B, Fig. 6.7A and B). These patients differ distinctly from patients with POHS, however, in that all had vitreous inflammatory cells and typically ran a chronic course consisting of multiple episodes of the development of new active lesions. The patients described in this series fit the clinical descriptions of several other authors. Nozik and Dorsch (84), Dreyer and Gass (85), Watzke et al. (86), and Morgan and Schatz (87) have described clinical series that may include patients with the same disease process.

The patients range in age from the adolescent to the elderly, but most are young adults. There is a slight female preponderance. Symptoms described by these patients include blurring, metamorphopsia, floaters, peripheral and central scotomata, and photopsias. Some patients described a viral or "flu-like" febrile illness just prior to developing ocular symptoms.

Physical findings in this syndrome include decreased visual acuity, ranging from 20/20 to light perception. Involvement may be bilateral or unilateral, and many unilateral cases subsequently become bilateral. The lesions in the fundus are discrete and vary in number from a few to several hundred. Acute lesions are described as yellow to gray at the level of the RPE. Shallow serous detachment of the neurosensory retina may occur over active lesions (Fig. 6.8). Inactive lesions appear as punched-out lesions with or without pigment. Lesions may occur in random lo-

cations throughout the posterior pole and the midperiphery or may occur in clusters or rows (Fig. 6.8). A mild papillitis may occur along with an afferent pupillary defect. In some patients, the finding of vitreous cells, and, in some, anterior chamber cells, has been noted in all series except that of Watzke and associates (86). None of the patients has remained systemically ill, but some have shown chronic lymphadenopathy, splenomegaly, hearing loss, and skin changes (83, 85).

Wong and associates (88) studied three patients with chronic, systemic Epstein-Barr infection and described bilateral anterior uveitis or panuveitis in all three. One patient was described as having multiple chorioretinal scars in the midperiphery. This scarring appears to be compatible with the scarring described in the previous series. Patients in the Wong series showed evidence of some improvement when treated with systemic and/or topical acyclovir.

Treatment

In addition to antiviral therapy, such as acyclovir as mentioned above, steroid treatment for inflammatory changes may be beneficial. Also, laser treatment has been found effective in some cases of this syndrome complicated by choroidal neovascularization (89).

In another report, Raymond and associates (90) described a case of punctate outer retinitis in a patient with acute infectious mononucleosis. This seven-year-old boy had punctate outer retinal lesions, pigment epithelial disturbance, and vitreous cells. His Epstein-Barr viral serology clearly demonstrated primary infection at the time of initial presentation, with retinitis as evidenced by the presence of VCA-IgM and absence of EBNA antibodies. In subsequent follow-up, he developed EBNA antibodies and a drop in VCA-IgM titer. The patient also had a *Toxoplasma* IgG antibody titer, but it remained unchanged during the period of follow-up.

Before ascribing a causative role to any agent, care must be taken that its presence

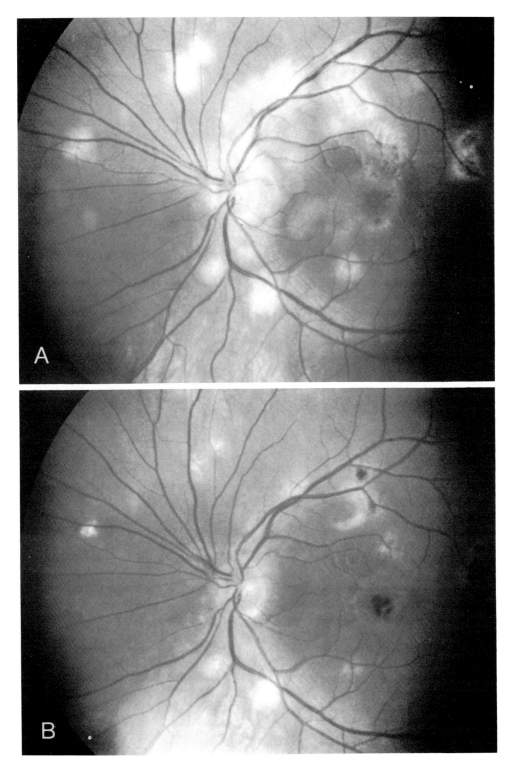

Figure 6.6. A. 23 year old had vision of 20/25. Note the punched out scars, peripapillary changes, and active macular lesions. **B**. The same patient as in Fig. 6.1A, 6 months later. The lesions are now inactive, the macula is heavily pigmented, and vision was 20/20.

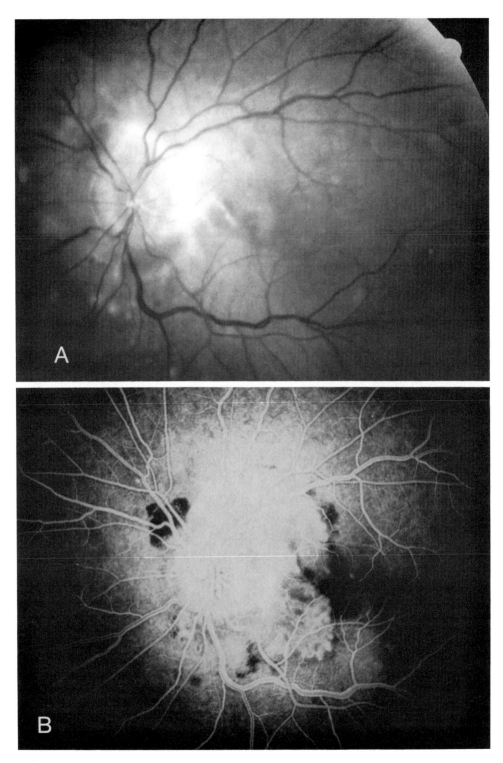

Figure 6.7. A. A patient with peripapillary scarring has developed a peripapillary choroidal neovascular membrane. **B**. The fluorescein angiogram shows the large peripapillary neovascular membrane more distinctly.

190

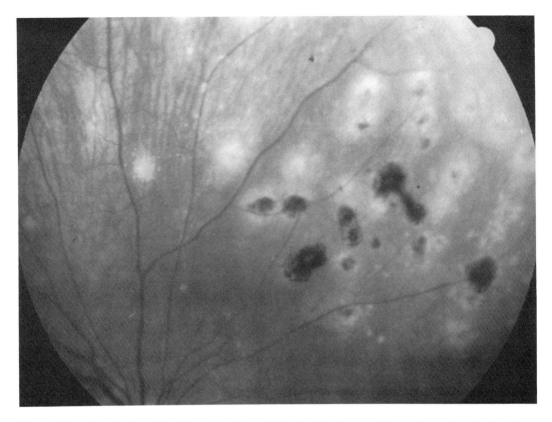

Figure 6.8. Lesions in the midperiphery in clusters. Note the differing age of the lesions. Acute lesions have overlying subretinal fluid.

can be demonstrated in actual diseased tissue. Clinical descriptions of patients with multiple chorioretinal lesions abound, and these cases are usually lumped together or given separate status based on clinically observable criteria. Many diseases thus split into separate groups on the basis of clinical appearances may indeed be the same etiologically, and some entities grouped together as one disease because of clinical similarities may have very different causes. Confusion may occur when a clinical picture has been ascribed to more than one cause, such as the case of Raymond et al. (90), in which the description is also consistent with punctate outer toxoplasmosis (91). The hazards of using serology to confirm a clinical diagnosis have been emphasized by Rothova et al. (92), who found a 100% prevalence of IgG *Toxoplasma* an-

tibodies using the ELISA technique in patients with definite ocular toxoplasmosis. They also found a 58% prevalence of antibodies in a control group without ocular toxoplasmosis. The level of titer did not correlate with ocular disease, nor did any rise in the titer occur during episodes of active ocular infection. Worley et al. (93) similarly demonstrated a prevalence of antibody to *Toxocara canis* (equal to or greater than 1:32 by the ELISA test) in 23.1% of kindergarten children who had no evidence of ocular toxocariasis. These examples demonstrate the high likelihood of a false-positive diagnosis using serological evidence in what appears to be an appropriate clinical picture.

Many questions regarding the relationship of the Epstein-Barr virus to chorioretinal disease remain unanswered. The virus may be able to infect RPE or neurosensory retina cells directly. Typically, the Epstein-Barr virus infects B lymphocytes, but evidence for the possibility that it infects epithelial cells also exists (94–96), and the association of the Epstein-Barr virus with nasopharyngeal carcinoma has been well established. Subretinal fibrosis has been ascribed to transformed B cell lines, and it could be speculated that this might be related to Epstein-Barr infection as well. Of course, the possibility of the antibody response being related to a more global abnormality of the immune system cannot be overlooked. The ultimate role of the Epstein-Barr virus in chorioretinal disease awaits further elucidation.

HERPES SIMPLEX VIRUS TYPE 1 (HSV-1)

Transmission

Infection of HSV-1 is transmitted by direct contact in children and adults.

Clinical Manifestations

Primary infection often is more severe than recurrent infection, but the latter is more common. The virus remains dormant in nerve ganglia until an event such as physical trauma, sunburn (ultraviolet energy), or stress stimulates a recurrence. The virus then travels to the dermatome of the involved nerve, causing a cold sore or vesicular eruption. Herpetic dendritic keratitis may also result from recurrent HSV-1 infections. Although HSV-1 rarely causes genital lesions, it may be transmitted to neonates and may result in systemic infection and chorioretinitis (97–98). Infection with this virus can also cause a severe encephalitis in children and adults that may be associated with retinal hemorrhages, vasculitis, retinitis, and/or exudative retinal detachment. Encephalitis is an uncommon but devastating disease that has a high morbidity and mortality (99–106). The incidence of retinitis associated with encephalitis is probably higher than reported because the patients are critically ill and examination of the retina may be overlooked.

Treatment

Antivirals administered intravenously have been successful in improving the prognosis in cases of encephalitis due to HSV-1 infection. Both adenosine arabinoside (Ara-A) and acyclovir have been shown to decrease mortality, especially when started early in the infection (100). Acyclovir has been shown to be beneficial for immunosuppressed patients with labial or oropharyngeal herpetic lesions (107).

HSV-1 has been cultured in cases of acute retinal necrosis (ARN) (108). (See the section on ARN, below.)

HERPES SIMPLEX VIRUS TYPE 2 (HSV-2)

Transmission

HSV-2 is transmitted by direct sexual contact and results in recurrent, painful genital ulcers (genital herpes). Genital-ocular transmission has been reported (109). The virus is transmitted to the neonate by contact with herpetic cervicitis in the mother during the infant's passage through the birth canal or by contact with infected maternal fluids when the membranes rupture prematurely (110). The risk of infection of the neonate is about 40% when the virus is present at the time of delivery (111). Transplacental transmission has been suspected in rare instances (112, 113). The diagnosis of neonatal herpes infection is usually made by demonstrating a history of recurrent genital herpes or recent exposure to genital herpes in the mother or father. Acute and convalescent viral titers may be helpful. Since 90% of the population have antibody titers to HSV-1 or 2, markedly high rising and/or falling titers may indicate active disease.

Clinical Manifestations

HSV-2 is rarely seen in labial or corneal lesions and is usually the cause of genital herpes. It is characterized by recurrent, painful genital ulcers. Transmission by direct contact from genital infection to the eye may result in conjunctivitis or keratitis (109). The neonatal infection is most often a disseminated infection, with the primary involvement being a severe encephalitis having a high morbidity and mortality (114–116). One-fifth of these encephalitis cases have ocular involvement (115) that may include conjunctivitis, keratitis, cataract, muscle palsies, and retinitis (97, 110, 117). The patient may develop retinal hemorrhages, cotton-wool patches, necrotizing retinitis, vasculitis, retinal detachment, and/or optic neuritis (110, 112–115, 117–127).

Acute Retinal Necrosis (ARN)

The retinitis described in some cases of HSV-2 infections is very similar to the retinitis that occurs in ARN in that they both may show vasculitis, retinal hemorrhage, and areas of retinal necrosis. (See the section on ARN, below.)

Follow-up ocular examinations of children who survive neonatal encephalitis are important to identify late changes such as strabismus, corneal changes, optic atrophy, macular changes, and late onset of cataract (112).

Treatment

Acyclovir has been successfully used to prevent recurrences of genital herpes (128, 129) and has been effective in treating immunosuppressed patients, as well (130). Antivirals have been shown to have a beneficial effect in neonatal herpes encephalitis, but some also have serious side effects. Acyclovir, which has been very beneficial in some viral infections, is specific only for the cells actually infected with the virus and has very few systemic side effects. Because treatment is most beneficial when started early, prompt diagnosis is important. Since the eye may be the route of entry for the virus, prophylactic topical ocular treatment with vidarabine has been recommended for infants born to infected mothers either vaginally or via cesarian

section 4 or more hours after rupture of the membranes (113). If signs of encephalitis occur, intravenous treatment with antivirals is indicated.

Histopathology

Histopathological studies of a case of HSV-2 endophthalmitis have revealed viral particles in the area of transition between normal and necrotic retina, suggesting that direct viral infection of the retina rather than an immune reaction was responsible for the retinal changes. These findings support treatment specific to the viral infection, as well as for the inflammatory reaction, rather than just for the inflammatory reaction (131).

VARICELLA ZOSTER VIRUS (VZV)

Chicken Pox and Herpes Zoster (Shingles)

Transmission

The primary infection known as chicken pox (varicella zoster virus) is transmitted by direct contact and is highly infectious in infancy and childhood. Reactivation of the virus resulting in herpes zoster, or shingles, occurs most frequently in the elderly but also occurs in adults and, rarely, in children. The virus is reactivated from a nerve ganglion and travels along the nerve to the cutaneous distribution or dermatome, resulting in a crop of painful vesicles. Immunosuppressed individuals are much more likely to contract varicella or develop zoster and are more likely to have disseminated disease. Congenital infection, though rare, has been reported when the mother has contracted varicella infection during pregnancy, thus infecting the fetus.

Clinical Manifestations

Chicken pox is usually a mild illness in children, who exhibit a typical vesicular rash, often over the whole body. The infection is often more serious in adults. The encephalitis produced by varicella is rare and usually more benign than that which occurs in measles, German measles, or influenza (132). In some cases, the headaches of encephalitis occur before the chicken pox rash appears, whereas in other cases, the encephalitis occurs after the rash has cleared (133). Optic neuritis may cause severe decrease in vision, but recovery usually occurs (132, 134). Transient, yellow-white macular lesions have been reported (134). Other ocular complications include involvement of the skin of the lids, conjunctivitis, keratitis, iridocyclitis, uveitis, optic atrophy, and/or cranial nerve palsies (135, 136). Disseminated chicken pox occurs most frequently in immunosuppressed individuals. Congenital infection may produce microphthalmos, chorioretinitis, cataract, limb deformities, cicatricial skin lesions, and/or brain damage in the fetus (137).

Adults with recurrent herpes zoster (shingles) develop vesicular skin lesions in the dermatome of the involved nerve after the virus is reactivated from the ganglion. These patients often have a few vesicles (like chicken pox) elsewhere on the body (138). The post-herpetic neuralgia is one of the most debilitating sequelae of the disease (135). The deep, boring pain located in the area previously affected by the vesicles is unresponsive to most treatment and is unbearable in some patients. Several investigators feel that the use of systemic steroids during the acute illness diminishes the frequency and severity of post-herpetic neuralgia (139–142). The use of steroids is controversial, however, because of the danger of generalized dissemination of the disease, which is thought to be caused by the immunosuppression induced by the steroids. The authors who have administered steroids to their patients have not seen this complication, but patients already receiving steroids for other systemic conditions appear to have an increased risk of disseminated zoster. Patients may have a predisposing condition, such as advanced age, stress, trauma, exposure to irradiation, surgery (especially of the trigeminal nerve), heavy metal poi-

soning, or pharmacological immunosuppression, which increases their likelihood of developing zoster (138, 143). Patients with predisposing systemic diseases also have an increased incidence of dissemination. These include leukemia, lymphoma, other malignant neoplastic diseases, tuberculosis, ileitis, syphilis, and immunodeficiency syndromes, especially HIV infection (138, 143–146). Disseminated disease, although it occurs infrequently, has been observed in 2% to 10% of cases that have been reported by referral centers where the more severe cases are seen (146, 147). Systemic evaluation for occult neoplasm or immunosuppression (HIV infection) should be considered in young patients who develop zoster and do not have an obvious predisposing condition (146–150). However, Lightman (151) has shown that most patients in his study were healthy; only 1.2% of the patients he observed had malignancies, all of which had been previously diagnosed. Hemorrhagic complications such as subdural and subarachnoid bleeding are possible in patients with zoster who are also taking coumadin (152, 153).

Herpes Zoster Ophthalmicus

Herpes zoster ophthalmicus occurs when the nasociliary nerve and the nerves in the distribution of the first and second division of the trigeminal nerve are involved (142). The inflammation ordinarily begins with a vesicular rash on one side of the face. When vesicles appear on the tip of the nose on the same side of the face as the other vesicles, this indicates the involvement of the nasociliary nerve and probably the involvement of the globe. The skin lesions around the eye may be severe. Cutaneous vesicles and ulcerations become virologically sterile within about a week and usually heal within about 2 weeks, but sometimes they require several weeks or months to heal. Secondary infection, usually with *Staphylococcus aureus* or *Streptococcus* may cause cicatrization with trichiasis, loss of lashes, entropion, ectropion, or stenosis or occlusion of the lacrimal puncta or canaliculi. Prolonged healing is usually due to secondary bacterial infection or to allergic contact dermatitis caused by topical medication. During and after the acute illness, neuralgic dysesthesia and pain are common (154, 155).

Ocular Manifestations

Ocular complications occur in 20% to 50% of the general population but in 57% of AIDS patients (150). The eye on the same side as the vesicular skin eruption may be affected with a severe iridocyclitis, secondary glaucoma, hypopyon, anterior segment ischemia, hyphema, scleritis, extraocular muscle palsies, cataract, and/or posterior segment involvement. Corneal pseudodendrites, mucous plaque keratitis, or late nummular or disciform corneal scarring may occur (154–157). Posterior uveitis and retinitis are rare but may include vasculitis, retinal necrosis, choroiditis, optic neuritis, and optic atrophy. Sometimes, retinal changes occur weeks or months after the skin eruption has resolved (135, 153, 154, 158, 159). The retinal findings can mimic those seen in acute retinal necrosis (Fig. 6.9; see also the section on ARN) (158). Uveitis may be so severe that the eye becomes phthisical. In the acute phase of the disease, phthisis is thought to be due to occlusive vasculitis and necrosis of the ciliary body (160). It is possible for ocular inflammation, including episcleritis, disciform and scleral keratitis, iritis, and glaucoma, to recur even 1 to 10 years after the acute episode (155). Myositis or neuritis may result in ptosis, motility problems, and pupillary abnormalities (Horner's syndrome, light-near dissociation, loss of accommodation). Nerve palsies include third, fourth, sixth, seventh, parasympathetic, or sympathetic nerves (154).

Treatment

Intravenous acyclovir lessened the severity and duration of acute symptoms in healthy adults with zoster of 3 days duration or less but did not prevent late pain (161). In other studies, acyclovir halted progression of zoster, speeded healing, and seemed to reduce early and late pain in immunocompromised patients, both when given early (<3 days of onset) and when given later to patients with disseminated disease (162–164). Acyclovir has been helpful in treating uveitis and cornea inflammation.

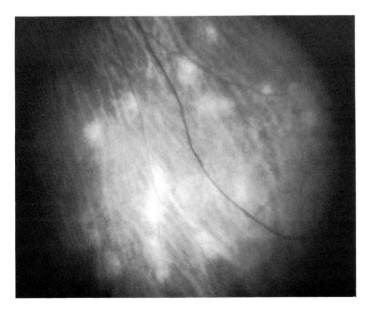

Figure 6.9. Multifocal zoster chorioretinitis in a patient who also had scleritis secondary to herpes zoster ophthalmicus. (Courtesy of WW Culbertson.)

Oral acyclovir in high doses (800 mg 5 times per day for 10 days) has been effective in halting progression and promoting healing of skin lesions, but some disagreement exists concerning the effectiveness for post-herpetic pain (165–167). Cobo (168, 169) showed that oral acyclovir administered within 72 hours of the appearance of the rash speeds resolution of the skin lesions, reduces post-herpetic neuralgia, and may decrease the severity of the ocular involvement. Oral steroids also help post-herpetic neuralgia but may lead to dissemination in immunocompromised hosts (see also treatment of herpes zoster above) (146). Wilson recommended not starting the administration of steroids for 3 to 5 days after the eruption, to allow the host's immune responses a chance to mobilize and reduce the risk of dissemination (135, 154). He did not find that this delay decreased the beneficial effect. However, if steroids were not given within about 2 weeks of onset, they were unlikely to have any beneficial effect on the neuralgia (154). Other investigators feel that starting steroid therapy as early as possible is very important, and for the best results, Scheie (142) recommended starting systemic steroids as soon as the diagnosis was made. Patients with proptosis, posterior scleritis, and optic neuritis may be helped by systemic steroids (155). Ara-A and interferon have been shown to be helpful in clinical studies and, in particular, for immunosuppressed patients (137, 170). Cytosine arabinoside has not been helpful in clinical trials (137). Carbamazepine tegretol and phenytoin dilantin, which are helpful in idiopathic trigeminal neuralgia, do not help zoster post-herpetic neuralgia (171). Patients should be observed for signs and symptoms of depression, which occurs fairly frequently in patients with zoster ophthalmicus and is probably related to the debilitating illness and severe post-herpetic pain. Antidepressants may be very helpful in treating the depression.

Passive immunization has been successfully used in treating high-risk, immunosuppressed individuals, such as children with malignancies who are receiving high-dose steroids. The frequency and severity of the primary infection with varicella virus (chicken pox) is decreased when a regimen of passive immunization is administered. Varicella zoster immunoglobulin may be given to individuals who have been exposed to the virus, but often the exposure is not recognized before the clinical infection is established. Immunization with live attenuated vaccine has also been successfully used to protect high-risk persons from severe primary infections (137, 172–174).

Topical Treatment

The skin lesions are treated palliatively. Cool compresses of saline or Burrow's solution are often helpful. Topical steroids should not be used in the first few days when replicating virus is present. Nor should the steroids be used alone, but, after a few days, they may be combined with topical antibiotics to speed healing and inhibit scarring. Highly sensitizing antibiotics (neomycin, gentamicin, tobramycin) should not be used for long periods. Drying preparations (calamine) should not be used because they prolong healing, produce confluence and necrosis of lesions, and may cause immobilization of the upper eyelid, causing ocular exposure (171). Applying flexible collodion to the skin has been said to relieve pain (175).

Many of the ocular manifestations respond to topical treatment, but topical idoxuridine, vidarabine (adenine arabinoside), and trifluridine have been of no value in clinical experience (154). Dendrites on the cornea often have a self-limited, benign course without treatment, but they have been successfully treated with simple cotton-swab debridement or with topical steroids alone (156, 157). McGill has found that topical acyclovir was more helpful than steroids for treating keratouveitis (176, 177). Keratitis, iritis, and scleritis usually respond promptly to topical steroids, but the dosage must be carefully titrated and may have to be maintained at low dosage (1 drop/day or every other day) for long periods (up to 2 years) to prevent recurrence (155). Nonhealing corneal epithelial lesions usually have a neurotropic component and should be managed as such. The secondary glaucoma that can accompany the keratouveitis may respond to topical steroids alone or to any of the available antiglaucoma drugs.

Topical treatment has no effect on postherpetic neuralgia. (See the section on systemic treatment under herpes zoster.)

The varicella zoster virus has been cultured from cases of acute retinal necrosis (ARN), and treatment in these cases is discussed in the section on ARN.

Histopathological changes may be seen in all tissues of eyes infected with herpes zoster ophthalmicus. Granulomatous inflammation may involve the choroid, retina, and sclera as noted clinically. A mild, chronic inflammatory reaction may be seen in the optic nerve, with cells usually located around vessels, verifying the vasculitis and optic neuritis seen clinically (178).

Acute Retinal Necrosis (ARN)

Acute retinal necrosis (ARN) represents a distinct clinical entity proven by culture to be caused by HSV-1 or VZV (179–181).

Transmission

In most cases, the route of transmission of the virus is unknown. Primary infection and recurrent infection appear to be possible means of transmission (182). Several authors have described indirect evidence of viral infection in ARN, including rising viral titers, coexisting herpes virus skin lesions, and viral particles seen histopathologically (183–192). Varicella zoster virus and HSV-1 have been cultured from the eyes of patients with ARN in the acute phase (182, 193).

Clinical Manifestations (179, 180, 194–204)

The patient is usually systemically healthy. The first symptoms are often ocular injection and a deep, boring pain in the eye. It is not uncommon for a diagnosis of conjunctivitis to be made at this stage. Most,

but not all, patients then develop an anterior granulomatous uveitis, and a transient elevation of intraocular pressure is sometimes seen (179). This condition is followed in a few days by posterior uveitis, vasculitis, and acute retinal necrosis. The necrotizing retinitis typically begins with multiple foci in the periphery that become confluent and spread to the posterior fundus (Figs. 6.10, 6.11). Individual patches of the retinitis may occur in the posterior pole. Inflammation of the arteries is more severe than that of the veins, and, in some patients, the walls of the vessels become opaque. Fluorescein angiography demonstrates decreased perfusion, vascular occlusion, choroidal inflammation, and retinal pigment epithelial damage (Fig. 6.12). Optic neuritis accompanied by swelling of the disc is often present. Vitreous cells are present early on and become worse as the retinal lesions begin to heal, due to sloughing of retina into the vitreous. This may obscure the clinician's view of the fundus. In some cases, the retinal lesions may clear within days, but in others, the lesions may persist for weeks. As the retinal lesions heal, a mild to moderate pigment mottling remains, sharply demarcating the areas of previous retinal necrosis (Fig. 6.13). Optic neuritis may develop as a result of vasculitis, vascular occlusion, and ischemia of the optic nerve; these three factors or the neuritis they cause may result in a sudden loss of vision to light perception or no light perception.

Retinal detachment is common and occurs in 50% to 75% of eyes, usually within 30 to 90 days of the onset of the disease (179, 180, 203). The vitreous becomes organized and contracts, resulting in retinal detachment with proliferative vitreoretinopathy and huge dehiscences in the retina. These breaks in the retina usually occur at the junction of the affected and normal retina (Fig. 6.14). Repairing the detachments is difficult. Retinal neovascularization may also be seen (Fig. 6.15).

In one-third of the patients, the second eye develops ARN, usually within 3 months of the onset of ARN in the first eye, but the second eye may become involved even

Figure 6.10 A and B. **A.** Multiple areas of retinal necrosis during the acute phase of the disease. **B.** Same eye as Fig. 6.10A, 6 weeks later. Note optic atrophy and mild pigmentary changes in areas of previous necrosis. Visual acuity was 20/30.

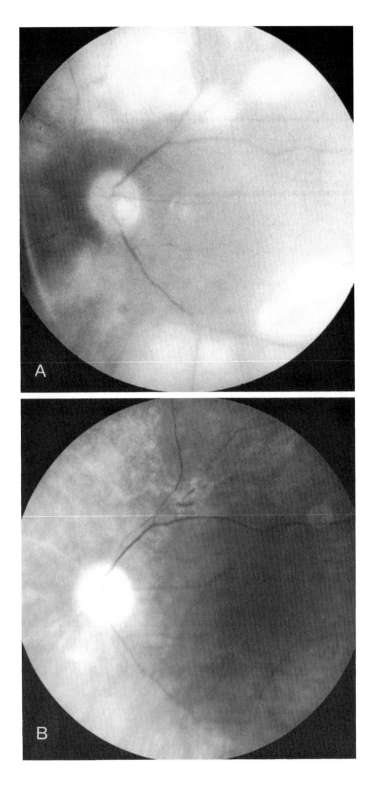

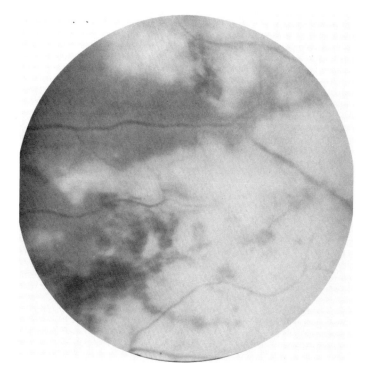

Figure 6.11. Confluent retinal necrosis in the peripheral retina.

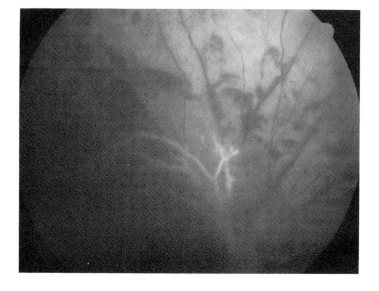

Figure 6.12. Fluorescein angiogram shows marked vascular occlusion in a patient with ARN.

Figure 6.13. Typical pigmentation with sharp borders between normal and affected retina.

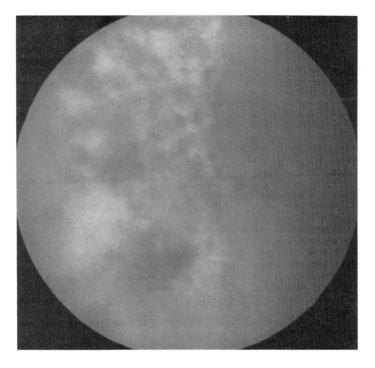

Figure 6.14. Typical large dehiscence in the retina with a retinal detachment.

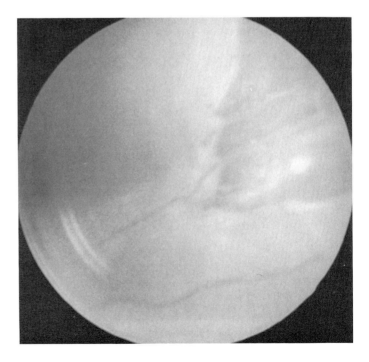

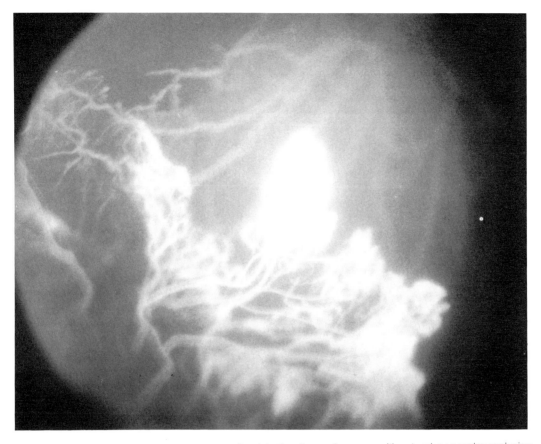

Figure 6.15. Massive neovascularization extending into the vitreous in an eye with extensive vascular occlusion and retinal detachment.

years later (179, 204). This devastating disease may lead to total blindness.

Asymptomatic central nervous system involvement has been documented in one case in which magnetic resonance imaging showed inflammation of the optic tracts and lateral geniculate bodies. This patient did experience malaise, but the neurological examination was otherwise normal (182).

Treatment

Topical steroids and cycloplegia are beneficial for treating anterior uveitis. Acyclovir, 1500 mg/m^2/24hr administered intravenously in three divided doses for 10–14 days, has been observed to halt progression of the disease (205). Twenty-four

to 48 hours after starting the treatment with the antiviral, systemic steroids may be given to prevent damage caused by the inflammatory reaction. Steroids in high intravenous doses are also used to treat optic neuritis that has produced a sudden, severe loss of vision.

Prophylactic treatment has been tried to prevent the frequent retinal detachments, but efficacy has been difficult to assess because of the small number of patients. Photocoagulation has been applied to the posterior edge of the involved peripheral retina to create a new ora serrata in order to prevent retinal detachment (189). However, photocoagulation is often impossible to perform because vitreous haze obscures the clinician's view. The benefit of photocoagulation has not been established because too few cases have been treated using this procedure. Prophylactic encircling scleral buckling procedures have also been tried to support the peripheral retina, thus preventing retinal detachment, and as with photocoagulation, there are too few cases to evaluate the effect. When detachment does occur, the surgical repair is often difficult. Detachment cases can sometimes be repaired by scleral buckling procedures alone, but they frequently require more than one procedure and often require vitrectomy (203). Some cases have been repaired without performing a scleral buckle procedure by using vitrectomy to release all traction on the retina and using air or gas injection to create an internal tamponade. Laser treatment is then performed to form a new ora (203).

Histopathology

Culbertson et al. (191) published a report of the histopathology of the acute phase of the disease. There was full-thickness retinal necrosis with intranuclear inclusions, consistent with a herpes virus, which was seen by electron microscopy at the juncture of normal and involved retina. Also noted were thromboses in retinal arteries and segmental necrotizing optic neuritis. All of these findings correlate with the clinical findings of the acute phase of ARN. In the later phases of the disease with retinal detachment, Topilow (206) showed that the preretinal membranes in an ARN patient with retinal detachment were derived from the retinal pigment epithelium.

RIFT VALLEY FEVER

Etiology

This disease is caused by an RNA virus and commonly affects livestock. It is spread to humans by the mosquito or tick vector and by direct contact with infected animals or their carcasses (207). It is endemic in the Rift Valley, which includes Egypt and East Africa, and generally is not seen in other parts of the world, except in patients who have traveled from the endemic areas.

Clinical Manifestations

In humans, Rift Valley fever is an acute febrile illness with biphasic temperature elevations mimicking dengue fever. Patients have muscle and joint pains, headaches, and occasionally, nausea and vomiting. Occasionally, encephalitis and fatal hemorrhagic illness have been reported (207–209).

Ocular Manifestations

At the onset, there is commonly conjunctivitis and photophobia. Visual loss may occur days or weeks after the fever subsides. In about 10% of patients, an acute necrotizing and hemorrhagic retinitis occurs in the macular and paramacular areas (207). Macular necrosis or exudate is yellow-white and resolves in weeks to months, leaving a chorioretinal scar (209–213). Following retinitis, 40% to 50% of patients have a permanent decrease in vision (209). Retinal detachments have been reported to develop in a few cases (211, 213).

POSTVIRAL SYNDROME

The postviral syndrome occurs during or immediately following an upper respiratory or flu-like viral illness. This syndrome involves an acute, bilateral decrease in vision associated with retinal periphlebitis and optic neuritis (214). Patients may have mild or marked papillitis, vasculitis, or anterior chamber and/or vitreous cells and may develop a macular star and retinal striae (Fig. 6.16). Vision usually returns to normal 2 to 6 weeks after the onset, and the findings in the fundus return to normal. Hartridge (215) and Cross (216) reported similar cases of optic neuritis and optic atrophy following viral infection with influenza.

CYTOMEGALOVIRUS (CMV)

See Chapter 5, AIDS.

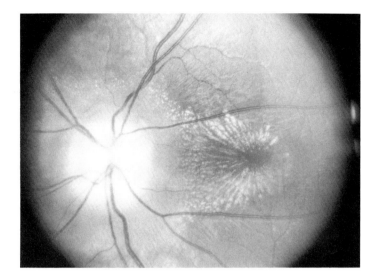

Figure 6.16. A papillitis and a macular star following a viral illness. (Courtesy of J Glaser.)

General References

1. Gass JDM. Stereoscopic atlas of macular diseases; diagnosis and treatment. 3rd. ed. St. Louis: CV Mosby, 1987.
2. Tabbara KF, Hyndiuk RA, eds. Infections of the eye. Boston: Little, Brown, 1986.
3. Darrell RW, ed. Viral diseases of the eye. Philadelphia: Lea & Febiger, 1985.
4. Boniuk M, ed. Rubella and other intraocular viral diseases in infancy. Int Ophthalmol Clin 1972;12(2).
5. Pavan-Langston D, ed. Ocular viral disease. Int Ophthalmol Clin 1975; 15(4).
6. Chamberlain WP Jr. Ocular findings in scrub typhus. Arch Ophthalmol 1952;48:313–321.
7. Scheie HG. Ocular changes associated with scrub typhus; a study of four hundred and fifty-one patients. Arch Ophthalmol 1948;40:245–267.
8. Fischer DH. Viral disease and the retina. In: Tabbara KF, Hyndiuk RA, eds. Infections of the eye. Boston: Little, Brown, 1986:487–497.

Rubeola
9. Duke-Elder S, ed. System of ophthalmology. Vol. X. Diseases of the retina. St. Louis: CV Mosby, 1967:261–266.
10. Scheie HG, Morse PH. Rubeola retinopathy. Arch Ophthalmol 1972;88:341–344.
11. Foxman SG, Heckenlively JR, Sinclair SH. Rubeola retinopathy and pigmented paravenous retinochoroidal atrophy. Am J Ophthalmol 1985;99:605–606.
12. Metz HS, Harkey ME. Pigmentary retinopathy following maternal measles (morbilli) infection. Am J Ophthalmol 1968;66:1107–1110.
13. Dawson JR Jr. Cellular inclusions in cerebral lesions of lethargic encephalitis. Am J Pathol 1933;9:7–15.

14. Van Bogaert L, De Busscher J. Sur la sclerose inflammatoire de la substance blanche des hemispheres (Spielmeyer) (Contribution a l'etude des scleroses diffuses non familiales). Rev Neurol 1939;71:679–701.
15. Pette H, Doring G. Uber einheimische Panencephalomyelitis von Charakter der Encephalitis japonica. Dtsch Z Nervenheilkd 1939;149:7–44.
16. Bouteille M, Fontaine C, Vedrenne C, Delarue J. Sur un cas d'encephalite subaigue a inclusions. Etude anatomo-clinique et ultra structurale. Rev Neurol 1965;113:454–458.
17. Connolly JH, Allen IV, Hurwitz LJ, Millar JHD. Measles-virus antibody and antigen in subacute sclerosing panencephalitis. Lancet 1967;1:542–544.
18. Horta Barbosa L, Fuccillo DA, Sever JL, Zeman W. Subacute sclerosing panencephalitis: isolation of measles virus from a brain biopsy. Nature 1969;221:974.
19. Payne FE, Baublis JV, Itabashi HH. Isolation of measles virus from cell cultures of brain from a patient with subacute sclerosing panencephalitis. N Engl J Med 1969;281:585–589.
20. Steele RW, Fuccillo DA, Hensem SA, et al. Specific inhibitory factors of cellular immunity in children with subacute sclerosing panencephalitis. J Pediatr 1976;88:56–62.
21. Aaby P, Bukh J, Lisse IM, Smits AJ. Risk factors in subacute sclerosing panencephalitis: age- and sex-dependent host reactions or intensive exposure? Rev Infect Dis 1984;6:239–250.
22. Modlin JF, Halsey NA, Eddins DL, et al. Epidemiology of subacute sclerosing panencephalitis. J Pediatr 1979;94:231–236.
23. Taylor WJ, DuRant RH, Dyken PR. Treatment of subacute sclerosing panencephalitis; an overview. Drug Intell Clin Pharm 1984;18:375–381.

24. Dyken PR. Subacute sclerosing panencephalitis; current status. Neurol Clin 1985;3:179–196.

25. Jabbour JT, Garcia JH, Lemmi H, et al. Subacute sclerosing panencephalitis; a multidisciplinary study of eight cases. JAMA 1969;207:2248–2254.

26. Hiatt RL, Grizzard HT, McNeer P, Jabbour JT. Ophthalmologic manifestations of subacute sclerosing panencephalitis (Dawson's encephalitis). Trans Am Acad Ophthalmol Otolaryngol 1971;75:344–350.

27. Sebestyen J, Strenger J. Die ophthalmologischen Beziehungen bei der subakuten progressiven Panenzephalitis. Klin Monatsbl Augenheilkd 1964;145:202–212.

28. Lund OE, Forster C, Rise K. Zerebral bedingte Sehstorungen als Erstsymptom bei subakuter sklerosierender Panenzephalitis (SSPE). Klin Monatsbl Augenheilkd 1983;182:290–293.

29. Cherry PMH, Faulkner JD. A case of subacute sclerosing panencephalitis with exophthalmos. Ann Ophthalmol 1975;7:1579–1586.

30. Glowacki J, Guazzi GC, Van Bogaert L. Pseudotumoural presentation of certain cases of subacute sclerosing leucoencephalitis. J Neurol Sci 1967;4:199–215.

31. Gass JDM. Stereoscopic atlas of macular diseases; diagnosis and treatment. 2nd ed. St. Louis: CV Mosby, 1977:302.

32. Otradovec J. Chorioretinitis centralis bei Leucoencephalitis subacuta sclerotisans Van Bogaert. Ophthalmologica 1963;146:65–73.

33. Brudet-Wickel CLM, Hogeweg M, de Wolff-Rouendaal D. Subacute sclerosing panencephalitis (SSPE); a case report. Doc Ophthalmol 1982;52:241–250.

34. Koniszewski G, Ruprecht KW, Flugel KA. Nekrotisierende Retinitis bei subakuter sklerosierender Panencephalitis (SSPE). Klin Monatsbl Augenheilkd 1984;184:99–103.

35. La Piana FG, Tso MOM, Jenis EH. The retinal lesions of subacute sclerosing panencephalitis. Ann Ophthalmol 1974;6:603–610.

36. De Laey JJ, Hanssens M, Colette P, et al. Subacute sclerosing panencephalitis: fundus changes and histopathologic correlations. Doc Ophthalmol 1983;56:11–21.

37. Nelson DA, Weiner A, Yanoff M, de Peralta J. Retinal lesions in subacute sclerosing panencephalitis. Arch Ophthalmol 1970;84:613–621.

38. Font RL, Jenis EH, Tuck KD. Measles maculopathy associated with subacute sclerosing panencephalitis; immunofluorescent and immunoultrastructural studies. Arch Pathol 1973;96:168–174.

39. Zilber N, Rannon L, Alter M, Kahana E. Measles, measles vaccination, and risk of subacute sclerosing panencephalitis (SSPE). Neurology 1983;33:1558–1564.

40. Dyken PR, Swift A, DuRant RH. Long-term follow-up of patients with subacute sclerosing panencephalitis treated with inosiplex. Ann Neurol 1982;11:359–364.

41. Panitch HS. Gomez-Plascencia J, Norris FH, et al. Subacute sclerosing panencephalitis: remission after treatment with intraventricular interferon. Neurology 1986;36:562–566.

Rubella

42. Freij BJ, South MA, Sever JL. Maternal rubella and the congenital rubella syndrome. Clin Perinatol 1988;15:247–257.

43. Wolff SM. The ocular manifestations of congenital rubella. Trans Am Ophthalmol Soc 1972;70:577–614.

44. Rawls WE. Virology and epidemiology of rubella virus. Int Ophthalmol Clin 1972;12(2):21–66.

45. Sever JL, South MA, Shaver KA. Delayed manifestations of congenital rubella. Rev Infect Dis 1985;7(suppl 1):S164–169.

46. Boniuk V. Systemic and ocular manifestations of the rubella syndrome. Int Ophthalmol Clin 1972;12(2):67–76.

47. Boniuk M, ed. Rubella and other intraocular viral diseases in infancy. Int Ophthalmol Clin 1972;12(2):1–234.

48. Boniuk V. Rubella. Int Ophthalmol Clin 1975;15(4):229–241.

49. Krill AE. The retinal disease of rubella. Arch Ophthalmol 1967;77:445–449.

50. Collis WJ, Cohen DN. Rubella retinopathy: a progressive disorder. Arch Ophthalmol 1970;84:33–35.

51. Deutman AF, Grizzard WS. Rubella retinopathy and subretinal neovascularization. Am J Ophthalmol 1978;85:82–87.

52. Orth DH, Fishman GA, Segall M, et al. Rubella maculopathy. Br J Ophthalmol 1980;64:201–205.

53. Rudolph AJ, Desmond MM. Clinical manifestations of the congenital rubella syndrome. Int Ophthalmol Clin 1972;12(2):3–19.

54. Gregg NM. Congenital cataract following German measles in the mother. Trans Ophthalmol Soc Aust 1941;3:35–46.

55. Krill AE. Retinopathy secondary to rubella. Int Ophthalmol Clin 1972;12(2):89–103.

56. LaPlane R, Bregeat P, Ossipovski B. Un cas d'embryopathie consecutive a une varicelle maternelle. Arch Fr Pediatr 1950;7:530.

Mumps

57. Darrell RW. Mumps virus ocular disease. In: Darrell RW, ed. Viral diseases of the eye. Philadelphia: Lea & Febiger, 1985:227–232.

58. Oh JO. Ocular virology. In: Tabbara KF, Hyndiuk RA, eds. Infections of the eye. Boston: Little, Brown, 1986:93–105.

59. deLuise VP. Viral conjunctivitis. In: Tabbara KF, Hyndiuk RA, eds. Infections of the eye. Boston: Little, Brown, 1986:437–460.

60. Vastine DW. Nonherpetic viral keratitis. In: Tabbara KF, Hyndiuk RA, eds. Infections of the eye. Boston: Little, Brown, 1986:387–411.

61. Meyer RF, Sullivan JH, Oh JO. Mumps conjunctivitis. Am J Ophthalmol 1974;78:1022–1024.

62. Riffenburgh RS. Ocular manifestations of mumps. Arch Ophthalmol 1961;66:739–743.

63. Young RC. Mumps encephalitis: report of a case with bilateral optic neuritis, rapid and complete blindness and complete recovery. N Orleans Med Surg J 1933–1934;86:25–26.

64. Swan JW, Penn RF. Scleritis following mumps; report of a case. Am J Ophthalmol 1962;53:366–368.

65. Fields J. Ocular manifestations of mumps; a case of mumps keratitis. Am J Ophthalmol 1947;30:591–595.

66. Danielson RW, Long JC. Keratitis due to mumps. Am J Ophthalmol 1941;24:655–657.

67. Katavisto M. Eye complications of epidemic parotitis. Acta Ophthalmol 1956;34:208–213.

68. North DP. Ocular complications of mumps. Br J Ophthalmol 1953;37:99–101.

69. Walsh FB, ed. Clinical neuro-ophthalmology. 2nd ed. Baltimore: Williams & Wilkins, 1957:474–476.

70. Woodward JH. The ocular complications of mumps. Ann Ophthalmol (St. Louis) 1907;16:7–38.

71. Swab CM. Encephalitic optic neuritis and atrophy due to mumps; report of a case. Arch Ophthalmol 1938;19:926–929.

72. Powell LS, Dunlap RL. Report of two cases with visual disturbance complicating epidemic parotitis. J Kansas Med Soc 1940;41:432–433.

73. Rogell G. Infectious and inflammatory diseases. In: Duane TD, ed. Clinical ophthalmology. Philadelphia: Lippincott, 1976: Vol 5, Chap 33, p 6.

74. Duke-Elder S, ed. System of ophthalmology. Vol. 15. Summary of systemic ophthalmology. St. Louis: CV Mosby, 1967:119.

75. Paufique L, Audibert J, Dorne, Bonnet-Gehin M. Uveite avec atteinte chorio-retinienne d'origine ourlienne. Bull Soc Ophtalmol Fr 1963;226–228.

76. Weskamp RL, Boccalandro C. Epidemic parotitis and choroiditis. Arch Oftalmol Buenos Aires 1939;14:193–202.

77. Holowach J, Thurston DL, Becker B. Congenital defects in infants following mumps during pregnancy. A review of the literature and a report of chorioretinitis due to fetal infection. J Pediatr 1957;50:689–694.

Epstein-Barr Virus

78. Fleisher GR. Epstein-Barr virus. In: Belshe RB, ed. Textbook of human virology. Littleton, Mass: PSG Publishing, 1984:853–886.

79. Henle W, Henle G. Epstein-Barr virus and infectious mononucleosis. N Engl J Med 1973;288:263–264.

80. Niederman JC, Evans AS, Subrahmanyan L, McCollum RW. Prevalence, incidence and persistence of EB virus antibody in young adults. N Engl J Med 1970;282:361–365.

81. Henle W, Henle GE, Horwitz CA. Epstein-Barr virus: specific diagnostic tests in infectious mononucleosis. Hum Pathol 1974;5:551–565.

82. Henle W, Henle G. Serodiagnosis of infectious mononucleosis. Resident Staff Physician 1981;27(1):37–43.

83. Tiedeman JS. Epstein-Barr viral antibodies in multifocal choroiditis and panuveitis. Am J Ophthalmol 1987;103:659–663.

84. Nozik RA, Dorsch W. A new chorioretinopathy associated with anterior uveitis. Am J Ophthalmol 1973;76:758–762.

85. Dreyer RF, Gass JDM. Multifocal choroiditis and panuveitis; a syndrome that mimics ocular histoplasmosis. Arch Ophthalmol 1984;102:1776–1784.

86. Watzke RC, Packer AJ, Folk JC, et al. Punctate inner choroidopathy. Am J Ophthalmol 1984;98:572–584.

87. Morgan CM, Schatz H. Recurrent multifocal choroiditis. Ophthalmology 1986;93:1138–1147.

88. Wong KW, D'Amico DJ, Hedges TR III, et al. Ocular involvement associated with chronic Epstein-Barr virus disease. Arch Ophthalmol 1987;105:788–792.

89. Singerman LJ. Discussion of Morgan CM, Schatz H. Recurrent multifocal choroiditis. Ophthalmology 1986;93:1143–1147.

90. Raymond LA, Wilson CA, Linnemann CC Jr, et al. Punctate outer retinitis in acute Epstein-Barr infection. Am J Ophthalmol 1987;104:424–426.

91. Doft BH, Gass JDM. Punctate outer retinal toxoplasmosis. Arch Ophthalmol 1985;103:1332–1336.

92. Rothova A, van Knapen F, Baarsma GS, et al. Serology in ocular toxoplasmosis. Br J Ophthalmol 1986;70:615–622.

93. Worley G, Green JA, Frothingham TE, et al. *Toxocara canis* infection: clinical and epidemiological associations with seropositivity in kindergarten children. J Infect Dis 1984;149:591–597.

94. Jondal M, Klein G. Surface markers on human B and T lymphocytes. II. Presence of Epstein-Barr virus receptors on B lymphocytes. J Exp Med 1973;138:1365–1378.

95. Young LS, Clark D, Sixbey JW, Rickinson AB. Epstein-Barr virus receptors on human pharyngeal epithelia. Lancet 1986;1:240–242.

96. Portnoy J, Ahronheim GA, Ghibu F, et al. Recovery of Epstein-Barr virus from genital ulcers. N Engl J Med 1984;311:966–968.

HSV-1

97. Hutchison DS, Smith RE, Haughton PB. Congenital herpetic keratitis. Arch Ophthalmol 1975;93:70–73.

98. Reerstad P, Hansen B. Chorioretinitis of the newborn with herpes simplex virus type 1; re-

port of a case. Acta Ophthalmol 1979;57:1096–1100.

99. Whitley RJ, Soong SJ, Linneman C Jr, et al. Herpes simplex encephalitis; clinical assessment. JAMA 1982;247:317–320.

100. Whitley RJ, Alford CA, Hirsch MS, et al. Vidarabine versus acyclovir therapy in herpes simplex encephalitis. N Engl J Med 1986; 314:144–149.

101. Minckler DS, McLean EB, Shaw CM, Hendrickson A. Herpesvirus hominis encephalitis and retinitis. Arch Ophthalmol 1976;94:89–95.

102. Bloom JN, Katz JI, Kaufman HE. Herpes simplex retinitis and encephalitis in an adult. Arch Ophthalmol 1977;95:1798–1799.

103. Johnson BL, Wisotzkey HM. Neuroretinitis associated with herpes simplex encephalitis in an adult. Am J Ophthalmol 1977;83:481–489.

104. Savir H, Grosswasser Z, Mendelson L. Herpes virus hominis encephalomyelitis and retinal vasculitis in adults. Ann Ophthalmol 1980;12:1369–1371.

105. Partamian LG, Morse PH, Klein HZ. Herpes simplex type 1 retinitis in an adult with systemic herpes zoster. Am J Ophthalmol 1981;92:215–220.

106. Pepose JS, Kreiger AE, Tomiyasu U, et al. Immunocytologic localization of herpes simplex type 1 viral antigens in herpetic retinitis and encephalitis in an adult. Ophthalmology 1985;92:160–166.

107. Mitchell CD, Bean B, Gentry SR, et al. Acyclovir therapy for mucocutaneous herpes simplex infections in immunocompromised patients. Lancet 1981;1:1389–1392.

108. Lewis ML, Culbertson WW, Post MJD, et al. Herpes simplex virus type 1; a cause of the acute retinal necrosis syndrome. Ophthalmology 1989;96:875–878.

HSV-2

109. Oh JO. Ocular infections of herpes simplex virus type 2 in adults. In: Darrell RW, ed. Viral diseases of the eye. Philadelphia: Lea & Febiger, 1985:59–62.

110. Nahmias AJ, Hagler WS. Ocular manifestations of herpes simplex in the newborn (neonatal ocular herpes). Int Ophthalmol Clin 1972; 12(2):192–213.

111. Nahmias AJ, Josey WE, Naib ZM, et al. Perinatal risk associated with maternal genital herpes simplex virus infection. Am J Obstet Gynecol 1971;110:825–837.

112. Mitchell JE, McCall FC. Transplacental infection by herpes simplex virus. Am J Dis Child 1963;106:207–209.

113. Gammon JA, Nahmias AJ. Herpes simplex ocular infections in the newborn. In: Darrell RW, ed. Viral diseases of the eye. Philadelphia: Lee & Febiger, 1985:46–58.

114. Pettay O, Leinikki P, Donner M, Lapinleimu K.

Herpes simplex virus infection in the newborn. Arch Dis Child 1972;47:97–103.

115. Nahmias AJ, Visintine AM, Caldwell DR, Wilson LA. Eye infections with herpes simplex viruses in neonates. Surv Ophthalmol 1976; 21:100–105.

116. Whitley RJ, Ch'ien LT, Alford CA Jr. Neonatal herpes simplex virus infection. Int Ophthalmol Clin 1975;15(4):141–149.

117. Pavan-Langston D, Brockhurst RJ. Herpes simplex panuveitis; a clinical report. Arch Ophthalmol 1969;81:783–787.

118. Florman AL, Mindlin RL. Generalized herpes simplex in an eleven-day-old premature infant. Am J Dis Child 1952;83:481–486.

119. Cogan DG, Kuwabara T, Young GF, Knox DL. Herpes simplex retinopathy in an infant. Arch Ophthalmol 1964;72:641–645.

120. Bahrani M, Boxerbaum B, Gilger AP, et al. Generalized herpes simplex and hypoadrenocorticism; a case associated with adrenocortical insufficiency in a prematurely born male: clinical, virologic, ophthalmological and metabolic studies. Am J Dis Child 1966;111:437–445.

121. Hagler WS, Walters PV, Nahmias AJ. Ocular involvement in neonatal herpes simplex virus infection. Arch Ophthalmol 1969;82:169–176.

122. Golden B, Bell WE, McKee AP. Disseminated herpes simplex with encephalitis in a neonate; treatment with idoxuridine. JAMA 1969; 209:1219–1221.

123. Cibis GW, Flynn JT, Davis EB. Herpes simplex retinitis. Arch Ophthalmol 1978;96:299–302.

124. Greer GH. Bilateral necrotizing retinitis complicating fatal encephalitis probably due to herpes simplex virus type 2. Ophthalmologica 1980;180:146–150.

125. Mousel DK, Missall SR. Pan uveitis and retinitis in neonatal herpes simplex infection. J Pediatr Ophthalmol Strabismus 1979;16:7–9.

126. Colin J, Bodereau X, Baikoff G. Encephalite et retinite herpetiques chez un adulte: a propos d'une observation. Bull Soc Ophtalmol Fr 1981;81:701–703.

127. Young GF, Knox DL, Dodge PR. Necrotizing encephalitis and chorioretinitis in a young infant; report of a case with rising herpes simplex antibody titers. Arch Neurol 1965;13:15–24.

128. Douglas JM, Critchlow C, Benedetti J, et al. A double-blind study of oral acyclovir for suppression of recurrences of genital herpes simplex virus infection. N Engl J Med 1984;310:1551–1556.

129. Straus SE, Takiff HE, Seidlin M, et al. Suppression of frequently recurring genital herpes; a placebo-controlled double-blind trial of oral acyclovir. N Engl J Med 1984;310:1545–1550.

130. Mitchell CD, Bean B, Gentry SR, et al. Acyclovir therapy for mucocutaneous herpes simplex infections in immunocompromised patients. Lancet 1981;1:1389–1392.

131. Yanoff M, Allman MI, Fine BS. Congenital herpes simplex virus, type 2, bilateral endophthalmitis. Trans Am Ophthalmol Soc 1977;75:325–338.

Varicella Zoster (VZV)

132. Applebaum E, Rachelson MH, Dolgopol VB. Varicella encephalitis. Am J Med 1953;15:223–230.

133. Walsh FB, ed. Clinical neuro-ophthalmology. 2nd ed. Baltimore: Williams & Wilkins, 1957: 474–476.

134. Copenhaver RM. Chickenpox with retinopathy. Arch Ophthalmol 1966;75:199–200.

135. Friedlaender MH. Allergy and immunology of the eye. Hagerstown: Harper & Row, 1979:152–156.

136. Strachman J. Uveitis associated with chicken pox. J Pediatr 1955;46:327–328.

137. Gershon AA. Varicella-zoster infections. In: Darrell RW, ed. Viral diseases of the eye. Philadelphia: Lea & Febiger, 1985:63–92.

138. Juel-Jensen BE, MacCallum FO. Herpes simplex, varicella and zoster; clinical manifestations and treatment. London: William Heinemann, 1972.

139. Eaglstein WH, Katz R, Brown JA. The effects of early corticosteroid therapy on the skin eruption and pain of herpes zoster. JAMA 1970;211:1681–1683.

140. Elliot FA. Treatment of herpes zoster with high doses of prednisone. Lancet 1964;2:610–611.

141. Keczkes K, Basheer AM. Do corticosteroids prevent postherpetic neuralgia? Br J Dermatol 1980;102:551–555.

142. Scheie HG. Herpes zoster ophthalmicus. Trans Ophthalmol Soc UK 1970;90:899–930.

143. Craver LF, Haagensen CD. A note on the occurrence of herpes zoster in Hodgkin's disease, lymphosarcoma, and the leukemias. Am J Cancer 1932;16:502–514.

144. Pavan-Langston D. Varicella-zoster ophthalmicus. Int Ophthalmol Clin 1975;15(4):171–185.

145. Weller TH. Varicella-herpes zoster virus. In: Evans AS, ed. Viral infections of humans; epidemiology and control. New York: Plenum, 1976:457–480.

146. Merselis JG Jr, Kaye D, Hook EW. Disseminated herpes zoster; a report of 17 cases. Arch Intern Med 1961;113:679–686.

147. Downie AW. Chickenpox and zoster. Br Med Bull 1959;15:197–200.

148. Cole EL, Meisler DM, Calabrese LH, et al. Herpes zoster ophthalmicus and acquired immune deficiency syndrome. Arch Ophthalmol 1984; 102:1027–1029.

149. Kestelyn P, Stevens AM, Bakkers E, et al. Severe herpes zoster ophthalmicus in young African adults: a marker for HTLV-III seropositivity. Br J Ophthalmol 1987;71:806–809.

150. Sandor EV, Millman A, Croxson TS, Mildvan D. Herpes zoster ophthalmicus in patients at risk for the acquired immune deficiency syndrome (AIDS). Am J Ophthalmol 1986;101:153–155.

151. Lightman S, Marsh RJ, Powell D. Herpes zoster ophthalmicus: a medical review. Br J Ophthalmol 1981;65:539–541.

152. Blumenkopf B, Lockhart WS Jr. Herpes zoster infection and use of oral anticoagulants; a potentially dangerous association. JAMA 1983;250:936–937.

153. Schwartz JN, Cashwell F, Hawkins HK, Klintworth GK. Necrotizing retinopathy with herpes zoster ophthalmicus; a light and electron microscopical study. Arch Pathol Lab Med 1976;100:386–391.

154. Wilson FM II. Varicella and herpes zoster ophthalmicus. In: Tabbara KF, Hyndiuk RA, eds. Infections of the eye. Boston: Little, Brown, 1986:369–386.

155. Marsh RJ. Ophthalmic herpes zoster. In: Darrell RW, ed. Viral diseases of the eye. Philadelphia: Lea & Febiger, 1985:78–89.

156. Pavan-Langston D, McCulley JP. Herpes zoster dendritic keratitis. Arch Ophthalmol 1973; 89:25–29.

157. Piebenga LW, Laibson PR. Dendritic lesions in herpes zoster ophthalmicus. Arch Ophthalmol 1973;90:268–270.

158. Brown RM, Mendis U. Retinal arteritis complicating herpes zoster ophthalmicus. Br J Ophthalmol 1973;57:344–346.

159. Jensen J. A case of herpes zoster ophthalmicus complicated with neuroretinitis. Acta Ophthalmol 1948;26:551–555.

160. Amanat LA, Cant JS, Green FD. Acute phthisis bulbi and external ophthalmoplegia in herpes zoster ophthalmicus. Ann Ophthalmol 1985;17:46–51.

161. Bean B, Braun C, Balfour HH Jr. Acyclovir therapy for acute herpes zoster. Lancet 1982;2:118–121.

162. Balfour HH Jr, Bean B, Laskin OL, et al. Acyclovir halts progression of herpes zoster in immunocompromised patients. N Engl J Med 1983;308:1448–1453.

163. Spector SA, Hintz M, Wyborny C, et al. Treatment of herpes virus infections in immunocompromised patients with acyclovir by continuous intravenous infusion. Am J Med 1982;73:275–280.

164. Peterslund NA, Seyer-Hansen K, Ipsen J, et al. Acyclovir in herpes zoster. Lancet 1981;2:827–830.

165. Huff JC, Bean B, Balfour HH Jr, et al. Therapy of herpes zoster with oral acyclovir. Am J Med 1988;85(2A):84–89.

166. Wood MJ, Ogan PH, McKendrick MW, et al. Efficacy of oral acyclovir treatment of acute herpes zoster. Am J Med 1988;85(2A):79–83.

167. Morton P, Thomson AN. Oral acyclovir in the treatment of herpes zoster in general practice. NZ Med J 1989;102(863):93–95.

168. Cobo LM, Foulks GN, Liesegang T, et al. Oral acyclovir in the therapy of acute herpes zoster ophthalmicus; an interim report. Ophthalmology 1985;92:1574–1583.

169. Cobo LM, Foulks GN, Liesegang T, et al. Oral acyclovir in treatment of acute herpes zoster ophthalmicus. Ophthalmology 1986;93:763–770.

170. Merigan TC, Rand KH, Pollard RB, et al. Human leuckocyte interferon for the treatment of herpes zoster in patients with cancer. N Engl J Med 1978;298:981–987.

171. Jones DB. Herpes zoster ophthalmicus. In: Golden B, ed. Ocular inflammatory disease. Springfield: Charles C Thomas, 1974:198–209.

172. Gershon AA. Live attenuated varicella-zoster vaccine. Rev Infect Dis 1980;2:393–407.

173. Gershon AA, Steinberg S, Borkowsky W, & NIH Collaboration Study Group. Varicella vaccine: use in children with leukemia. Pediatr Res 1982;16(Pt 2):241A.

174. Gershon AA, Steinberg S, Gelb L, et al. A multicentre trial of live attenuated varicella vaccine in children with leukemia in remission. Postgrad Med J 1985;61(suppl 4):73–78.

175. Krulig L, Jacobs PH. Flexible collodion. Arch Dermatol 1974;110:446–467.

176. McGill J. Acyclovir treatment of herpes zoster infection. In: ACTA: XXIV International Congress of Ophthalmology, San Francisco, 1982. Philadelphia: Lippincott, 1983;1:235–237.

177. McGill J. Topical acyclovir in herpes zoster ocular involvement. Br J Ophthalmol 1981;65:542–545.

178. Naumann G, Gass JDM, Font RL. Histopathology of herpes zoster ophthalmicus. Am J Ophthalmol 1968;65:533–541.

Acute Retinal Necrosis

179. Fisher JP, Lewis ML, Blumenkranz M, et al. The acute retinal necrosis syndrome. Part 1: Clinical manifestations. Ophthalmology 1982;89:1309–1316.

180. Gass JDM. Acute herpetic thrombotic retinal angiitis and necrotizing neuroretinitis ("acute retinal necrosis syndrome"). In: Symposium on Medical and Surgical Diseases of the Retina and Vitreous; Transactions of the New Orleans Academy of Ophthalmology. St. Louis: CV Mosby, 1983:97–107.

181. Culbertson WW, Blumenkranz MS, The acute retinal necrosis syndrome. In: Blodi FC, ed. Herpes simplex infections of the eye. New York: Churchill Livingstone, 1984:77–89.

182. Lewis ML, Culbertson WW, Post MJD, et al. Herpes simplex virus type 1; a cause of the acute retinal necrosis syndrome. Ophthalmology 1989;96:875–878.

183. Saari KM, Boke W, Manthey KF, et al. Bilateral acute retinal necrosis. Am J Ophthalmol 1982;93:403–411.

184. Saari KM. Association of acute retinal necrosis with herpetic infection. In: Saari KM, ed. Uveitis update; Proceedings of the First International Symposium on Uveitis held in Hanasaari, Espoo, Finland on May 16–19, 1984. Amsterdam, New York: Elsevier, 1984:223–249.

185. Matsuo T, Nakayama T, Matsuo N, Koide N. Immunological studies of uveitis. 1. Immune complex containing herpes virus antigens in four patients with acute retinal necrosis syndrome. Jpn J Ophthalmol 1986;30:472–479.

186. Sarkies N, Gregor Z, Forsey T, Darougar S. Antibodies to herpes simplex virus type I in intraocular fluids of patients with acute retinal necrosis. Br J Ophthalmol 1986;70:81–84.

187. Reese L, Sheu MM, Lee F, et al. Intraocular antibody production suggests herpes zoster is only one cause of acute retinal necrosis (ARN). ARVO Abstracts. Invest Ophthalmol Vis Sci 1986;27(suppl):12.

188. Peyman GA, Goldberg MF, Uninsky E, et al. Vitrectomy and intravitreal antiviral drug therapy in acute retinal necrosis syndrome; report of two cases. Arch Ophthalmol 1984;102:1618–1621.

189. Han DP, Lewis H, Williams GA, et al. Laser photocoagulation in the acute retinal necrosis syndrome. Arch Ophthalmol 1987;105:1051–1054.

190. Jampol LM. Acute retinal necrosis. Am J Ophthalmol 1982;93:254–255.

191. Culbertson WW, Blumenkranz MS, Haines H, et al. The acute retinal necrosis syndrome. Part 2. Histopathology and etiology. Ophthalmology 1982;89:1317–1325.

192. Freeman WR, Thomas EL, Rao NA, et al. Demonstration of herpes group virus in acute retinal necrosis syndrome. Ophthalmology 1986;102:701–709.

193. Culbertson WW, Blumenkranz MS, Pepose JS, et al. Varicella zoster virus is a cause of the acute retinal necrosis syndrome. Ophthalmology 1986;93:559–569.

194. Urayama A, Yamada N, Sasaki T, et al. Unilateral acute uveitis with retinal periarteritis and detachment. Jpn J Clin Ophthalmol 1971;25:607–619.

195. Willerson D Jr, Aaberg TM, Reeser FH. Necrotizing vaso-occlusive retinitis. Am J Ophthalmol 1977;84:209–219.

196. Young NJA, Bird AC. Bilateral acute retinal necrosis. Br J Ophthalmol 1978;62:581–590.

197. Bando K, Kinoshita A, Mimura Y. Six cases of so-called "Kirisawa Type" uveitis. Jpn J Clin Ophthalmol 1979;33:1515–1521.

198. Okinami S, Tsukahara I. Acute severe uveitis with retinal vasculitis and retinal detachment. Ophthalmologica 1979;179:276–285.

199. Price FW Jr, Schlaegel TF Jr. Bilateral acute retinal necrosis. Am J Ophthalmol 1980;89:419–424.

200. Gorman BD, Nadel AJ, Coles RS. Acute retinal necrosis. Ophthalmology 1982;89:809–814.

201. Sternberg P Jr, Knox DL, Finkelstein D, et al. Acute retinal necrosis syndrome. Retina 1982;2:145–151.

202. Saga U, Ozawa H, Soshi S, et al. Acute retinal necrosis (Kirisawa's uveitis). Jpn J Ophthalmol 1983;27:353–361.

203. Clarkson JG, Blumenkranz MS, Culbertson WW, et al. Retinal detachment following the acute retinal necrosis syndrome. Ophthalmology 1984;91:1665–1668.

204. Martenet AC. Frequence et aspects cliniques

des complications retiniennes de l'uveite intermediare. Bull Mem Soc Fr Ophtalmol 1980;92:40–42.

205. Blumenkranz MS, Culbertson WW, Clarkson JG, Dix R. Treatment of the acute retinal necrosis syndrome with intravenous acyclovir. Ophthalmology 1986;93:296–300.

206. Topilow HW, Nussbaum JJ, Freeman HM, et al. Bilateral acute retinal necrosis; clinical and ultrastructural study. Arch Ophthalmol 1982; 100:1901–1908.

Rift Valley Fever

207. Gear JHS. Clinical aspects of African viral hemorrhagic fevers. Rev Infect Dis 1989;11 (suppl 4):S777–782.

208. Meegan JM. The Rift Valley fever epizootic in Egypt 1977–78. 1. Description of the epizootic and virological studies. Trans R Soc Trop Med Hyg 1979;73:618–623.

209. Siam AL, Meegan JM, Gharbawi KF. Rift Valley fever ocular manifestations: observations during the 1977 epidemic in Egypt. Br J Ophthalmol 1980;64:366–374.

210. Gass JDM. Stereoscopic atlas of macular diseases; diagnosis and treatment. 3rd ed. St. Louis: CV Mosby, 1987:502.

211. Deutman AF, Klomp HJ. Rift Valley fever retinitis. Am J Ophthalmol 1981;92:38–42.

212. Freed I. Rift Valley fever in man complicated by retinal changes and loss of vision. S Afr Med J 1951;25:930–932.

213. Schrire L. Macular changes in Rift Valley fever. S Afr Med J 1951;25:926–930.

Postviral Syndrome

214. Gass JDM. Fluorescein angiography in endogenous intraocular inflammation. In: Aronson SB, Gamble CN, Goodner EK, O'Connor GR, eds. Clinical methods in uveitis; the Fourth Sloan Symposium of Uveitis. St. Louis: CV Mosby, 1968:202–229.

215. Hartridge G. A case of double optic neuro-retinitis after influenza. Trans Ophthalmol Soc UK 1893;13:77–79.

216. Cross FR. Four cases of neuritis after influenza. Trans Ophthalmol Soc UK 1893;13:79–82.

CHAPTER 7

Retinal-Choroidal Toxicity

Howard Schatz, Ronald E. Carr, Brian P. Conway, Travis A. Meredith,
H. Richard McDonald, and Robert N. Johnson

INTRODUCTION

Various chemicals, drugs, and metabolic by-products may have deleterious effects on the retina, retinal pigment epithelium, or choroid. Such agents may come in contact with retinal and choroidal tissues following oral ingestion or intravenous, intracarotid, or intravitreal injection, or they may be produced through metabolic pathways. For example, the drug abuser who injects crushed chemical tablets that are diluted with talc may cause talc damage to the retina. Therapeutic drugs also may be retinotoxic. Finally, ocular toxicity may develop from drugs injected directly into the vitreous, for example, toxicity resulting from intravitreous gentamicin.

All physicians should be aware of the toxic effects of the drugs they prescribe, and all ophthalmologists should be knowledgeable about the retinal, retinal pigment epithelial, and choroidal manifestations of toxicity caused by such chemicals.

In this chapter, we discuss the characteristic fundus lesions caused by a variety of agents that adversely affect the retina.

TALC RETINOPATHY

Talc retinopathy occurs in some intravenous drug abusers, especially those who inject crushed methylphenidate hydrochloride (Ritalin) tablets (1–17). The filler in Ritalin is talc. However, drug dealers are also known to dilute (or "cut") other powdered drugs with talc.

Because talc particles are inert, intravenous administration of talc results in talc deposits in the lungs, where the fine capillaries filter out the talc particles. For a time this filtering mechanism will prevent the talc from entering the systemic (arterial) circulation because the diameter or lumen of the pulmonary capillaries is smaller than that of the talc particles. Over the course of many months or years of intravenous drug abuse, however, collateral vessels form in the lungs, secondary to clogging of the pulmonary capillaries. Blood then flows from the right ventricle, through the collaterals in the lungs, bypassing the obstructed pulmonary capillaries, into the left side of the heart, carrying talc particles to the systemic circulation. The inert talc particles can then lodge in the vessels of any organ in the body, including the retina and choroid.

Ophthalmoscopically, talc deposits can be seen outside the foveal avascular zone in retinal capillaries or in the tissues of the inner retina, particularly in the macular area (8, 14, 17). Vision is usually normal. Talc may cause hemorrhages and cotton-wool spots due to microocclusions of retinal capillaries and even precapillary arterioles. In some cases, occlusion of the macular capillaries can cause infarction and visual loss. The deposition of talc in the peripheral retinal vessels can cause non-perfusion, followed by retinal neovascularization, vitreous hemorrhage, and traction retinal detachment.

Histopathogically, talc particles may also be found in the choriocapillaris, but there they probably do not cause any visual problems (16).

There is no treatment that will clear the talc from the eye. Proliferative retinopathy can be treated with laser photocoagulation. Users of Ritalin and other powdered drugs that may contain talc must be educated about the harmful, often irreversible effects of the illicit intravenous administration of these agents.

CANTHAXANTHINE RETINOPATHY

Canthaxanthine, a naturally occurring carotenoid, is used to color foods and drug products. It has also been distributed as an oral tanning agent in countries other than the United States.

Canthaxanthine ingestion causes bilateral deposits of fine, light-colored crystals in the inner retina, especially surrounding the central fovea. These deposits may be found outside the fovea (18–25). Patients who have taken over 20 g of canthaxanthine appear to be at risk for developing retinopathy. In one report, over 50% of patients taking 30 g or more had retinal crystalline changes. Other studies show that almost all patients taking over 60 g of canthaxanthine will have retinal changes. These changes are probably related not only to the total dose but also to multiple factors such as patient age and individual susceptibility.

Patients with retinal canthaxanthine deposits are generally asymptomatic. Fluorescein angiography is usually normal, except when the crystals are so numerous that they cause hypofluorescence by blocking (masking) choroidal fluorescence. Canthaxanthine maculopathy may be associated with very mildly abnormal electrophysiological testing. Studies have shown that patients with canthaxanthine maculopathy tend to have a lower sensitivity on static perimetry tests than do normal control subjects. Dark adaptation may be delayed, and electro-oculography (EOG) and electroretinography (ERG) may be reduced. Most of these changes, however, are mild.

Some studies have indicated that the crystalline deposition is irreversible, but recent reports have shown a minimal decrease in the number of crystals following cessation of canthaxanthine ingestion.

Daicker et al. (21) reported an autopsy case of a patient who had ingested canthaxanthine. The crystals were red, birefringent, lipid soluble, and 4 μm to 25 μm in size. They were particularly large and numerous in the perifoveal area. The crystals were also deposited in the inner layers of the retina, in rows, between the nerve fibers or near small retinal vessels. They were also seen peripherally. None was seen in the choroid or retinal pigment epithelium (RPE). Atrophic and degenerative changes of the inner retina appeared to be related to the crystalline deposits.

The crystals appeared to be identical to unaltered canthaxanthine crystals available for oral usage, although Daicker et al. (21) thought that the retinal crystals represented a canthaxanthine-like lipoprotein complex rather than pure canthaxanthine.

Because of possible retinal damage and the electrophysiological changes that may occur, patients are advised not to take this drug for tanning. Restrictions have also been imposed on the use of the drug as a food additive.

OXALOSIS AND OXALATE RETINOPATHY

Oxalate is an end product of normal metabolism and is removed from the body by the kidney. Oxalosis, a systemic condition that results from the tissue storage of excess oxalate, can affect the eye and produce a "flecked retina." It can also result in renal failure and death, usually in the first or second decade (26–36).

There are two kinds of oxalosis: primary and secondary. Primary oxalosis can be subdivided into Types I and II, each caused by a rare autosomal recessive inborn error of metabolism. There is no abnormality seen in the presumed heterozygote. Type I primary hyperoxaluria is due to a deficiency of α-ketogluturate glyoxylate carboligase. The deficiency of this enzyme results in increased production of oxalic acid. Urinary excretion of oxalate and glycolate increases in patients before the onset of renal failure (32). Type II primary oxalosis is caused by a deficiency of D-glyceric dehydrogenase, resulting in an increased urinary excretion of oxalate and glycerate. Primary oxaluria is a serious disease leading to renal insufficiency, uremia, and death, usually before the age of 20 (34). There may be a family history of recurrent renal calculi and early death from renal failure (27).

Secondary oxalosis occurs from increased ingestion of oxalate or its precursors, such as rhubarb or ethylene glycol (antifreeze). It may also occur after methoxyflurane anesthesia or as a result of hyperabsorption of oxalate following small bowel resection. It may also be seen in patients with renal failure, sarcoidosis, cirrhosis of the liver, or heart failure (29).

Oxalosis is diagnosed by detecting increased urinary excretion of oxalic acid. This increased excretion may include other acids, such as glycolic and glyoxylic acids. In both primary and secondary oxalosis, oxalate crystals can deposit in many tissues of the body: the eyes, kidneys, bone, liver, thyroid, testes, and heart. When crystals deposit in the heart conduction areas, heart block can occur.

In the eye, oxalate crystals may deposit in any vascular tissue, including the choroid, retina, iris, ciliary body, conjunctiva, and episclera (35). In particular, oxalate crystals deposit between Bruch's membrane and the pigment epithelium or within the pigment epithelium. As a result, pigment epithelial hyperplasia can occur,

causing large, black, pigmented lesions in the macula. In the retina, oxalate crystals may be seen in the retinal vasculature or in the inner half of the retina; they are not found in the outer retina.

Histopathology shows crystalline, birefringent, colorless, calcium oxalate deposits in the retinal pigment epithelium. The smaller crystals are intracellular; the large extracellular crystals cause disruption and degenerative changes of the retinal pigment epithelium.

Oxalosis produces a flecked retinopathy (30, 31, 33). The white flecks are caused by oxalate deposits at the level of the pigment epithelium, though white flecks may also be seen in the retina and in the retinal vessels. The oxalate crystals appear as small, refractile, crystalline dots scattered diffusely throughout the fundus, especially in the posterior pole and midperiphery. In some cases, the crystals may be large and occlude the retinal vessels, causing cotton-wool spots, retinal vascular nonperfusion, neovascularization, vitreous hemorrhage, and visual loss. Multiple, round, highly refractile, crystalline deposits of various sizes may lodge in the perifoveal macular region. Hypertrophy of retinal pigment epithelium may occur around some of the deeper crystalline lesions (36).

The treatment of primary oxalosis is not satisfactory. After renal transplantation, one form of treatment designed to reduce the oxalate load, oxalate crystals will form in the new kidney. A permanent reduction in oxalate formation is almost impossible to attain, because it is the defective metabolism that causes the condition. If the kidneys do not excrete oxalate properly, it remains in the body. Hemodialysis is neither practical nor effective, but it may prolong life if used in association with a high fluid intake and a diet high in magnesium oxide and pyridoxine.

Oxalate crystals may also be found in tissues of the eye as part of severe degenerative ocular disease, unrelated to systemic oxalate metabolism. Crystals have been found in mature cataracts, under long-standing retinal detachments, and in diabetic patients, especially in association with trauma (28).

PHENOTHIAZINE TOXICITY

The fact that certain phenothiazines are retinotoxic was recognized initially in 1956 (37) when a newly developed drug, NP 207, was found to cause subjective problems with dark adaptation and result in the ophthalmoscopic picture of pigmentary retinopathy. Subsequent studies (38) demonstrated that the retinal changes were indicative of widespread photoreceptor disease, and findings similar to those noted in man were later reproduced in cats (39). The drug was removed from the market, but in 1958 a new phenothiazine, thioridazine (Mellaril), was introduced, and in 1960 (39) four cases of pigmentary retinopathy following a high dosage of this medication were described.

The retinal changes caused by thioridazine include pigment clumping, initially in the periphery and later in the posterior pole, with subsequent coalescence of some pigmented areas into flat, pigmented plaques. Other regions show pigment loss, which enhances visualization of the choroidal vessels. Several patients have also developed acute and transient retinal edema in the posterior pole, with subsequent pigment clumping and atrophy. A late fundus change, seen with long-term administration (in some cases several years after cessation of the drug), is the development of multiple, round or nummular areas of retinal pigment epithelial and choriocapillaris atrophy (40). These sharply delimited lesions seem to evolve from areas of prior pigmentary clumping and can extend from the posterior pole to the midperiphery. Fluorescein angiography demonstrates loss of the RPE as well as the choriocapillaris. These areas of atrophy may expand and coalesce and produce a fundus appearance like that of choroideremia.

One histologic study (41) demonstrated that the initial problem pathologically is in the photoreceptor outer segments and is accompanied by a later loss of RPE cells and choriocapillaris. Such a sequence correlates well with the progressive ophthalmoscopic changes noted above.

Phenothiazines show a high uptake by pigmented cells, particularly in the uvea (42), which may be the reason for the toxic retinopathy. The retinotoxic phenothiazine NP 207 is structurally different from other drugs in this class, having a piperidine ring present on the carbon side chain. Both NP 207 and thioridazine have been shown to inhibit the oxidation of retinol (43), which may be the inciting pathological event.

The relationship between the amount of thioridazine ingested and the occurrence of pigmentary retinopathy is unclear, but for many years 800 mg/day was suggested as a safe upper limit. However, in one case report a patient took 700 mg/day up to a total dose of 500 g and developed pigmentary stippling (44). This case is considered unusual; two subsequent reports showed no cases of retinopathy in patients on regimens not exceeding 600 mg/day (45, 46). It seems that the total dosage is not as important as an excessive *daily* dose. Retinal changes have been noted following a total dosage of as little as 27 g with a very high daily dose of 1800 mg (47).

However, there have been several reports of patients who used a low daily dosage of thioridazine for a long period of time and who also developed retinopathy. In one, the daily dosage was 100–400 mg/day, but the total dosage was 752 g (48). In another, the daily dosage was no higher than 300 mg/day. Twenty percent of thioridazine retinopathy cases occur at a dosage less than 800 mg/day (49).

The phenothiazine that causes pigmentary retinopathy most commonly is thioridazine. However, chlorpromazine (Thorazine) has been convincingly implicated in at least four cases as a cause of pigmentary retinopathy in patients using dosages exceeding 2400 mg/day (50). Additionally, retinal toxicity has been reported in one patient taking trifluoperazine (Stelazine) at a dosage of 15 mg/day. This case may well have been idiosyncratic, since 159 other patients in the same study showed no adverse retinal changes (51).

CHLOROQUINE AND HYDROXYCHLOROQUINE TOXICITY

In 1957 Cambiaggi (52) described a bull's-eye macular lesion that he called an "unusual ocular lesion" of systemic lupus erythematosus. It became clear, however, as later studies were published (53, 54), that this was a manifestation of a chloroquine-induced macular change.

Chloroquine and hydroxychloroquine were drugs initially developed as replacements for the more toxic drug, quinacrine, used to treat malaria. Later, these drugs also were used in place of quinacrine to treat lupus erythematosus, rheumatoid arthritis, and other collagen diseases (55). Both of these drugs are substituted 4-aminoquinoline compounds, and they differ only by a hydroxyl group. Substantial binding of these drugs to plasma proteins occurs, with a very high accumulation in pigmented cells, particularly in the uvea and retinal pigment epithelium (56). The binding of these drugs is so strong that trace amounts can be found in the plasma or urine of patients up to 5 years following cessation of medication.

While a bull's-eye maculopathy was the initial retinal change to be described, later studies (57) showed that the initial change in chloroquine-induced retinopathy was a mottling of the foveal and parafoveal RPE, which can evolve into a bull's-eye maculopathy even if therapy is discontinued (58). Several cases have been reported in which a generalized degeneration of the retina developed (53, 59). This is presumably due to the continuing toxic effects of RPE-bound chloroquine.

The specific drug-dose relationship for the production of chloroquine-induced retinopathy is unknown. It is known that excessive dosages—over 250 mg/day of chloroquine and 400 mg/day of hydroxychloroquine—are toxic. Although several hundred cases of chloroquine retinopathy have been described, the more severe cases are usually seen with higher daily doses.

Hydroxychloroquine is purported to have much less toxicity at therapeutic levels (60).

However, a significant number of patients receiving the recommended daily dose of each drug have developed retinopathy (61, 62). This implies that, aside from a dose-related toxicity, some other predisposing factor (possibly idiosyncratic) may play a part. For unknown reasons, certain individuals are more susceptible, and toxicity has occurred when the dosage was below recommended levels, even at the level used in malarial prevention (100 mg/day) (63, 64).

Because the early macular changes may be reversible or may not progress if medication is stopped (57, 65, 66), periodic ocular evaluations are now suggested for patients taking these medications. A number of different psychophysical and electrophysiological tests have been used in attempts to detect the early stages of this disease; all these tests must be interpreted with the knowledge that the 4-aminoquinolines are toxic to the retina. Following prolonged intake of such drugs, even at approved therapeutic dosages, measurable changes in retinal function are always present, irrespective of a lack of ophthalmoscopic change (67). These facts do not imply, however, that all such patients will develop maculopathy, but they indicate that a retinotoxic effect is evident if a sensitive test is used. When evaluating such patients, it is important to separate those with mild psychophysical changes but no retinopathy from those with visible retinal changes.

Electrophysiological testing with the electroretinogram (ERG) and electro-oculogram (EOG) is so variable that it is of no real use (68). Tangent screen testing with a red stimulus, though capable of demonstrating paracentral scotomas, is not a reliable predictor of retinal disease although it can demonstrate a loss of retinal sensitivity. Furthermore, such testing is unreliable because 6% of the normal population will show scotomas (69). Amsler grid testing in such patients can show scotomatous areas before static and kinetic field abnormalities (70), but this finding in no way implies that such patients will develop macular changes. It would seem that the most reliable method of following such patients is with fundus photographs of the macular area to look for the earliest changes of macular granularity and loss of the foveal reflex (68, 71). Unlike the more refined psychophysical tests, which often show an abnormality after prolonged drug intake, photography will identify the patient who develops maculopathy.

CARBAMAZEPINE TOXICITY

Carbamazepine (Tegretol) has been used in the treatment of epilepsy and certain neuralgias, but it has only recently been shown to be retinotoxic (72). This drug is pharmacologically similar to thioridazine, and since it is lipophilic, it easily crosses cell membranes and the blood-ocular barriers. The single report on retinotoxicity describes two female patients who had taken more than 2000 g of Tegretol over a period of 7 or 10 years. Both patients showed changes in the retinal pigment epithelium in the posterior pole, with associated mild reductions in vision and paracentral scotomas. Cessation of the drug led in both cases to a disappearance of symptoms with no or little change in the abnormal appearance of the RPE.

TOXICITY OF INTRAVITREAL DRUG INJECTION

Gentamicin

As the concepts of antimicrobial therapy with antibiotics evolved, it was suggested that direct intraocular injection might be the most effective way of treating infectious endophthalmitis (73). As more and more antimicrobial agents became available, many were tested for intraocular toxicity. Because of its broad spectrum of activity, particularly for Gram-negative organisms such as *Pseudomonas*, gentamicin became an intravitreal antibiotic of choice. Toxicity studies, mostly in rabbit models, were performed to ascertain the

safe intravitreal dose (74). Although there was some disagreement (75), a dose of 100–400 µg of gentamicin was thought to be safe for intravitreal injection. The initial reports of clinical experience using this dose were favorable (76).

In a review of the visual results after direct intraocular antibiotic injection for endophthalmitis, Peyman and associates (77) noted two cases of gentamicin injection with poor outcomes that were associated with "cilio-retinal artery occlusion." The occasional occurrence of this fundus picture, which has also been termed "macular infarction," became more difficult to attribute to damage from the infection when it was seen after relatively mild endophthalmitis (78) or when intravitreal antibiotics were given for infectious prophylaxis after penetrating injuries (79). The suspicion that gentamicin toxicity might cause this macular infarction was supported by the publication of cases showing similar but more severe retinal damage after the accidental intraocular injection of undiluted gentamicin (79, 80).

Following the accidental intraocular injection of undiluted aminoglycoside antibiotics, a dense white opacification of the retina with complete shutdown of the retinal vascular supply may develop within 24 hours (79–81). Gentamicin may be mistaken for Miochol or balanced salt solution, leading to its intraocular injection. Inadvertent scleral perforation may occur as the surgeon attempts a sub-Tenon's injection of gentamicin. In moderate cases, which are often seen after rapid injection of appropriate therapeutic doses of gentamicin for suspected endophthalmitis or as prophylaxis in penetrating injury, a less fulminant picture develops (78, 79). The initial finding is a white opacification of the macula. If the eye still sees, the patient complains of a central scotoma. At first, the capillary perfusion of the macula may be intact, but if the damage is sufficiently severe, the picture of "macular infarction" develops, with a distinctive shutdown of the capillary circulation. In the mild cases, in which infarction apparently does not develop, there can be recovery of useful

(20/50) vision. More severe cases show no recovery, and the blood supply to the macula remains permanently occluded.

Injection of large doses (3000 µg) of gentamicin into the vitreous cavity of primate eyes duplicates the clinical appearance (82). Massive swelling of the retina is seen at 24 hours, with patent but leaking retinal vessels. By 72 hours, capillary perfusion is absent. Histopathological studies demonstrate that the major vessels and the capillaries are normal, while the retina is massively swollen and necrotic. From these observations, it has been concluded that the primary event is a toxic reaction in the neural tissue of the retina, which results in massive swelling. The shutdown of the capillary bed and infarction seem to be secondary phenomena, perhaps initiated or maintained by some mechanism such as "granulocytic plugging" (83). This pathogenetic hypothesis is supported by the observation that lower doses of intravitreal gentamicin cause an isolated swelling of the macula with no infarction (84, 85).

Amphotericin B

Systemic administration of effective doses of amphotericin B often causes significant renal toxicity. The intravenous and subconjunctival administration of amphotericin B results in almost no penetration into the vitreous cavity in normal eyes and minimal to moderate penetration in inflamed eyes (86). Axelrod and co-workers (87) found retinal necrosis and detachment after injection of 25 µg of amphotericin B into the center of the vitreous of rabbits, but no observable changes by serial ophthalmoscopy after doses of 5 µg and 10 µg. Electroretinography and light microscopy at 4 weeks showed no changes. However, Souri and Green (88) found histopathologic evidence of retinal necrosis at all dose levels (except for 1 of the 3 eyes receiving only 1.0 µg). Some of the discrepancies between these 2 reports are probably due to differences in injection technique.

A number of reports indicated that eyes injected with 10 µg of amphotericin B into the vitreous may have ultimate recovery of good vision. There is experimental evidence suggesting that primate eyes are more tolerant of intravitreal amphotericin B than are rabbit eyes.

A pharmacokinetic study of amphotericin B in rabbit eyes found marked differences in the half-life of the drug depending on whether or not the lens and vitreous were intact (89). The half-life was 9.1 days in the intact eye, 8.6 days in infected intact eyes, 4.7 days in eyes in which the lens had been removed, and 1.4 days in eyes in which the lens and vitreous had been removed. Clinical experience supports the concept that eyes that lack a lens and vitreous tolerate multiple injections of 10 µg of amphotericin B at intervals as frequent as every 3 days (90).

There are few descriptions of the retinal toxic effects of amphotericin B. One eye obtained for study 7 weeks after a single intravitreal injection of 5 µg of amphotericin B for *Candida albicans* endophthalmitis showed only autolytic changes in the retina (91), which were not thought to be the result of amphotericin B toxicity.

Experiments in rabbit eyes (92) and in rhesus monkey eyes (93) have indicated that the amount of amphotericin B tolerated by both species (before the development of retinal toxicity) can be quadrupled by liposomal encapsulation. Interestingly, these studies also show that the primate eye tolerates 6 times as much amphotericin B as the rabbit eye does before developing histopathologic changes. This difference is somewhat greater than would be expected from the difference in the vitreous volume and may indicate a species difference in sensitivity to toxic effects.

Other Antibiotics

Intravitreal injection of cephalosporin derivatives is popular because of their high toxic-therapeutic ratio and their broad spectrum of activity. One of the first of these tried, cephaloridine, was found to cause a distinct retinal toxicity (94), perhaps by the same vascular irritant mechanism that is seen systemically. The greatest experience with cephalosporin derivatives has been with cefazolin. Recently, however, some authors (95) have advocated substituting vancomycin because of a problem with *Staphylococcus epidermidis* specifically resistant to cefazolin.

Antiviral Agents

The recent description of two types of viral retinitis, the acute retinal necrosis syndrome (ARN) and cytomegalovirus retinitis associated with AIDS, has increased interest in the direct intravitreal injection of antiviral agents. Vidarabine (ara-A) and acyclovir were investigated for their intraocular toxicity (96). No toxicity was seen with 80 μg of vidarabine, but a 400 μg/ml vitrectomy infusion fluid of acyclovir resulted in "disorganization of the outer layer of the retina." Forty μg/ml has been suggested for vitrectomy performed for retinal detachment associated with ARN. Ganciclovir, an agent especially useful for treatment of cytomegalovirus retinitis, has shown no retinal toxicity when infused into rabbit eyes (97). The repetitive direct intravitreal injection of 200 μg of ganciclovir for CMV retinitis in patients with AIDS appears safe (98).

Vitreous Substitutes

Vitreous substitutes and cytotoxic agents have been injected into the vitreous cavity to manage complicated retinal detachments, particularly those with proliferative vitreoretinopathy (PVR).

Gas

Many types of inert gas have been studied because of their ability to tamponade retinal breaks. Sulphur hexafluoride (SF_6) and perfluoropropane (C_3F_8) have found the widest clinical use. Animal studies show no specific retinal toxicity. The expansile property of such gases has been used experimentally for vitreous compression, collapsing the vitreous gel to simulate posterior vitreous separation or to improve the results of pars plana vitrectomy in humans (99). Intravitreal gas may create new retinal breaks, which may be detected soon after pneumatic retinopexy (100).

Silicone Oil

At present, there is disagreement about the retinal toxicity of intravitreous silicone oil. Most of the eyes into which the material is injected have preexisting severe pathology, making it difficult to ascertain how much of the retinal atrophy detected later is due to the preexisting pathology and how much is due to the effects of the silicone oil. One histopathological study (101) showed silicone oil infiltrating the retina. However, other studies showed no specific histopathological or electroretinographic findings attributable to the silicone that were not also seen in saline-injected control rabbit eyes. The controversy has continued (102), with the recent presentation of clinical evidence of retinal infiltration with silicone (103) and of damage to retinal cellular components in primate eyes chronically exposed to silicone (104).

Antiproliferative Agents

The realization that cellular proliferation is a crucial event in preretinal membrane formation that causes the majority of failures of retinal detachment surgery (105) led to a search for agents that could control the proliferation. Among the first groups to be studied were the corticosteroids. Although intravitreal injection of corticosteroids proved disappointing in the control of proliferative vitreoretinopathy, the experimental work provided information about the tolerance of these agents when injected into the eye. It became clear (106) that most of the toxicity associated with injecting the depo forms of these agents into the eye comes from the vehicles and preservatives, not from the corticosteroids themselves. Inadvertent injection of depot corticosteroids into the eye has occurred, causing effects similar to those seen in the animal models (107).

The next drugs screened for PVR were the cytotoxic and cytostatic agents. A large number of agents were assessed for toxicity and for their value in prevention of membrane formation. In experimental animals the retinal toxicity is most evident in the highly metabolically active outer retinal layers: the photoreceptor layer, and the retinal pigment epithelium. Of the many agents screened, fluorouracil has seen the most use clinically (108). The relatively short half-life of fluorouracil in the eye has led to work with liposome encapsulation in the hope of increasing the dose that can be injected and of prolonging its half-life (109).

The other antiproliferative agent used clinically is daunomycin (daunorubicin). Although the toxic-therapeutic ratio of this agent is small (110) because of photoreceptor toxicity, it has been reported to be useful in the prophylaxis of traumatic PVR (111) when used as a 7.5 μg/ml wash that is evacuated after 10 minutes by the instillation of a gas or silicone bubble.

More recently, agents having more specific antimetabolic effects have been investigated for use in the treatment of PVR. Microtubule action may be important in the contraction of membranes in PVR. Since colchicine inhibits microtubule function, it has been suggested as a therapy. Systemic administration of colchicine in an animal model of PVR appeared promising (112), but intravitreal administration has been shown to cause severe toxicity even in doses as low as 1.0 μg (113). The toxic changes occur primarily in the nerve fiber layer, which is not surprising since microtubule function is necessary for axonal transport. The agent taxol, an antineoplastic drug whose primary effect is on tubulin aggregation, has also been advocated (114). At high doses, it causes optic atrophy.

QUININE TOXICITY

Quinine is a naturally occurring alkaloid used for the oral treatment of malaria and muscle cramps. Acute toxicity (cinchonism) may occur following oral ingestion in an attempted abortion or suicide or in accidental poisoning. The visual problems, including acute blindness associated with quinine overdose, have been recognized for many years, but the pathogenesis of the disorder remains unclear.

The visual signs and symptoms in the affected patient vary, depending on the time that has elapsed between the quinine ingestion and when the patient is seen. Acutely, the vision is reduced, in some instances to no light perception. The retina and retinal vessels appear normal, the pupils are dilated and nonreactive, and the visual fields are constricted. Over the next several days, variable degrees of retinal edema may appear, although the retinal vessels remain normal. The visual acuity and the visual field deficits gradually improve. Over time, the edema resolves and the visual acuity returns to normal. The visual fields improve but always show some degree of constriction. The optic nerve becomes white, and the retinal arteries remain narrowed. This improvement in the visual acuity despite severe narrowing of the retinal vessels and disc pallor is called "the paradox of quinine."

The reports in the literature evaluating the electrophysiologic changes associated with quinine toxicity have been sufficiently contradictory to cause some confusion in understanding the pathogenesis of this disorder. Clinical and experimental studies show that the oscillatory potentials and the a- and b-wave amplitudes of the ERG are reduced during the first several hours after quinine toxicity (115). Within 24 hours, the ERG demonstrates a normal a-wave, a reduced b-wave, and continued loss of oscillatory potentials. The EOG and the visual evoked response (VER) are abnormal. The ERG usually returns to normal over the next several weeks, but it often will show a steady decrease in the b-wave and an increase in the a-wave. The EOG and VER remain abnormal. These morphological and electrophysiologic changes point to a diffuse toxic effect on multiple retinal elements, including ganglion cells, bipolar and amacrine cells, photoreceptors, and the retinal pigment epithelium.

The acute and chronic changes vary according to the degree of toxicity. Constant morphological and electrophysiological changes in late cases of quinine toxicity include the following:

1. Destruction of ganglion cells as indicated by optic atrophy and an abnormal VER.
2. Bipolar cell loss, probably due to trans-synaptic degeneration, as indicated by a loss of the ERG b-wave.
3. Amacrine cell dysfunction as manifested by a loss of the ERG oscillations.
4. Early photoreceptor changes as manifested by the initial ERG a-wave abnormalities. These changes are reversible, since the a-wave becomes normal. This rapid repair may indicate a transient disruption of the photoreceptor membrane.
5. Retinal pigment eptihelial damage as demonstrated by persistent EOG abnormalities. Whether the entire RPE is affected has not yet been studied, but a normal ERG a-wave associated with an abnormal EOG would point to a dysfunction of the basal portion of the RPE cells.

TOXICITY OF CANCER CHEMOTHERAPEUTIC AGENTS

Cancer chemotherapeutic agents may be given orally, intravenously, intramuscularly, or by intracarotid injection. In general, agents given by the oral route have less serious side effects than do those given by the intracarotid route.

Tamoxifen

Tamoxifen, an antiestrogen drug that attaches to estrogen receptors in the cytoplasm of cells, is used to treat metastatic breast carcinoma. Many patients with ocular changes present with modestly decreased vision (116–118). Corneal changes consisting of whorl-like subepithelial

changes are present in some eyes (116–118). In the macula, multiple white refractile deposits accumulate in the superficial retina, and yellow-white lesions are seen at the level of the retinal pigment epithelium (116, 118). Cystoid macular edema has also been noted (118).

The retinal lesions are usually observed after months of drug exposure and have been reported at doses of 20 mg/day (116, 117, 119, 120). One patient had ingested a total dose of 90 g over 8 months at the time the ocular changes were first noted (119).

On electron microscopy, small intracellular deposits, 3–10 μm in size, are present in the macular area; in the perimacular area the lesions are 30–50 μm and are extracellular (119). These lesions are located in the inner retina and stain positively for glycosaminoglycans. They may represent products of axonal degeneration.

Mitotane

Mitotane (o,p'DDD), an oral agent used to treat adrenal carcinoma, causes blurred vision and diplopia in some patients. One report noted a "toxic retinopathy with papilledema and retinal hemorrhages" (121).

Tilorone Hydrochloride

Tilorone hydrochloride is an experimental oral antitumor agent that can produce several ocular complications. Vision is often normal, but the cornea demonstrates diffuse clouding due to subepithelial infiltrates. Histological findings include clouding, swelling, and intracytoplasmic inclusions in the corneal and conjunctival epithelium (122). One patient developed a fine pigment mottling of the peripheral retina and macula with mild arterial narrowing. Goldmann visual fields disclosed marked peripheral constriction. The ERG and EOG were both abnormal. A second patient developed severe bilateral arterial narrowing, mild pigment mottling of the macula, and reduction of the EOG and ERG. In these patients, complications occurred at the normal dosage of 500 mg/day; the first patient had received a total dose of 152 g, and the second 189 g (123). Since the drug is an antioxidant that affects the free radical mechanism of the retinal pigment epithelium and has other similarities to chloroquine, the authors postulated that the mechanisms of damage may be the same (123).

Procarbazine

Retinal hemorrhages and papilledema have been reported after treatment with procarbazine (124).

Chlorambucil

In a case report of a 16-year-old with nephrotic syndrome, retinal hemorrhages and papilledema were reported (125).

Intracarotid Agents

In order to attain higher intracranial drug levels to treat central nervous system tumors, anticancer agents may be given by the intracarotid route. Compared with oral administration, intracarotid administration increases the likelihood of serious retinal complications.

Nitrogen Mustard

Nitrogen mustard is an alkylating agent that is parasympathomimetic and radiomimetic. In a review of 12 patients treated with carotid injection, 3 developed problems in the ipsilateral eye. In the early phase, a severe iritis with synechiae developed, accompanied by lid swelling and conjunctival chemosis. The retina could not be seen. As the anterior problems cleared, retinal edema, arterial narrowing, and hard exudates were found. Choroidal atrophy developed as a late effect. Two cases showed thrombi in the choroidal vessels and a significant necrotic vasculitis. Subretinal exudate was present in one case, but the retina showed only a few inflammatory foci (126).

Methotrexate

Methotrexate has been given for CNS tumors by the intracarotid route following injection of mannitol and cyclophosphamide to break down the blood-brain barrier. In a few reported patients, a mild visual loss was noted after treatment. Macular changes were noted, consisting of focal retinal pigment epithelial hyperplasia with smaller areas of retinal pigment epithelial atrophy. The average dose given to these patients was 8239 mg (127).

Cis-platinum
(cis-dichlorodiaminoplatinum II)

Cis-platinum causes ocular side effects after being given by the intracarotid route either alone or in combination with BCNU (carmustine). Rarely, complications have been reported after intravenous use alone.

In one study, 35 patients were treated with intracarotid injections of cis-platinum for progressive malignant brain tumors following cranial irradiation, and in some cases, prior chemotherapy. After preliminary treatment with intravenous mannitol, cis-platinum was infused via the carotid route in doses of 60–120 mg/m². Patients were thought to tolerate a monthly dose of 60–75 mg/m² reasonably well. Five of these patients developed visual blurring; in 2 patients, this was evaluated and attributed to papilledema and ischemic optic neuropathy (128).

In a second study, 11 patients were treated with cis-platinum and whole brain irradiation of 6020 rads. When the cis-platinum was injected above the bifurcation of the ophthalmic artery, no abnormalities developed. Of 5 patients treated with infusion below the ophthalmic artery, 4 developed complications. One eye had a retinal infarct and 1 an abnormal scotopic ERG. One eye had a severe loss of retinal pigment epithelium and was noted on fluorescein angiography to have loss of retinal and choroidal capillaries. Optic atrophy developed in one eye. The authors postulated induction of ischemic damage (129). Pigmentary retinopathy, optic atrophy, and vessel narrowing was noted in another reported patient (130).

Three patients were reported to have developed papilledema or retrobulbar neuritis after intravenous doses of *cis*-platinum alone or in combination with other chemotherapeutic agents. Optic neuropathy is also caused by systemic administration of other heavy metals (129, 130).

Nitrosoureas

Nitrosoureas used in cancer chemotherapy are BCNU (carmustine), CCNU (lomustine), and methyl-CCNU. BCNU has been given alone or in combination with *cis*-platinum.

Kupersmith et al. (129) reported no visual loss when BCNU was given by infusion above the ophthalmic artery. When the drug was given below the ophthalmic artery, all patients developed rod system dysfunction in the ipsilateral eye and one patient developed an abnormal ERG in the contralateral eye, suggesting that the drug crossed through the anterior communicating pathway to the contralateral carotid-ophthalmic arterial system.

Miller et al. (131) reported that after treatment with 600 to 800 mg of BCNU alone or in combination with *cis*-platinum, many eyes developed severe visual loss and fundus abnormalities. Severe pigmentary disturbances were noted in the posterior pole. Fluorescein angiography demonstrated periarterial and perivenous leakage with patchy hypo- and hyperfluorescence in the macula as a later finding. Shingleton et al. (132) noted retinal vessel narrowing, intraretinal hemorrhages, and nerve fiber layer infarcts in their patients. Fluorescein angiography demonstrated segmental perivascular staining, widespread capillary leakage, and optic disc hypofluorescence. Complications developed 2 to 14 weeks after intra-arterial injection in 7 of 10 patients. The cumulative minimum dose was 450 mg/kg in 2 treatments.

Although "optic neuroretinitis" has been reported in association with intravenous BCNU and procarbazine therapy (133), a review of clinical experience with reported ocular complications caused by intravenous BCNU, CCNU, or methyl-CCNU found that all cases had significant complications of the disease or concomitant radiotherapy or chemotherapy. The authors thought that there was no conclusive evidence of drug-related ocular lesions caused by this route of administration (134).

ACKNOWLEDGMENT

Supported by the Retina Research Fund of St. Mary's Hospital and Medical Center, San Francisco, California.

References

Talc Retinopathy
1. Hahn HH, Schweid AI, Beaty HN. Complications of injecting dissolved methylphenidate tablets. Arch Intern Med 1969;123:656–659.
2. Hopkins GB, Taylor DG. Pulmonary talc granulomatosis; a complication of drug abuse. Am Rev Respir Dis 1970;101:101–104.
3. Atlee WE Jr. Talc and cornstarch emboli in eyes of drug users. JAMA 1972;219:49–51.
4. Marschke G, Haber L, Feinberg M. Pulmonary talc embolization. Chest 1975;68:824–826.
5. Hildick-Smith GY. The biology of talc. Br J Ind Med 1976;33:217–229.
6. Murphy SB, Jackson WB, Pare JAP. Talc retinopathy. Can J Ophthalmol 1978;13:152–156.
7. Brucker AJ. Disk and peripheral retinal neovascularization secondary to talc and cornstarch emboli. Am J Ophthalmol 1979;88:864–867.
8. Friberg TR, Gragoudas ES, Regan CDJ. Talc emboli and macular ischemia in intravenous drug abuse. Arch Ophthalmol 1979;97:1089–1091.
9. Kresca LJ, Goldberg MF, Jampol LM. Talc emboli and retinal neovascularization in a drug abuser. Am J Ophthalmol 1979;87:334–339.
10. Schatz H. Methylphenidate abuse produces retinopathy. JAMA 1979;241:256.
11. Schatz H, Drake M. Self-injected retinal emboli. Ophthalmology 1979;86:468–483.
12. Tse DT, Ober RR. Talc retinopathy. Am J Ophthalmol 1980;90:624–640.
13. Bluth LL, Hanscom TA. Retinal detachment and vitreous hemorrhage due to talc emboli. JAMA 1981;246:980–981.
14. Jampol LM, Setogawa T, Rednam KRV, Tso MOM. Talc retinopathy in primates: a model of ischemic retinopathy. I. Clinical studies. Arch Ophthalmol 1981;99:1273–1280.
15. Keane JR. Embolic retinopathy from carotid artery self-injection. A case of true "mainline"

talc retinopathy. J Clin Neuro Ophthalmol 1981;1:119–121.

16. Kaga N, Tso MOM, Jampol LM, Setogawa T, Rednam KRV. Talc retinopathy in primates: a model of ischemic retinopathy. II. A histopathologic study. Arch Ophthalmol 1982;100:1644–1648.

17. Kaga N, Tso MOM, Jampol LM. Talc retinopathy in primates: a model of ischemic retinopathy. III. An electron microscopic study. Arch Ophthalmol 1982;100:1649–1652.

Canthaxanthine Retinopathy

18. Rousseau A. Canthaxanthine deposits in the eye. J Am Acad Dermatol 1983;8:123–124.

19. McGuiness R, Beaumont P. Gold dust retinopathy after the ingestion of canthaxanthine to produce skin-bronzing. Med J Aust 1985;143:622–623.

20. Ros AM, Leyon H, Wennersten G. Crystalline retinopathy in patients taking an oral drug containing canthaxanthine. Photodermatology 1985;2:183–185.

21. Daicker B, Schiedt K, Adnet JJ, Bermond P. Canthaxanthine retinopathy; an investigation by light and electron microscopy and physiochemical analysis. Graefes Arch Clin Exp Ophthalmol 1987;225:189–197.

22. Lonn LI. Canthaxanthine retinopathy. Arch Ophthalmol 1987;105:1590–1591.

23. Weber U, Kern W, Novotny GEK, Goerz G, Hanappel S. Experimental carotenoid retinopathy. I. Functional and morphological alterations of the rabbit retina after 11 months' dietary carotenoid application. Graefes Arch Clin Exp Ophthalmol 1987;225:198–205.

24. Weber U, Michaelis L, Kern W, Goerz G. Experimental carotenoid retinopathy. II. Functional and morphological alterations of the rabbit retina after acute canthaxanthine application with small unilamellar phospholipid liposomes. Graefes Arch Clin Exp Ophthalmol 1987; 225:346–350.

25. Harnois C, Cortin P, Samson J, Boudreault G, Malenfant M, Rousseau A. Static perimetry in canthaxanthine maculopathy. Arch Ophthalmol 1988;106:58–60.

Oxalosis and Oxalate Retinopathy

26. Scowen EF, Stansfeld AG, Watts RWE. Oxalosis and primary hyperoxaluria. J Pathol Bacteriol 1959;77:195–205.

27. Shepard TH II, Lee LW, Krebs EG. Primary hyperoxaluria. II. Genetic studies in a family. Pediatrics 1960;25:869–871.

28. Friedman AH, Charles NC. Retinal oxalosis in two diabetic patients. Am J Ophthalmol 1974;78:189–195.

29. Albert DM, Bullock JD, Lahav M, Caine R. Flecked retina secondary to oxalate crystals from methoxyflurane anesthesia: clinical and experimental studies. Trans Am Acad Ophthalmol Otolaryngol 1975;79:OP817–826.

30. Bullock JD, Albert DM. Flecked retina; appearance secondary to oxalate crystals from methoxyflurane anesthesia. Arch Ophthalmol 1975;93:26–31.

31. Gottlieb RP, Ritter JA. "Flecked retina"—an association with primary hyperoxaluria. J Pediatr 1977;90:939–942.

32. Holmgren G, Hornstrom T, Johansson S, Samuelson G. Primary hyperoxaluria (glycolic acid variant): a clinical and genetical investigation of eight cases. Ups J Med Sci 1978;83:65–70.

33. Fiedler AR, Garner A, Chambers TL. Ophthalmic manifestations of primary oxalosis. Br J Ophthalmol 1980;64:782–788.

34. Helin I. Primary hyperoxaluria: an analysis of 17 Scandinavian patients. Scand J Urol Nephrol 1980;14:61–64.

35. Zak TA, Buncic R. Primary hereditary oxalosis retinopathy. Arch Ophthalmol 1983;101:78–80.

36. Meredith TA, Wright JD, Gammon JA, Fellner SK, Warshaw BL, Maio M. Ocular involvement in primary hyperoxaluria. Arch Ophthalmol 1984;102:584–587.

Phenothiazine Toxicity

37. Goar EL, Fletcher MC. Toxic chorioretinopathy following the use of NP 207. Trans Am Ophthalmol Soc 1956;54:129–139.

38. Burian HM, Fletcher MC. Visual functions in patients with retinal pigmentary degeneration following the use of NP 207. Arch Ophthalmol 1958;60:612–629.

39. Weekley RD, Potts AM, Reboton J, May RH. Pigmentary retinopathy in patients receiving high doses of a new phenothiazine. Arch Ophthalmol 1960;64:65–76.

40. Meredith TA, Aaberg TM, Willerson WD. Progressive chorioretinopathy after receiving thioridazine. Arch Ophthalmol 1978;96:1172–1176.

41. Miller FS III, Bunt-Milam AH, Kalina RE. Clinical-ultrastructural study of thioridazine retinopathy. Ophthalmology 1982;89:1478–1488.

42. Kimbrough BO, Campbell RJ. Thioridazine levels in the human eye. Arch Ophthalmol 1981;99:2188–2189.

43. Meier-Ruge W, Cerletti A. Experimental pathology of chloroquine and phenothiazine retinopathy. Concilium Ophthalmologicum, 20th, 1966, Germany. 1967;2:1129–1136.

44. Heshe J, Engelstoft FH, Kirk L. Retinal injury developing under thioridazine treatment. Nord Psykiat T 1961;15:442–447.

45. Appelbaum A. An ophthalmoscopic study of patients under treatment with thioridazine. Arch Ophthalmol 1963;69:578–580.

46. Forrest FM, Snow HL. Prognosis of eye complications caused by phenothiazines. Dis Nerv Syst 1968;29(suppl):26–28.

47. Hagopian V, Stratton DB, Busiek RD. Five cases of pigmentary retinopathy associated with thioridazine administration. Am J Psychiatry 1966;123:97–100.

48. Lam RW, Remick RA. Pigmentary retinopathy associated with low-dose thioridazine treatment. Can Med Assoc J 1985;132:737.
49. Ball WA, Caroff SN. Retinopathy, tardive dyskinesia, and low-dose thioridazine. Am J Psychiatry 1986;143:256—257.
50. Siddall JR. Ocular toxic changes associated with chlorpromazine and thioridazine. Can J Ophthalmol 1966;1:190–198.
51. Reboton J Jr, Weekly RD, Bylenga ND, May RH. Pigmentary retinopathy and iridocycloplegia in psychiatric patients. J Neuropsychiatry 1962;3:311–316.

Chloroquine and Hydroxychloroquine Toxicity
52. Cambiaggi A. Unusual ocular lesions in a case of systemic lupus erythematosus. Arch Ophthalmol 1957;57:451–453.
53. Hobbs HE, Sorsby A, Freedman A. Retinopathy following chloroquine therapy. Lancet 1959;2:478–480.
54. Richards RD, Wilson WR. Retinopathy associated with chloroquine phosphate therapy. Am J Med 1961;31:141–143.
55. Page F. Treatment of lupus erythematosus with mepacrine. Lancet 1951;2:755–758.
56. Rubin M, Bernstein HN, Zvaifler NJ. Studies on the pharmacology of chloroquine; recommendations for the treatment of chloroquine retinopathy. Arch Ophthalmol 1963;70:474–481.
57. Carr RE, Henkind P, Rothfield N, Siegel IM. Ocular toxicity of antimalarial drugs; long-term follow-up. Am J Ophthalmol 1968;66:738–744.
58. Burns RP. Delayed onset of chloroquine retinopathy. N Engl J Med 1966;275:693–696.
59. Crews SJ. Chloroquine retinopathy with recovery in early stages. Lancet 1964;2:436–438.
60. Shearer RV, Dubois EL. Ocular changes induced by long-term hydroxychloroquine (Plaquenil) therapy. Am J Ophthalmol 1967;64:245–252.
61. Rynes RI. Ophthalmologic safety of long-term hydroxychloroquine sulfate treatment. Am J Med 1983;75:35–39.
62. Easterbrook M. Dose relationships in patients with early chloroquine retinopathy. J Rheumatol 1987;14:472–475.
63. Metge P, Rodor F, Chovet M, Montabone M, Llavador M. A propos de 6 cas de retinopathie chloroquinique consecutive a une prophylaxie antipalustre. Bull Soc Ophtalmol Fr 1979;79:347–351.
64. Verin P, Comte P. Retinopathie chloroquinique et prophylaxie du paludisme. Bull Soc Ophtalmol Fr 1986;86:975–979.
65. Carr RE, Gouras P, Gunkel RD. Chloroquine retinopathy: early detection by retinal threshold test. Arch Ophthalmol 1966;75:171–178.
66. Brinkley JR Jr, Dubois EL, Ryan SJ. Long-term course of chloroquine retinopathy after cessation of medication. Am J Ophthalmol 1979;88:1–11.
67. Mills PV, Beck M, Power BJ. Assessment of the retinal toxicity of hydroxychloroquine. Trans Ophthalmol Soc UK 1981;101:109–113.
68. Henkind P, Carr RE, Siegel IM. Early chloroquine retinopathy: clinical and functional findings. Arch Ophthalmol 1964;71:157–165.
69. Percival SPB, Behrman J. Ophthalmological safety of chloroquine. Br J Ophthalmol 1969;53:101–109.
70. Easterbrook M. The sensitivity of Amsler grid testing in early chloroquine retinopathy. Trans Ophthalmol Soc UK 1985;104:204–207.
71. Cruess AF, Schachat AP, Nicholl J, Augsburger JJ. Chloroquine retinopathy. Is fluorescein angiography necessary? Ophthalmology 1985;92:1127–1129.

Carbamazepine Toxicity
72. Nielsen NV, Syversen K. Possible retinotoxic effect of carbamazepine. Acta Ophthalmol 1986;64:287–290.

Toxicity of Intravitreal Drug Injection
73. Von Sallmann L. Controversial points in ocular penicillin therapy. Trans Am Ophthalmol Soc 1947;45:570–636.
74. Peyman GA, May DR, Ericson ES, Apple D. Intraocular injection of gentamicin: toxic effects and clearance. Arch Ophthalmol 1974;92:42–47.
75. Zachary IG, Forster RK. Experimental intravitreal gentamicin. Am J Ophthalmol 1976;82:604–611.
76. Peyman GA, Vastine DW, Raichand M. Postoperative endophthalmitis: experimental aspects and their clinical application. Ophthalmology 1978;85:374–385.
77. Vastine DW, Peyman GA, Guth SB. Visual prognosis in bacterial endophthalmitis treated with intravitreal antibiotics. Ophthalmic Surg 1979;10:76–83.
78. Conway BP, Campochiaro PA. Macular infarction after endophthalmitis treated with vitrectomy and intravitreal gentamicin. Arch Ophthalmol 1986;104:367–371.
79. McDonald HR, Schatz H, Allen AW, et al. Retinal toxicity secondary to intraocular gentamicin injection. Ophthalmology 1986;93:871–877.
80. Snider JD III, Cohen HB, Chenoweth RG. Acute ischemic retinopathy secondary to intraocular injection of gentamicin. In: Ryan SJ, Dawson AK, Little HL, eds. Retinal diseases. Orlando, FL: Grune & Stratton, 1985:227–232.
81. Balian JV. Accidental intraocular tobramycin injection: a case report. Ophthalmic Surg 1983;14:353–354.
82. Conway BP, Tabatabay CA, Campochiaro PA, D'Amico DJ, Hanninen LA, Kenyon KR. Gentamicin toxicity in the primate retina. Arch Ophthalmol 1989;107:107–112.
83. Schmid-Schoenbein GW. Capillary plugging by granulocytes and the no-reflow phenomenon in

the microcirculation. Fed Proc 1987;46:2397–2401.

84. Maurice DM. Injection of drugs into the vitreous body. In: Leopold IH, Burns RP, eds. Symposium on ocular therapy. Vol 9. New York: Wiley & Sons, 1976:59–72.

85. Barza M. Antibacterial agents in the treatment of ocular infections. Infect Dis Clin North Am 1989;3:533–551.

86. Green WR, Bennett JE, Goos RD. Ocular penetration of amphotericin B; a report of laboratory studies and a case report of postsurgical cephalosporium endophthalmitis. Arch Ophthalmol 1965;73:769–775.

87. Axelrod AJ, Peyman GA, Apple DJ. Toxicity of intravitreal injection of amphotericin B. Am J Ophthalmol 1973;76:578–583.

88. Souri EN, Green WR. Intravitreal amphotericin B toxicity. Am J Ophthalmol 1974;78:77–81.

89. Doft BH, Weiskopf J, Nilsson-Ehle I, Wingard LB Jr. Amphotericin clearance in vitrectomized versus nonvitrectomized eyes. Ophthalmology 1985;92:1601–1605.

90. Pflugfelder SC, Flynn HW Jr, Zwickey TA, et al. Exogenous fungal endophthalmitis. Ophthalmology 1988;95:19–30.

91. Stern GA, Fetkenhour CL, O'Grady RB. Intravitreal amphotericin B treatment of *Candida* endophthalmitis. Arch Ophthalmol 1977;95:89–93.

92. Tremblay C, Barza M, Szoka F, Lahav M, Baum J. Reduced toxicity of liposome-associated amphotericin B injected intravitreally in rabbits. Invest Ophthalmol Vis Sci 1985;26:711–718.

93. Barza M, Baum J, Tremblay C, Szoka F, D'Amico DJ. Ocular toxicity of intravitreally injected liposomal amphotericin B in rhesus monkeys. Am J Ophthalmol 1985;100:259–263.

94. Vlchek JK, Peyman GA. Cephaloridine-induced retinopathy by intravitreal injection: an ultrastructural study. Ann Ophthalmol 1975;7:903–914.

95. Pflugfelder SC, Hernandez E, Fliesler SJ, Alvarez J, Pflugfelder ME, Forster RK. Intravitreal vancomycin. Retinal toxicity, clearance, and interaction with gentamicin. Arch Ophthalmol 1987;105:831–837.

96. Pulido JS, Palacio M, Peyman GA, Fiscella R, Greenberg D, Stelmack T. Toxicity of intravitreal antiviral drugs. Ophthalmic Surg 1984;15:666–669.

97. Kao GW, Peyman GA, Fiscella R, House B. Retinal toxicity of ganciclovir in vitrectomy infusion solution. Retina 1987;7:80–83.

98. Henry K, Cantrill H, Fletcher C, Chinnock BJ, Balfour HH Jr. Use of intravitreal ganciclovir (dihydroxy propoxymethyl guanine) for cytomegalovirus retinitis in a patient with AIDS. Am J Ophthalmol 1987;103:17–23.

99. Thresher RJ, Ehrenberg M, Machemer R. Gas-mediated vitreous compression: an experimental alternative to mechanized vitrectomy. Graefes Arch Clin Exp Ophthalmol 1984;221:192–198.

100. McAllister IL, Meyers SM, Zegarra H, Gutman FA, Zakov ZN, Beck GJ. Comparison of pneumatic retinopexy with alternative surgical techniques. Ophthalmology 1988;95:877–883.

101. Lee PF, Donovan RH, Mukal N, et al. Intravitreous injection of silicone: an experimental study: I. Clinical picture and histology of the eye. Ann Ophthalmol 1969;1:15–25.

102. Ober RR, Blanks JC, Ogden TC, Pickford M, Minckler DS, Ryan SJ. Experimental retinal tolerance to liquid silicone. Retina 1983;3:77–85.

103. Jalkh AE, McMeel JW, Kozlowski IMD, Schepens CL. Silicone oil retinopathy. Arch Ophthalmol 1986;104:178–179.

104. Sebag J, Zucker CL, Pankratov MM, et al. Silicone oil induced changes in squirrel monkey retinal morphology. ARVO Abstracts. Invest Ophthalmol Vis Sci 1988;29(suppl):403.

105. Laqua H, Machemer R. Clinical-pathological correlation in massive periretinal proliferation. Am J Ophthalmol 1975;80:913–929.

106. Hida T, Chandler D, Arena JE, Machemer R. Experimental and clinical observations of the intraocular toxicity of commercial corticosteroid preparations. Am J Ophthalmol 1986;101:190–195.

107. Price NC, Cooling RJ, Andrew NC. The role of vitrectomy following accidental intraocular injection of deposteroid preparations. Trans Ophthalmol Soc UK 1986;105:469–472.

108. Blumenkranz M, Hernandez E, Ophir A, Norton EWD. 5-Fluorouracil: new applications in complicated retinal detachment for an established antimetabolite. Ophthalmology 1984;91:122–130.

109. Joondeph BC, Peyman GA, Khoobehi B, Yue BY. Liposome-encapsulated 5-fluorouracil in the treatment of proliferative vitreoretinopathy. Ophthalmic Surg 1988;19:252–256.

110. Santana M, Wiedemann P, Kirmani M, et al. Daunomycin in the treatment of experimental proliferative vitreoretinopathy: retinal toxicity of intravitreal daunomycin in the rabbit. Graefes Arch Clin Exp Ophthalmol 1984;221:210–213.

111. Wiedemann P, Lemmen K, Schmiedl R, Heimann K. Intraocular daunorubicin for the treatment and prophylaxis of traumatic proliferative vitreoretinopathy. Am J Ophthalmol 1987; 104:10–14.

112. Lemor M, Yeo JH, Glaser BM. Oral colchicine for the treatment of experimental retinal detachment. Arch Ophthalmol 1986;104:1226–1229.

113. Davidson C, Green WR, Wong VG. Retinal atrophy induced by intravitreous colchicine. Invest Ophthalmol Vis Sci 1983;24:301–311.

114. Van Bochxmeer FM, Martin CE, Thompson DE, Constable TS. Taxol for the treatment of proliferative vitreoretinopathy. Invest Ophthalmol Vis Sci 1985;26:1140–1147.

Quinine Toxicity
115. Cibis GW, Burian HM, Blodi FC. Electroretinogram changes in acute quinine poisoning. Arch Ophthalmol 1973;90:307–309.

Toxicity of Cancer Chemotherapeutic Agents

116. Kaiser-Kupfer MI, Lippman ME. Tamoxifen retinopathy. Cancer Treat Rep 1978;62:315–320.

117. Griffiths MF. Tamoxifen retinopathy at low dosage. Am J Ophthalmol 1987;104:185–186.

118. McKeown CA, Swartz M, Blom J, Maggiano JM. Tamoxifen retinopathy. Br J Ophthalmol 1981;65:177–179.

119. Kaiser-Kupfer MI, Kupfer C, Rodrigues MM. Tamoxifen retinopathy: a clinicopathologic report. Ophthalmology 1981;88:89–93.

120. Vinding T, Nielsen NV. Retinopathy caused by treatment with tamoxifen in low dosage. Acta Ophthalmol 1983;61:45–50.

121. Hutter AM Jr, Kayhoe DE. Adrenal cortical carcinoma; results of treatment with o, p'DDD in 138 patients. Am J Med 1966;41:581–592.

122. Weiss JN, Weinberg RS, Regelson W. Keratopathy after oral administration of tilorone hydrochloride. Am J Ophthalmol 1980;89:46–53.

123. Weiss JN, Ochs AL, Abedi S, Selhorst JB. Retinopathy after tilorone hydrochloride. Am J Ophthalmol 1980;90:846–853.

124. Fraunfelder FT. Drug-induced ocular side effects and drug interactions. Philadelphia: Lea & Febiger, 1976:220–231.

125. Saraux H, Laplane F, Béqué H. Oedeme papillaire spontanement curable au cous d'un traitement par le chlorambucil. Bull Soc Belge Ophtalmol 1972;160:567–569.

126. Anderson B, Anderson B Jr. Necrotizing uveitis incident to perfusion of intracranial malignancies with nitrogen mustard or related compounds. Trans Am Ophthalmol Soc 1960;58:95–105.

127. Millay RH, Klein ML, Shults WT, Dahlborg SA, Neuwelt EA. Maculopathy associated with combination chemotherapy and osmotic opening of the blood-brain barrier. Am J Ophthalmol 1986;102:626–632.

128. Feun LG, Wallace S, Stewart DJ, et al. Intracarotid infusion of *cis*-diamminedichloroplatinum in the treatment of recurrent malignant brain tumors. Cancer 1984;54:794–799.

129. Kupersmith MJ, Frohman LP, Choi IF, et al. Visual system toxicity following intra-arterial chemotherapy. Neurology 1988;38:284–289.

130. Ostrow S, Hahn D, Wiernik PH, Richards RD. Ophthalmologic toxicity after *cis*-dichlorodiammineplatonum (II) therapy. Cancer Treat Rep 1978;62:1591–1594.

131. Miller DF, Bay JW, Lederman RJ, Purvis JD, Roger LR, Tomsak RL. Ocular and orbital toxicity following intracarotid injection of BCNU (carmustine) and *cis*platinum for malignant gliomas. Ophthalmology 1985;92:402–406.

132. Shingleton BJ, Bienfang DC, Albert DM, Ensminger WD, Chandler WE, Greenberg HS. Ocular toxicity associated with high-dose carmustine. Arch Ophthalmol 1982;100:1766–1772.

133. McLennan R, Taylor HR. Optic neuroretinitis in association with BCNU and procarbazine therapy. Med Pediatr Oncol 1978;4:43–48.

134. Louie AC, Turrisi AT, Muggia FM, Bono VH Jr. Visual abnormalities following nitrosourea treatment. Med Pediatr Oncol 1978;5:245–247.

CHAPTER 8

Optic Nerve Toxicity: A Classification

Russell S. Sobel and Lawrence A. Yannuzzi

Optic nerve atrophy (ONA) is a general term for the end-stage of a number of processes that result in a reduction of the quantity or the size of nerve fibers within the optic nerve. The nerve fibers comprising the optic nerve are axonal projections from the ganglion cells of the retina, and, hence, any process or substance that adversely affects the ganglion cells will affect the optic nerve. Likewise, ischemia, demyelination, or compression of the intraorbital, intracanalicular, or intracranial portion of the optic nerve may also cause atrophy, because damage to optic nerve fibers ultimately leads to ganglion cell death via retrograde degeneration.

Grant (1) and Fraunfelder (2) list 67 and 155 substances, respectively, that have been associated with optic nerve atrophy or toxicity. Many substances listed in each report are incidentally or questionably associated with the resulting pathology, and these data are often based on single case reports. This ambiguity creates difficulty in the assessment of a substance's toxicity. A substance is toxic if it affects a target cell or organism to the extent that function is impaired or death ensues (3). Toxic agents may be classified in many ways; for example, by their intended use, by the particular cell or organ to be targeted, or by the effect of the agent on a particular cell or organ.

Neurotoxins specifically exert their toxic effects on neural cells. The ganglion cells and their axonal projections fall into the category of susceptible cells, as do the supportive astrocytes and oligodendroglial cells. Anoxia and direct cytotoxicity are two important mechanisms by which neurotoxins affect neurons. Anoxic effects may be further subdivided as to the mechanism of anoxia. Because of their high metabolic rate and diminished capacity for anaerobic respiration (4), neural cells are especially sensitive to a lack of oxygen. Anoxia may result from diminished blood flow to the neuron or from lowered blood oxygen tension. However, metabolic inhibition of neuronal use of oxygen via disruption of oxidative phosphorylation is the most common phenomenon seen with the neurotoxins. This situation creates what is termed cytotoxic or histotoxic anoxia.

The histopathological effects of cytotoxic anoxia are well characterized. They include the swelling of the neuron, its intracellular components, and its nucleolus and the dispersion of the rough endoplasmic reticulum. These effects are secondary to a shutdown in mitochondrial production of adenosine triphosphate (ATP), an oxygen-dependent process. Without ATP, maintenance of ionic equilibrium is disrupted. Sodium accumulates within the cell, drawing in water, which leads to swelling of the cell and its organelles. These conditions destroy the cell (5). These histological signs are commonly seen with cytoanoxic neurotoxicity and often precede optic atrophy.

Direct toxicity to the neuron often results in a loss of myelin. The myelinoclastic effect is secondary to damage to the oligodendroglial cells responsible for producing the insulating material. Demyelination is another common histopathological finding in neurotoxicity.

It would be helpful to know which drugs and chemicals are definitely neurotoxic and are clearly associated with ONA. Because ONA is irreversible, histopathological evidence of direct damage to the ganglion cells or optic nerve fibers is the best criterion for establishing a definitive relationship between a suspected toxin and the pathology. The histopathological approach to categorizing drug toxicity is valuable because it helps to reveal the mechanisms by which substances exert their toxic effect. The microscopic findings often unveil the cellular basis for the clinical and biochemical findings that relate to adverse drug reactions (6).

In this review, 67 specific drugs and toxins were selected from the reviews of Grant and Fraunfelder. These particular substances were chosen based on the number of reports implicating their toxicity and on the probability of toxicity based on their chemical nature. We categorized these substances into four groups based on the documented histopathology following administration of the substance and the extent of neurotoxic effect.

Group I
Definitive Neurotoxins Causing Optic Nerve Atrophy

A drug or other substance in this group is associated with histopathological evidence of direct damage to the optic nerve and/or ganglion cells. The neurotoxic mechanism of action is mediated through cytoanoxia or myelin degeneration.

Group II
Other Definitive Toxic Substances Causing Optic Nerve Atrophy

A drug or other substance in this group is associated with similar histopathological evidence of damage to the optic nerve and/or ganglion cells, but the mechanism of action is neither cytoanoxia nor myelin degeneration. Instead, optic atrophy may occur through neuronal inhibition of protein synthesis, disruption of neurofilaments, interference with synaptic transmission, or enzyme inhibition. Substances that cause ONA secondary to nerve compression are also included in this group.

Group III
Toxic Substances Highly Suspected of Causing Optic Nerve Atrophy

A drug or substance in this group is associated with optic nerve atrophy without histopathological evidence of direct damage to the optic nerve and/or ganglion cells. Toxicity is assumed through clinical, laboratory, and electrophysiological tests confirming direct or indirect damage to these structures. Substances that behave as neurotoxins or are otherwise known to be toxic are included in this group.

Group IV
Neurotoxins and Other Toxins Possibly Causing Optic Nerve Atrophy

A drug or substance in this group is presumptively associated with ONA. Little supporting clinical or laboratory evidence exists despite recognition of the substance's chemical toxicity. Association with ONA is usually based on a single case report.

In the text, the description of a substance will include the following: the customary use of the substance, the ophthalmological findings other than ONA, and the purported mechanism of action.

Group I
Definitive Neurotoxins Causing Optic Nerve Atrophy

Arsacetin
Carbon monoxide
Clioquinol
Cyanide
Ethambutol
Hexachlorophene
Isoniazid
Lead
Methanol
Plasmocid
Triethyl tin

Anti-infective
1. Arsacetin (arsenilic acid) is an arsenic compound formerly used in the treatment of syphilis. Optic neuritis and optic nerve atrophy have been reported following rapidly constricting visual fields. Histopathological evidence confirms damage to the retinal ganglion cells and optic nerve (7–9). Inorganic arsenic has not been associated with ONA; however, there are several reports of hemorrhagic retinopathy following exposure to the inorganic form of the molecule (10). The toxic effects of inorganic arsenic are partly related to its binding to sulfhydryl groups. Especially susceptible is the enzyme pyruvate dehydrogenase, a key enzyme in the glycolytic pathway (11). The special propensity of arsacetin and arsenilic acid to damage the ganglion cells and optic nerve appears to be related to the presence of an amino group in the molecule (8, 9). Arsenilic acid uncouples oxidative phosphorylation by substituting for inorganic phosphate (11).

Miscellaneous (Gas)
2. Carbon monoxide (CO) is a product of incomplete combustion. Carbon monoxide poisoning manifests itself in the eye as a retinopathy with flame-shaped and peripapillary hemorrhages and cotton-wool exudates (12). These symptoms usually clear after exposure to CO has stopped. Papilledema and clinical ONA have been reported in man. The cat demonstrates degeneration of optic fibers following carbon monoxide poisoning (13), and electron microscopy of CO-poisoned rat optic nerves show degenerative changes in the astrocytes (14).

Carbon monoxide binds with hemoglobin more strongly than oxygen does. This results in less oxygen binding with hemoglobin in the lungs and reduced dissociation of oxygen from oxyhemoglobin in the tissues, creating hypoxia. The hypoxia damages cerebral vessels and increases leakage from these vessels, raising intracranial pressure and causing papilledema. Furthermore, carbon monoxide has a direct inhibitory effect on cellular cytochromes, creating cytoanoxia (15).

Anti-infective
3. Clioquinol is a halogenated hydroxyquinoline, formerly used to treat acrodermatitis enteropathica and now to treat diarrhea of amoebic origin. Use of clioquinol has resulted in subacute myelo-optic neuropathy (SMON), a syndrome of the central and peripheral neuropathic symptoms. Because of these severe effects, the drug has been used infrequently since 1970. Of persons exposed, 5% developed optic atrophy (16). Autopsies show that the most severe damage to the ON occurs near the geniculate nuclei, which exhibit retrograde damage, and that there is loss of some retinal ganglion cells (17). Axonal degeneration is followed by demyelination. Rats exposed to clioquinol demonstrate loss of neurofilaments and myelin ovoids (18). Clioquinol is known to uncouple oxidative phosphorylation and cause mitochondrial swelling (19).

Miscellaneous (Cleaning agent, lacrimant)
4. Cyanide is an acute, lethal poison. Despite evidence of direct damage to the

optic nerve in animals, human evidence is lacking. Retinal edema and pupillary mydriasis have been reported following acute poisoning (20). Animals show definite damage to the ON following daily exposure to cyanide (21). Chronic cyanide poisoning has been hypothesized to be associated with tobacco amblyopia, Leber's hereditary optic neuropathy, and excessive eating of cassava root. In all cases, the inability to detoxify cyanide is the suspected risk factor (22). Detoxification is normally achieved by two routes: conversion to thiocyanate or binding with hydroxocobalamin. Tobacco smokers demonstrate elevated plasma thiocyanate levels, and symptoms of toxic amblyopia may be related to an inability to handle the excess cyanide stress. Patients with Leber's hereditary optic neuropathy have been shown to have decreased plasma thiocyanate, perhaps as a result of abnormal activity of rhodanese, the enzyme responsible for the conversion of cyanide to thiocyanate (23). Cyanide specifically inhibits cytochrome oxidase, resulting in cytotoxic anoxia.

Anti-infective

5. Ethambutol is a tuberculostatic drug shown to cause demyelination of the optic nerve at the level of the chiasm in humans and monkeys (24, 25). While retinal pathology is rare, retinal hemorrhages have been associated with ethambutol (26). Fortunately, toxicity is dose-related (the optimal nontoxic dose is 20 mg/kg). The mechanism of ethambutol's myelinoclastic action is unknown. There is some suggestion, however, that a chelating effect on zinc may play a role in the drug's toxicity. Chemicals similar in structure to ethambutol can chelate zinc. Cats and dogs do not demonstrate ONA, but the tapetum lucidum becomes depleted of zinc when ethambutol is given (27). Although the relationship between zinc and ethambutol toxicity is not clear,

some investigators suggest that low plasma zinc levels prior to initiation of treatment places the patient at greater risk of toxicity (28).

Anti-infective

6. Hexachlorophene was widely used until its toxic effects became more evident, and the drug currently is available only by prescription. Topical overapplication of the drug has caused papilledema, retinal hemorrhages, and pupillary mydriasis (29). Hexachlorophene is toxic to the entire visual system, from the retina to the cerebral cortex. Both human and animal autopsies have demonstrated severe damage to the white matter of the entire CNS and extensive demyelination and necrosis of the optic nerve and chiasm (30, 31). The retinal ganglion cells are also destroyed in a retrograde fashion (32). The mechanism of action of hexachlorophene toxicity is probably related to its polychlorinated phenolic rings, which may facilitate inhibition of oxidative phosphorylation (33).

Anti-infective

7. Isoniazid is currently used in the treatment of tuberculosis and causes several neurological side effects, including ONA. Most cases of vision loss are acute and are often associated with papilledema (34, 35). Dogs treated with isoniazid demonstrate pathological changes to the optic nerve, including demyelination (36). Administration of pyridoxine, 25 mg to 100 mg/day, is reported to be prophylactic during isoniazid treatment (34). Isoniazid is thought to inhibit the elongation of fatty acids, a process mediated in part by pyridoxine and essential for myelin production (37).

Miscellaneous (Metal)

8. Lead contained in auto emissions and paint chips, among other sources, is a serious pollutant of our environment. The primary ocular sites of lead tox-

icity are the visual cortex, suprageniculate pathways, optic nerve, and retina. Optic neuritis and papilledema precede nerve atrophy in 10% to 30% of cases (20, 38). Other retinal signs include turbidity of the retina, distension of the retinal veins (20), glial proliferation around the nerve head blood vessels, and stippling around the disc (39). The optic nerve may be affected secondary to elevated intracranial pressure or may be affected by a direct pathway. Elevated intracranial pressure is due to breakdown of the blood-brain barrier and is accompanied by leakage from the cerebral vasculature. There are reports of inflammation within the optic nerve as well (38). Studies of the developing optic nerve show a direct effect on oligodendroglial cells and myelin-producing enzymes (40). Lead toxicity probably results both from a vascular insult to the nerve, leading to ischemia and inflammation, and from a direct toxic effect on the oligodendrocytes. Compression of the nerve probably exacerbates the ischemia.

Miscellaneous (Alcohol)
9. Methanol is the simplest of the alcohols and is used industrially as a solvent and as an additive to ethanol in the denaturation process, which renders the ethanol toxic. Most cases of poisoning occur in alcoholics unaware of or unconcerned with the potentially lethal consequences of consumption. Accidental consumption of denatured ethanol accounted for 6% of all cases of blindness among the American armed forces during World War II (41). Because methanol has become more attractive as a fuel, the number of cases of methanol poisoning may increase.

   The association of ingested methanol with blindness and optic atrophy is well established. Ingestion of as little as 4 ml may lead to serious poisoning (42). Because catabolism of methanol proceeds more slowly than that of ethanol, ophthalmological signs usually appear from 18 to 48 hours after ingestion. Prior to this period, nausea and vomiting are the primary symptoms. Reduced visual acuity and central scotomata are first noted; ophthalmoscopically, the discs appear hyperemic (43). Mild retinal edema and blurring of the disc margins usually follow in the next 24 hours if the patient survives. In most cases, the edema appears within the nerve fiber layer. At this stage, some patients have demonstrated partial to complete resolution of visual symptoms, depending on the quantity of methanol consumed and the treatment initiated. However, many patients develop some optic atrophy and loss of visual field. Lack of a pupillary response to light and widespread retinal edema are poor prognostic signs and indicate that there is little chance of regaining normal vision (44).

   Electroretinography (ERG) demonstrates no early or late abnormalities, suggesting that the damage is to the retinal ganglion cells and the nerve. This suggestion is supported by histopathology in human cases, in which the nerve fibers and ganglion cells were found to be severely degenerated (43). In cases in which patients die within 1 to 2 days of intoxication, the ganglion cells demonstrate little or no change (45). One patient, in whom death ensued 30 hours after admission, demonstrated demyelination of the retrolaminar nerve, which was accompanied by intact ganglion cells and a normal retina (46). In another patient, 18 days after ingestion of methanol, the ganglion cells remained intact and the retrolaminar nerve again demonstrated severe demyelination. This finding suggests that ganglion cell death is secondary to retrograde degeneration (47, 48) and that methanol exerts its primary effect on the optic nerve.

   Although the mechanism of methanol toxicity on the nerve is not completely understood, formic acid, not methanol, is known to be the toxin involved (42). This acid is formed following hepatic oxidation of formaldehyde, the primary metabolite of methanol. Although acidosis from formate production is important, it is known not to cause the neuropathy. Studies with primates have shown that maintenance of acid-base balance following introduction of formic acid does not prevent the formation of optic lesions (42). The same situation is found in humans in whom contemporary treatment saves lives yet has no bearing on ensuing optic atrophy. Rapid treatment with ethanol, which competes with methanol for alcohol dehydrogenase, is the treatment of choice and should be performed along with hemodialysis and maintenance of acid-base balance.

Formate appears to have a direct effect on the retrolaminar portion of the optic nerve, a section of the nerve that, due to microvascular overlap, creates a basin in which the formate accumulates (49). The acid inhibits cytochrome oxidase, thereby inhibiting oxidative phosphorylation. The resultant histotoxic anoxia contributes to a myelinoclastic effect at this vulnerable segment of the nerve (50).

Anti-infective
10. Plasmocid, an antimalarial drug, is a quinoline derivative that has been associated with up to 90 cases of ONA (51). Reduced visual acuity with normal-appearing fundi is typical. Histopathological studies show a direct toxic effect on the optic nerve of rabbits, dogs, and cats (52). Ultrastructural findings of the effects of plasmocid, like those of the effects of clioquinol and iodoquinol, have demonstrated that plasmocid has a direct toxic effect on neuronal mitochondria (53), probably via uncoupling of oxidative phosphorylation.

Miscellaneous (Tin compound)
11. Triethyl tin was accidentally added to the formulation of an antibiotic used

in France in the 1950s (54). In persons treated with the antibiotic, photophobia and optic atrophy were usually preceded by severe headache, although permanent blindness was not common (55). Optic atrophy was partly the result of papilledema secondary to elevated intracranial pressure. Brain edema was demonstrated (56).

Animal studies have demonstrated the same results (54). Specifically, rabbits and monkeys poisoned with triethyl tin demonstrate swollen proximal optic nerves (57, 58). Triethyl tin appears to have a direct toxic effect on the nerve and retina, directly inhibiting glial ATPase (59). Although information in humans is lacking, the toxin appears to have an uncoupling effect on oxidative phosphorylation, resulting in an inhibition of oxygen uptake by in vitro brain slices (58, 60).

Group II
Other Definitive Toxic Substances Causing Optic Nerve Atrophy

Amyl acetate
Aspidium
Carbon dioxide
Carbon disulfide
Chloramphenicol
Ergot
Ethyl hydrocuprein hydrochloride
Pheniprazine
Quinine
Thallium
Tryparsamide
Vincristine

Miscellaneous (Solvent)
1. Amyl acetate is used as an industrial solvent. In patients exposed to amyl acetate, the disc shows blurring and dilated vessels. Animals exposed to the vapors demonstrate ONA (61). The mechanism of toxicity in amyl acetate poisoning is unknown.

Anti-infective
2. Aspidium, an extract from a male fern, is an antihelminthic formerly used for

the treatment of tapeworm infestations. In the several cases of toxicity that have been reported, retinal pigmentary disturbances and retinal edema have been noted (62). Experimental ONA has been reported in dogs and rabbits treated with this drug (63). The mechanism of optic nerve damage is unknown.

Miscellaneous (Gas)

3. Carbon dioxide is a chemical present in dry ice and carbonated beverages. If inhaled for prolonged periods, it can cause severe damage to the CNS and retinal ganglion cells (64). In patients with prolonged pulmonary insufficiency, papilledema is the most common ocular sign of hypercapnia and is often the cause for subsequent optic atrophy (65). Peripheral retinal microaneurysms, retinal hemorrhages, and soft exudates have also been reported (66). There is also histopathological evidence of a direct effect on retinal ganglion cells (64).

   The mechanism of hypercapnic optic atrophy associated with papilledema is related to anoxia as well as to a direct vasodilating effect of CO_2 on the cerebral blood vessels. Vasodilation and increased vascular permeability lead to increased intracranial pressure and compression of the optic nerve. The mechanisms of the direct effect upon retinal ganglion cells is unknown.

Miscellaneous (Industrial product)

4. Carbon disulfide is a substance used in the rubber and rayon industries. Optic neuritis, retinal microaneurysms, dot hemorrhages, and nystagmus are common ophthalmological findings along with ONA (67). Histopathological evidence of direct degeneration of ganglion cells and the optic nerve comes from studies of rabbits, mice, and monkeys (68, 69). The central retinal ganglion cells of the monkey appear to be most susceptible (69). Carbon disulfide damages neurons by

targeting and specifically binding to neurofilaments (70). Mice deficient in thiamine show enhanced susceptibility to carbon disulfide poisoning (71).

Anti-infective

5. Chloramphenicol is an antibiotic associated with neuritis and optic atrophy. Atrophy usually appears bilaterally, and peripapillary edema and retinal venous congestion are common signs (72). Histopathology in human cadaver specimens has revealed a loss of ganglion cells in the macular and paramacular area with anterograde degeneration to the level of the chiasm (73). Chloramphenicol's toxicity is related to its reactivity with the 50S subunit of the ribosome, inhibiting protein synthesis (74). Chloramphenicol also interacts with pyridoxine (75), and this interaction probably also plays a role in its toxicity.

Miscellaneous (Migraine treatment)

6. Ergot (ergot alkaloids, ergotin) is produced by a fungus that attacks rye plants. Its ability to cause severe convulsions, tissue damage, and gangrene has been known since the Middle Ages, yet its use as an inducer of labor and abortions has persisted into the 20th century. Currently, its approved use is limited to the treatment of migraines (ergotamine), suppression of prolactin secretion (bromocriptine), treatment for Parkinsonism (methysergide), and controlled uterine stimulation (ergonovine). The ocular fundus appears relatively normal in patients with acute ergot poisoning. Mild retinal edema and narrowing of retinal arterioles have been reported (20, 38, 76, 77). One case of optic atrophy has been reported (78), and animal studies have demonstrated degeneration of retinal ganglion cells (79).

   Ergot alkaloids probably exert their effect through agonistic and antagonistic interactions with adrenergic, dopaminergic, and serotonergic receptors (77). Vascular damage is secondary to vasoconstriction and lesions to the intimal lining (80). Narrowing of the retinal arteries in both humans and animals suggests that vascular damage may be the primary mechanism and that ischemia may be the immediate insult to the ON. Likewise, ergot potentiation or alteration of normal neural transmission between amacrine cells and ganglion cells may also cause ganglion cell damage because amacrine cells utilize adrenergic, serotonergic, and dopaminergic receptors (81–83).

Anti-infective
7. Ethyl hydrocuprein hydrochloride is a quinine derivative that formerly was used for the treatment of pneumonia. Like quinine, ethyl hydrocuprein causes retinal edema, narrowing of retinal arteries, and some pigmentary disturbances (78). Autopsies of patients poisoned with this drug demonstrate degeneration of retinal ganglion cells and optic nerve axons. Likewise, animal studies demonstrate damage to the ganglion cells as well as to other retinal layers (84). The mechanism of action of ethyl hydrocuprein, as well as quinine, is unknown.

Antidepressant
8. Pheniprazine is no longer used as an antidepressant because of the visual disturbances it produces. The drug blocks the action of monoamine oxidase (MAO), a catabolic enzyme devoted to the deactivation of catecholaminergic molecules (85). A human autopsy has demonstrated demyelination of the optic nerve (86); however, animal studies suggest an effect of the drug at the level of the retina (87). Red-green color vision is severely damaged in most cases, indicating a toxic effect on the nerve. The mechanism of action is presumably related to the inhibition of MAO. However, reactivity of the drug with the flavin prosthetic group of MAO and perhaps with other enzymes may also contribute to the drug's toxicity.

Anti-infective
9. Quinine is noted for damaging the visual system. Used predominantly for the treatment of malaria and nocturnal leg cramps, the drug is also used for attempted abortions and suicides. Clinical signs of quinine poisoning include narrowed retinal vessels, a hyperemic disc, and an edematous retina and macula (88). These signs are not always present, and blind patients have presented with normal fundi, although pallor of the nerve head is almost always present.

Electro-oculograms (EOGs) performed late in the course of treatment of patients poisoned with quinine demonstrate distinct abnormalities (89), and acute electrophysiological testing in humans and rabbits suggests a direct toxic effect on the ganglion cells and nerve (90). Histopathological evidence of direct damage to the optic nerve has been shown in dogs and humans (90, 91). The question of whether or not vascular damage is involved in the toxic effect of quinine is still unanswered. Vascular alteration often appears after prolonged periods of time and concurrent with improvements in vision (1). How quinine exerts its toxic effects is still unknown. It is termed a general protoplasmic toxin and may interfere with acetylcholine metabolism (88).

Miscellaneous (Rat poison)
10. Thallium, a heavy metal, in the form thallium sulfate is used as a rat poison. However, it is not selectively toxic to rodents, so many cases of human poisoning do occur. Chronic poisoning usually presents with visual symptoms. Blurred vision and central scotomata with pale discs are the most common features. Histopathological evidence of a highly selective loss of retinal ganglion cells with atrophy of

the nerve has been reported in man and monkeys (92, 93). Myelin was also lost to a smaller extent.

Thallium has been shown to collect in the lens of mice (94), and its uptake is thought to be related to potassium exchange. In fact, thallium has been shown to replace potassium in sodium/potassium ATPase (95). This replacement has devastating consequences for the retinal ganglion cells and oligodendroglial cells, because a normal, intracellular ionic milieu cannot be maintained. Thallium toxicity probably also involves the reaction of this heavy metal with one or more biological ligands, reactive groups essential for macromolecule function. However, because chelating therapy, used frequently for other heavy metal toxicities, is ineffectual with thallium poisoning (96), other mechanisms may be involved in this reaction.

Anti-infective
11. Tryparsamide is no longer used to treat syphilis or trypanosomal infections because of the high incidence of optic neuritis and atrophy. Visual field reduction is the hallmark; abnormalities of the fundus do not occur until later. None of the abnormalities is well documented. Experimental work demonstrates damage to the optic nerve in monkeys (97) and peripapillary edema and loss of retinal ganglion cells in rabbits (98). Tryparsamide is a derivative of arsenilic acid and much of its toxicity is probably related to the toxicity of arsenic. (See arsacetin, Group I.)

Antineoplastic
12. Vincristine is more toxic than vinblastine, another neoplastic drug, and has been associated with ONA in several cases. Central scotomata, dyschromatopsia, and papillitis are clinical signs of vincristine toxicity. Experimental poisoning in the monkey, as well as autopsy specimens in man, have demonstrated a loss of ganglion cells and damage to the optic nerve (99, 100). Vincristine (and vinblastine) are known to block cellular mitosis by specifically binding with tubulin protein. By binding in this fashion, the drug creates intracellular neurofibrillar tangles (101) that arrest intracellular mobile processes and stop axonal transport.

Group III
Toxic Substances Highly Suspected of Causing Optic Nerve Atrophy

Acetarsone
Broxyquinoline
Carbon tetrachloride
Cassava
Dapsone
Dinitrobenzene
Dinitrochlorobenzene
Dynamite
Ethylene glycol
Ethyl mercury toluene sulfonanilide
Formic acid
Halquinol
Iodoquinol
Linamarin
Methyl acetate
Methyl bromide
n-Hexane
Orsudan
Suramin
Trichloroethylene
Vitamin D2, Vitamin D3

Anti-infective
1. Acetarsone has been used for the treatment of syphilis. Reports of optic neuritis and ONA have been cited. Like other arsenic-containing drugs, acetarsone's action is probably related to its ability to bind and render ineffective any enzymes that contain sulfhydryl groups. Patients have been treated successfully with dimercaprol (102), suggesting a sulfhydryl blocking effect rather than a cytoanoxic effect, as found with arsacetin. (See Group I.)

Antiseptic

2. Broxyquinoline has been used as an intestinal antiseptic. A patient demonstrated optic atrophy and bull's-eye maculopathy following long-term self-medication (103). The mechanism of action is probably similar to that of other halogenated quinolines. (See Group I.)

Miscellaneous (Industrial solvent)

3. Carbon tetrachloride is used in industry and as a household spot remover. Patients exposed to carbon tetrachloride have demonstrated optic neuritis and visual field losses indicative of damage to the optic nerve, and a single report of optic atrophy has also been cited (104). However, there is no histopathological evidence of direct damage to the optic nerve or ganglion cells. Severely hepatotoxic, a metabolite of carbon tetrachloride is suspected to be the actual toxin (105). This metabolite (a free radical) is especially reactive with membrane lipids, releasing additional free radicals. This destructive lipid peroxidation leads to membrane degradation and subsequent cellular death (105, 106).

Miscellaneous (Tropical plant)

4. Cassava is a dietary staple in many areas of the world. Long-term consumption has been associated with a slow decrease in visual acuity, retrobulbar neuritis, and ONA. Linamarin, a glycoside found in the plant, releases cyanide when hydrolyzed. Serum cyanide and thiocyanate are elevated in patients who consume large quantities of the root (107). Cyanide inhibits cellular respiration by blocking the cytochrome system and preventing the utilization of oxygen. (See Group I.)

Anti-infective

5. Dapsone, a sulphur-containing drug somewhat similar to the sulfonamides, is used for the treatment of leprosy. Only patients who accidentally or intentionally take large doses demonstrate any ophthalmological signs. Retinal damage is vascular in origin and includes hemorrhages, exudates, and capillary drop-out. Intravascular hemolysis has been noted (108). Optic atrophy is probably the result of ischemia to the glial cells of the nerve and/or to the retinal ganglion cells. Dapsone-induced hemolysis is thought to be related to an inherent deficiency in the enzyme glucose 6-phosphate dehydrogenase (G6-PD), which is necessary for handling the oxidizing effect of the drug. Individuals with a red blood cell G6-PD deficiency cannot produce enough NADPH, the reducing agent necessary to counter the oxidizing effects of the drug. This results in damaged RBCs and hemolysis. Those individuals without a deficiency of G6-PD demonstrate no hemolysis as long as doses remain below 100 mg/day. Above this dosage, hemolysis is dose-related (109).

Miscellaneous (Explosives production)

6. Dinitrobenzene, used in weapons production, is absorbed through the skin and the respiratory and GI tracts. A case of partial ONA has been reported (110), as have retinal hemorrhages. Effects seem to be the result of long-term exposure. Mechanism of action is unknown; however, the substance is very lipophilic, which may contribute to its toxicity.

Miscellaneous (Explosives production)

7. Dinitrochlorobenzene, like dinitrobenzene, is used in the production of weapons and may, in conjunction with dinitrobenzene or by itself, be responsible for some isolated cases of optic atrophy (110). There are no other retinal signs associated with dinitrochlorobenzene toxicity, and the mechanism of damage is unknown, although this toxin is also very lipophilic.

Miscellaneous (Explosive)

8. Dynamite, when used to excavate an enclosed area, will leave carbon monoxide. The gas, rather than the explosive, is thought to be the agent responsible for causing ONA. Several patients developed ONA following variable periods of papilledema (112). The mechanism of action of carbon monoxide is described under Group I substances.

Miscellaneous (Antifreeze)

9. Ethylene glycol, when accidentally or purposely ingested, can be lethal within hours if treatment is not initiated. Although the chemistry and toxicology of ethylene glycol is somewhat similar to that of methyl alcohol, the ophthalmological side effects are not nearly as severe. Reports of blurred or swollen discs, dilated retinal veins, and nystagmus have been reported; however, only a single report exists of the chemical inducing ONA (113). Animal studies do not address visual effects and, in general, it is difficult to make a close association of ONA with ethylene glycol ingestion (114).

   The damage from ethylene glycol includes cerebral edema, scattered cerebral hemorrhages, and cortical cell loss (115). These effects are caused by severe acidosis, created by the metabolite glyoxylic acid. Because ethylene glycol is metabolized and excreted in the urine much more quickly than is methanol, the eyes may be spared from severe damage (1).

Miscellaneous (Fungicide)

10. Ethyl mercury toluene sulfonanilide is used to treat fungus-infected grains. When the grain is ingested, severe vision loss and optic atrophy may result. Twenty-six cases have been reported (116). The mechanism of action is unknown, but the mercurial moiety in the compound may be responsible for the severe toxicity. Mercury reacts strongly with many biological ligands (carboxyl, amine, phosphoryl groups) and renders them and the associated macromolecule ineffective.

Miscellaneous (Ant venom)

11. Formic acid is the predominant toxin found in ant venom and is also used in the treatment of livestock fodder. An animal study implicated formic acid in degeneration of the retina and optic nerve (117), but in vitro studies do not support this. There are no reports of human ONA secondary to formic acid exposure. Formic acid, however, plays a central role in methanol toxicity. (See Group I.)

Anti-infective

12. Halquinol, similar to clioquinol, has been reported to cause ONA in two patients (118). Other neurological signs appear similar to the subacute myelo-optic neuropathology seen in clioquinol toxicity. There is no histopathological evidence to support a direct neurotoxic effect, but the purported mechanism of damage is probably similar to that of clioquinol (Group I).

Anti-infective

13. Iodoquinol is an iodinated 8-hydroxyquinoline and, like clioquinol, has caused optic nerve atrophy in children. While no histopathological evidence supports a direct effect upon the visual apparatus, patients demonstrate nerve head pallor, edema, pigmentary changes to the retina, narrowing of the arterioles, and bilateral ERG reduction (119, 120, 121). Iodoquinol is not as well absorbed as clioquinol and hence its toxicity is reduced (122).

Miscellaneous (Plant toxin)

14. Linamarin is the compound in cassava root that releases cyanide when metabolized. (See Cyanide, Group I.) Excessive eating of cassava has been associated with ONA (107).

Miscellaneous (Solvent)

15. Methyl acetate is very irritating to the eyes, nose, and throat and has been associated with a single case of optic atrophy following inhalation of its vapors. Metabolism of methyl acetate produces methanol, which is neurotoxic (123). (See Methanol, Group I.)

Miscellaneous (Fumigant)

16. Methyl bromide is one of the most poisonous of the organophosphate insecticides and is particularly dangerous due to its lack of odor, color, or irritating effect. A strong stimulator of lacrimation, chloropicrin is sometimes added as an early warning sign of exposure to methyl bromide (124). There are two reports of optic atrophy (125, 126). Diplopia and blurred vision are common early symptoms of toxicity. Hyperemia of the discs, retinal venous tortuosity, and dilation have been seen, along with retinal hemorrhages. Histopathology in animals and humans does not demonstrate optic nerve atrophy (127), but abnormal findings on the EOG in a particular case suggest damage to the nerve. Controversy exists as to whether methyl bromide exerts its toxic effects via intraocular conversion to methanol, but there is no formate formed as in methanol poisoning. (See Methanol, Group I.) In vitro studies suggest that methyl bromide is directly toxic to mammalian cells (124), and its lipophilicity facilitates its uptake into the fatty myelin sheath. Methyl bromide also has a high affinity for sulfhydryl groups, which may also contribute to its toxic action (124).

Miscellaneous (Solvent)

17. A major component of glues, n-hexane, has been reported to cause optic nerve atrophy in 5% of patients exposed to the substance (123). Macular edema is another ophthalmological sign, along with abnormal visual evoked potentials (VEPs), in workers exposed to n-hexane. Other hexacarbon neurotoxins are known to cause peripheral polyneuropathy (129), and their toxicity is related to the length of the target nerve fibers. The optic nerve may be affected at later phases. The mechanism of n-hexane toxicity is related to its conversion to 2,5 hexanedione, which causes disruption of neurofilaments (128).

Anti-infective

18. Orsudan is a derivative of arsenilic acid. A single case of ONA has been documented (130). The mechanism of action is related to the presence of arsenic. (See Arsacetin, Group I.)

Anti-infective

19. Suramin is used to treat trypanosomiasis and has caused optic atrophy in patients treated with the drug. In the cited study, however, some patients with onchocerciasis who were not treated with suramin also developed ONA, suggesting a toxic effect of the microfilaria. It is hypothesized that destroyed microfilaria may cause local inflammation and secondary atrophy of the nerve. Tryparsamide (Group I), another antitrypanosomic, antionchocerciatic drug, may create a similar inflammatory situation, initiating or aggravating atrophy of the nerve (131).

Anesthetic

20. Trichloroethylene was formerly used as an anesthetic. Its volatile and labile properties have removed it from the anesthesia market and into the degreasing and dry cleaning industries. The substance is clearly toxic in large quantities, yet there is much confusion as to whether it or a decomposition product is responsible for the toxic effects elicited. Visual symptoms include decreased vision, central scotomata, temporal pallor of the disc, and peripapillary hemorrhages (132). Visual field defects and lack of association with any other probable cause suggest that either the substance or one of its by-products can cause

atrophy of the optic nerve. Negative histopathological evidence from canine experiments has added to the speculation (133). Rabbit studies demonstrate a reduction in retinal ATP content but no visible damage to the retina (134). While the mechanism of trichloroethylene toxicity is unknown, its high lipophilicity may play a role in its penetration and toxicity.

Vitamin (Vitamin D2 or Vitamin D3)
21. Optic atrophy in cases of Vitamin D toxicity is primarily seen in infants and is due to hypercalcemia created by these vitamins. Calcium deposits in and around the optic foramina create a narrowing and subsequent pressure on the developing optic nerve (135).

Group IV
Neurotoxins and Other Toxins Possibly Causing Optic Nerve Atrophy

Antimony potassium tartrate
Bee stings
Brayera
Bromiosovalum
Carbromal
Castor beans
Catha edulis
Chenopodium oil
Clindamycin
Cortex granati
Dinitrotoluene
Glibenclamide
Hexamethonium
Iodoform
Lindane
Methylene blue
Minoxidil
Octamoxin
Phenazone
Sodium salicylate
Streptomycin
Thioridazine hydrochloride
Warfarin

Anti-infective
1. Antimony potassium tartrate has been used for the treatment of schistosomi-asis. Patients have developed papilledema and ONA following its use. Antimony reacts with sulfhydryl (SH) groups, possibly rendering ineffective sulfhydryl-containing enzymes, such as pyruvate dehydrogenase (136).

Miscellaneous (Animal toxin)
2. Bee stings have been reported to cause optic atrophy. Retinal vascular sheathing and narrowing of retinal arterioles were concomitant findings. Other reports associate bee stings with optic neuritis (93). Bee venom often contains one or more kinins, initiators of inflammation, and ONA may be secondary to the inflammation.

Anti-infective
3. Brayera is an extract from the kosso plant. This antitapeworm drug has been reported to cause optic atrophy, although the mechanism is unknown (137).

Sedative
4. Bromiosovalum is a sedative and hypnotic drug. Patients may show papillary abnormalities, nystagmus, or diplopia. A case of optic atrophy has been reported (138). The mechanism is unknown.

Sedative
5. Carbromal has caused visual disturbances in some individuals. Retrobulbar neuritis, nerve head hyperemia, and retinal edema have also been reported. A single report of ONA is cited, yet no direct evidence of change to the nerve or ganglion cells has been noted. The mechanism of action is unknown (139).

Miscellaneous (Plant beans)
6. When pressed, whole castor beans yield castor oil. The beans have been reported to cause optic atrophy in a single case of large ingestion of the beans (140). The bean covering and residue after pressing contains a toxin, ricin, which is especially irritating. Ricin is

one of the more toxic natural plant substances and is known to inhibit protein synthesis by binding and inhibiting the 60S ribosomal subunit (141).

Miscellaneous (Plant)
7. *Catha edulis*, also known as the khat plant, has been used in eastern Africa and southern Saudi Arabia as a natural mental stimulant. ONA has been reported in two patients who consumed the leaves of the plant. Both patients had decreased vision, central scotomata, pigmentary abnormalities at the disc, and thinning of the papillomacular bundle. Both patients demonstrated gross optic atrophy and one demonstrated a reduced ERG. Khat contains two alkaloids, cathine and cathinone, which are structurally similar to amphetamine. The mechanism of toxicity is unknown (142).

Anti-infective
8. Chenopodium oil is an antihelminthic. It has been associated with papilledema and, in a single case, with ONA (143). The mechanism of action is unknown.

Anti-infective
9. Clindamycin has been associated with a single case of ONA. In concentrations of more than 10 μg/ml, the drug causes severe retinal damage when injected into the vitreous of the rabbit.

Papillitis has been noted in conjunction with atrophy, appearing in one of two patients treated with retrobulbar injection of clindamycin for ocular toxoplasmosis (144). Clindamycin reacts with the 50S subunit of the ribosome, inhibiting protein synthesis and, thereby, possibly exerting its toxic effect (145).

Anti-infective
10. Cortex granati, a derivative of pomegranate bark, contains pelletierine tannate, a drug used for treating tapeworm infections. Visual loss with disc

pallor is the only reported sign of clinical toxicity. Some reports of optic atrophy coincided with adjunctive use of aspidium (Group II), but some did not (20).

Miscellaneous (Explosives production)
11. Dinitrotoluene is a compound used in the production of TNT. A single case of ONA accompanied by narrowing of the retinal vessels has been reported (146). The mechanism of action is unknown, but the ocular and peripheral symptoms resemble those of dinitrochlorobenzene and dinitrobenzene (Group III).

Hypoglycemic agent
12. Glibenclamide is used to treat diabetes. A single case of ONA following its use has been reported. The association is probably secondary to hypoglycemic encephalopathy. Glibenclamide, like the other sulfonylureas, stimulates insulin secretion from the pancreatic beta cells, perhaps through a calcium-mediated influx (148) or by inhibiting release of catecholamine (149).

Ganglionic blocker
13. Hexamethonium is no longer used in the United States as a ganglionic blocking agent. It has been associated with three cases of ONA. The fundi of these patients also exhibited narrowed retinal arterioles, macular edema, and a hypertensive retinopathy that includes exudates and hemorrhages (150, 151). Hexamethonium blocks cholinergic nicotinic receptors in the autonomic ganglia.

Antiseptic
14. Iodoform is no longer used as a topical or intravitreal antiseptic, but several cases of partial or complete ONA have been reported. Occasionally, retinal hemorrhages have been seen as well (38). Iodoform is a triiodomethane compound and does not show the same retinotoxic characteristics as iodate and

iodoacetic acid. The mechanism of action is unknown.

Miscellaneous (Scabicide, pediculicide)
15. Lindane is used to treat crab lice infections. Reports of systemic poisoning include a single report of optic atrophy with no concomitant ocular findings. The mechanism of action is unknown (152).

Miscellaneous (Dye)
16. Methylene blue has been associated with a single case of ONA that occurred after diagnostic injection of the drug into the lumbar subarachnoid space. Blurring of the disc margins and hydrocephalus were concomitant signs (93). The mechanism of action is unknown, but an alteration in cerebral vascular permeability is likely, resulting in secondary ON compression.

Antihypertensive
17. Minoxidil, in a single case, when combined with prednisone and azathioprine, was associated with ONA. Decreased vision and swollen, hyperemic discs were noted, as well as a yellow scar in the macula. The mechanism is unknown (153). Minoxidil is commonly used as an antihypertensive, because of its ability to relax vascular smooth muscle. It is used topically to treat baldness.

Antidepressant
18. Octamoxin has been reported to cause ONA in several individuals using the drug for treatment of depression. Reduced visual acuity has been the only symptom with progressive atrophy of the nerve (154). The drug works by inhibition of monoamine oxidase (MAO), which is a mitochondrial enzyme responsible for the degradation of the catecholamines in neural and other target tissues. The MAO inhibitors irreversibly block the enzyme and hence create a pool of unmetabolized active neurotransmitters. The activity of this group of transmitters may con-

tribute to the drug's toxicity. (See pheniprazine, Group II).

Analgesic
19. Phenazone is no longer used in the United States, but it is maintained as an analgesic in other countries. A derivative of phenylbutazone, the drug has been associated with a single case of ONA. Visual symptoms occur only after chronic or excessive usage of the drug (155). The mechanism of action is unknown.

20. Sodium salicylate, the medicinal predecessor of aspirin, has been associated with several cases of optic atrophy. Since the introduction of aspirin, no additional cases have been reported. Various abnormalities of the fundus have been noted, including narrowing and widening of the retinal vessels, edematous optic disc and retina, retinal hemorrhage, and nystagmus (156). Sodium salicylate works via inhibition of prostaglandin biosynthesis by specifically inhibiting cyclo-oxygenase, the enzyme responsible for the conversion of arachidonic acid into the prostaglandin precursor PGG2.

Anti-infective
21. Streptomycin, when administered intrathecally, has been known to cause ONA. Central scotomata, optic neuritis, and atrophy have all been reported (157). The association of intravitreal streptomycin with retinal damage is well known (158). Streptomycin, like other aminoglycosides, disrupts protein synthesis and transport across the cell membrane (159, 160).

Antipsychotic
22. Thioridazine hydrochloride (Mellaril) is strongly associated with pigmentary disturbances and retinopathy, yet only a single case of optic nerve atrophy has been reported. The 12-year-

old patient had consumed large doses of the drug (up to 1600 mg/day) and developed ONA as well as bilateral chorioretinal pigmentary disturbances (161). Dosages of 600 mg/day have been shown to be safe (162). Other retinal signs include retinal edema, accumulation of pigment, atrophy of the retinal pigment epithelium (RPE), and choroidal atrophy. Animal studies demonstrate an affinity of the drug for melanin and a toxic effect on retinal enzymes (163). While the mechanism of thioridazine's effects (and those of other phenothiazines) is not known, it is suspected that they interfere with the activity of dopamine, a key neurotransmitter in the retina (164).

Anticoagulant
23. Warfarin produces multiple retinal hemorrhages in toxic situations, and one case of bilateral optic atrophy has been reported in a newborn (165). The fetus seems to be particularly susceptible to warfarin following use by the mother. Almost half of one series of infants demonstrated ocular abnormalities, including optic atrophy. Warfarin (Coumadin) blocks the action of vitamin K in the production of prothrombin, thereby causing a clotting defect (164).

Drugs and substances associated with optic nerve atrophy have been classified according to their association with direct histopathological damage to the retinal ganglion cells or the optic nerve and to their mechanisms of neurotoxic damage. This approach should serve to classify the long lists of drugs and toxins associated with ONA into a focused hierarchy that can distinguish "definite" from "possible" toxic substances.

Histopathological evidence was selected as a benchmark for toxicity. In contrast, findings derived from clinical and electrophysiological testing are less definitive. The most common clinical signs of optic atrophy are reduction in visual acuity, constriction of visual fields, central scotomata, red-green dyschromatopsia, optic nerve head pallor, and mydriasis. Retinal signs are variable and may be absent as further deterioration of the nerve occurs, a situation that occurs particularly in cases of methanol poisoning.

Because optic nerve atrophy reflects the existence of damage to neural components, whether the site of initial damage is ganglion cells, nerves, or associated astrocytes and oligodendroglia, further classification of the drugs according to their demonstration of classic neurotoxic behavior seemed appropriate (Table 1). Because neurons are especially sensitive to anoxia, one mechanism of action chosen in the classification process was cytotoxic anoxia, the anoxia occurring at the cellular level due to an uncoupling or blocking of oxidative phosphorylation. Demyelination accompanied by the disruption of axonal conduction was a second mechanism chosen. Blockage of synaptic transmission, inhibition of protein synthesis, and neurofilament inhibition and general enzyme inhibition are other common, direct neurotoxic mechanisms, but they are often reversible, in contrast to the terminal damage resulting from anoxia and demyelination.

The substances in Group I, which comprise about 15% of the list, are well-established neurotoxins, and there is substantial human and/or animal histopathological evidence of their toxicity. In these cases, further corroboration of the neurotoxic effect is sometimes noted by specific histopathological reports of swollen axons and mitochondria, as well as by distinct loss of myelin, for example, in cases involving clioquinol, plasmocid, and triethyl tin (19, 53, 57, 58) and ethambutol, hexachlorophene, isoniazid, and methanol (24, 30, 36, 46).

Within Group II, which comprised almost 18% of the substances reviewed, histopathological evidence supports a direct effect of these toxins on the visual apparatus. The primary mechanisms exhibited by these substances are inhibition of protein synthesis (chloramphenicol (74)), disruption of neurofilaments (vincristine and

Table 8.1. Toxic Mechanisms Resulting in Optic Nerve Atrophy

Direct Mechanisms	
1. Cytotoxic or Histotoxic Anoxia	Interference with oxidative phosphorylation in ganglion or supportive cells
2. Demyelination	Interference with fatty acid elongation and myelin production in oligodendroglial cells
3. Inhibition of Protein Synthesis	Interference with ribosomal subunits, inhibiting cellular protein synthesis
4. Neurofilament Inhibition	Interference with tubulin protein, resulting in abnormal neurofilament production and inhibition of cellular transport
5. Synaptic Transmission Defects	Interference with neurotransmitter synthesis, degradation, or postsynaptic receptors
6. General Enzyme Inhibition	Interference with intracellular enzymes through ligand reactivity
Indirect Mechanisms	
1. Optic Nerve Compression	Secondary to cerebral edema or narrowing of optic foraminae
2. Optic Nerve Inflammation	Secondary to destroyed parasites, production of kinins

carbon disulfide (101, 70)), possible interference with neurotransmitter activity (ergot alkaloids (77)), and compression of the nerve due to elevation of intracranial pressure secondary to cerebral edema (carbon dioxide (64)). A summary of the most hazardous Group I and Group II compounds is presented in Table 8.2.

Many drugs in Group III share purported mechanisms with those in Group I, but those in Group III either do not induce histopathologically evident optic atrophy, or such evidence has not yet been collected. However, there is clinical and electrophysiological evidence that supports the notion that these Group III drugs induce atrophy of the nerve. There may be several reasons for this discrepancy. The Group I compounds may be more toxic due to enhanced absorption (e.g., clioquinol, Group I, vs. iodoquinol, Group III (122)), or they may contain a reactive group (e.g., NH_2) in a different position that causes greater toxicity (e.g., arsacetin vs. acetarsone (68)). Furthermore, an active component or metabolite of a Group III substance (e.g., linamarin, cassava) may not be present in sufficient amounts to cause acute atrophy. In addition, much experimental work is often done with parent compounds (Group I), leaving a paucity of experimental evidence for secondary compounds (Groups III and IV).

Although Group IV drugs share common mechanisms with some of the more serious toxins, reports of ONA associated with these drugs have rarely been substantiated. Little information has been gathered because the exposure to these substances is relatively rare, because many of them have been replaced by newer and safer drugs. Of interest are the toxins found in the kosso and khat plants and castor beans. Cathine (found in the khat plant), brayera (from kosso), and ricin (from castor beans) have been associated with a few cases of atrophy, but not many researchers are motivated to conduct experimentation, hence the paucity of data. However, although not much is known about cathine or brayera, ricin is known to be very toxic, because it actively inhibits protein synthesis (141). Therefore, these and other potentially toxic substances are included in Group IV.

In reviewing the literature describing ONA, a recurrent and interesting theme is noted: there seems to be a relationship between particular toxins causing ONA and the deficiency of certain vitamins, particularly vitamin B1 (thiamine) and vitamin B6 (pyridoxine). Specifically, carbon di-

Table 8.2. Definitive Neurotoxins Capable of Causing Histologically Confirmed Optic Nerve Atrophy

Groups of Toxic Substances Associated with Optic Nerve Atrophy	
GROUP I	**GROUP II**
Arsacetin	Amyl acetate
Carbon monoxide	Aspidium
Clioquinol	Carbon dioxide
Cyanide	Carbon disulfide
Ethambutol	Chloramphenicol
Hexachlorophene	Ergot
Isoniazid	Ethyl hydrocuprein hydrochloride
Lead	Pheniprazine
Methanol	Quinine
Plasmocid	Thallium
Triethyl tin	Tryparsamide
	Vincristine
GROUP III	**GROUP IV**
Acetarsone	Antimony potassium tartrate
Broxyquinoline	Bee stings
Carbon tetrachloride	Brayera
Cassava	Bromiosovalum
Dapsone	Carbromal
Dinitrobenzene	Castor beans
Dinitrochlorobenzene	Catha edulis
Dynamite	Chenopodium oil
Ethylene glycol	Clindamycin
Ethyl mercury toluene sulfonanilide	Cortex granati
Formic acid	Dinitrotoluene
Halquinol	Glibenclamide
Iodoquinol	Hexamethonium
Linamarin	Iodoform
Methyl acetate	Lindane
Methyl bromide	Methylene blue
n-Hexane	Minoxidil
Orsudan	Octamoxin
Suramin	Phenazone
Trichloroethylene	Sodium salicylate
Vitamin D2, Vitamin D3	Streptomycin
	Thioridazine hydrochloride
	Warfarin

Toxic Substances Associated with Optic Nerve Atrophy	
Toxin	**Group**
Acetarsone	Group III
Amyl acetate	Group II
Antimony potassium tartrate	Group IV
Arsacetin	Group I
Aspidium	Group II
Bee stings	Group IV
Brayera	Group IV
Bromiosovalum	Group IV
Broxyquinoline	Group III
Carbon dioxide	Group II
Carbon disulfide	Group II
Carbon monoxide	Group I
Carbon tetrachloride	Group III
Carbromal	Group IV
Cassava	Group III

Table 8.2. Definitive Neurotoxins Capable of Causing Histologically Confirmed Optic Nerve Atrophy (Continued)

Toxic Substances Associated with Optic Nerve Atrophy	
Toxin	**Group**
Castor beans	Group IV
Catha edulis	Group IV
Chenopodium oil	Group IV
Chloramphenicol	Group II
Clindamycin	Group IV
Clioquinol	Group I
Cortex granati	Group IV
Cyanide	Group I
Dapsone	Group III
Dinitrobenzene	Group III
Dinitrochlorobenzene	Group III
Dinitrotoluene	Group IV
Dynamite	Group III
Ergot	Group II
Ethambutol	Group I
Ethyl hydrocuprein hydrochloride	Group II
Ethyl mercury toluene sulfonanilide	Group III
Ethylene glycol	Group III
Formic acid	Group III
Glibenclamide	Group IV
Halquinol	Group III
Hexachlorophene	Group I
Hexamethonium	Group IV
Iodoform	Group IV
Iodoquinol	Group III
Isoniazid	Group I
Lead	Group I
Linamarin	Group III
Lindane	Group IV
Methanol	Group I
Methyl acetate	Group III
Methyl bromide	Group III
Methylene blue	Group IV
Minoxidil	Group IV
n-Hexane	Group III
Octamoxin	Group IV
Orsudan	Group III
Phenazone	Group IV
Pheniprazine	Group II
Plasmocid	Group I
Quinine	Group II
Sodium salicylate	Group IV
Streptomycin	Group IV
Suramin	Group III
Thallium	Group II
Thioridazine hydrochloride	Group IV
Trichloroethylene	Group III
Triethyl tin	Group I
Tryparsamide	Group II
Vincristine	Group II
Vitamin D2	Group III
Vitamin D3	Group III
Warfarin	Group IV

sulfide, cyanide, and the halogenated hydroxyquinolines are associated with vitamin B1 to the extent that a deficiency in the vitamin often exacerbates the toxicity. Likewise, pyridoxine is often given before isoniazid treatment is begun in order to alleviate any adverse effects. Clearly, some of the drugs may exert some of their toxic effects by inhibiting vitamin activity or production.

In cases of thiamine deficiency, axonal degeneration has been reported (167), and myelin degeneration has been noted in pyridoxine deficiencies (168). Isoniazid and chloramphenicol are known to bind with pyridoxine and may exert an effect by reducing vitamin availability. In particular, isoniazid, which has a documented myelinoclastic effect, is thought to inhibit elongation of fatty acids (32), a process that is mediated in part through pyridoxine.

Another example of the association between ONA and vitamins is tobacco-alcohol amblyopia. An autopsy demonstrated the loss of up to 50% of optic nerve fibers in a man in whom the disorder was diagnosed (75). The etiology of tobacco-alcohol amblyopia is suspected to involve the inability to process the excess cyanide stress induced by cigarette smoke. Likewise, the poor nutritional status of most alcoholics creates a vitamin deficiency (e.g., vitamin B12, hydroxycobalamin). Because most individuals presenting with tobacco-alcohol amblyopia are both heavy drinkers and smokers, delineating the precise risk factors is difficult (75), but the best treatment has been discontinuation of smoking and drinking, with dietary supplementation of hydroxycobalamin (169).

Given the number of definitive and potential toxic substances that can cause ONA, further research into the mechanisms of actions of these substances is clearly warranted. Attention should also be given to some of the less notorious toxins. Understanding the toxicity of these compounds can lead to safer and more rigorous controls over environmental and occupational exposures, and further elucidation of the mechanisms of action can lead to more rational intervention therapies following exposure. Certainly, given the known associations between particular vitamins and some of the more serious toxins, more work needs to be done in this important area.

ACKNOWLEDGMENTS

The author would like to acknowledge Ms. Virginia Franklin for typing the manuscript and Ms. Dede Silverstone for assistance in library research.

References

1. Grant WM. Toxicology of the eye. 3rd ed. Springfield: CC Thomas, 1986:34–54, 75–99.
2. Fraunfelder FT. Drug-induced ocular side effects and drug interactions. 2d ed. Philadelphia: Lea & Febiger, 1982:591–593.
3. Klaassen CD. Principles of toxicology. In: Klaassen CD, Amdur MO, Doull J, eds. Casarett & Doull's toxicology: the basic science of poisons. 3rd ed. New York: Macmillan Press, 1986:11–33.
4. Ruscak M, Ruscakova D, Hager H. The role of the neuronal cell in the metabolism of the rat cerebral cortex. Physiol Bohemoslov 1968; 17:113–121.
5. Doull J. Systemic toxicology. In: Klaassen CD, Amdur MO, Doull J, eds. Casarett and Doull's toxicology: the basic science of poisons. 3rd ed. New York: Macmillan Press, 1986:350–385.
6. Mullick FG, Drake RM, Irey NS. Morphologic changes in adverse drug reactions in infants and children. Hum Pathol 1977;8:361–378.
7. Prickman LE, Hollenhorst RW, Ammermann EO. Toxic retinopathy with vascular proliferation and hemorrhage into the vitreous in an asthmatic patient being treated with arsenic. Am J Ophthalmol 1960;50:64–70.
8. Young AG, Loevenhart AS. The relation of chemical constitution of certain organic arsenical compounds to their action on the optic tract. J Pharmacol Exp Ther 1923;21:197–198.
9. Klaassen CD. Heavy metals and heavy-metal antagonists. In: Gilman AG, Goodman LS, Rall TW, Murad F, eds. Goodman and Gilman's The pharmacological basis of therapeutics. 7th ed. New York: Macmillan Publishing, 1985:1605–1627.
10. Longley BJ, Clausen NM, Tatum AL. The experimental production of primary optic atrophy in monkeys by administration of organic arsenical compounds. J Pharmacol Exp Ther 1942;76:202–206.
11. Freedman A, Sevel D. The cerebro-ocular effects of carbon dioxide poisoning. Arch Ophthalmol 1966;76:59–65.
12. Bilchik RC, Muller-Bergh HA, Freshman ME. Ischemic retinopathy due to carbon monoxide poisoning. Arch Ophthalmol 1971;86:142–144.
13. Ikeda T. Experimental carbon monoxide poisoning: its electrophysiological effects on the

visual pathway in cats. Folia Psychiatr Neurol Jpn 1969;23:135–142.

14. Ohara M. The electron microscopic studies on the optic nerves of mice poisoned with carbon monoxide gas or potassium cyanide solution. Folia Ophthalmol Jpn 1968;19:99–123.

15. Gutierrez G. Carbon monoxide toxicity. In: McGrath JJ, Barnes CD, eds. Air pollution physiological effects. New York: Academic Press, 1982:127–147.

16. Aron JJ, Lebuisson DA, Guidi M. La nevrite optique aux derives due clioquinol chez l'enfant. (A propos de 2 cas). Bull Soc Ophtalmol Fr 1977;77:409–411.

17. Okuda K, Matsuo H, Ueno H. Ocular disorders in SMON (subacute myelo-optico neuropathy), especially neuro-retinal lesions. Acta Soc Ophthalmol Jpn 1971;75:1937–1943.

18. Ozawa K, Saida K, Saida T. Experimental clioquinol intoxication in rats: abnormalities in optic nerves and small nerve cells of dorsal root ganglia. Acta Neuropathol 1986;69:272–277.

19. Yamanaka N, Imanari T, Tamura Z, Yagi K. Uncoupling of oxidative phosphorylation of rat liver mitochondria by chinoform. J Biochem (Tokyo) 1973;73:993–998.

20. Lewin L, Guillery H. Die Wirkungen von Arzneimitteln und Giften auf das Auge; Handbuch fur die gesamte arztliche Praxis. 2nd ed. Berlin: August Hirschwald, 1913:138–203.

21. Pentschew A. Intoxikationen. In: Lubarsch O, Henke F, Rossle R. Handbuch der speziellen Pathologischen, Anatomie und Histologie. Bd 13, t.2. Nervensystem. Erkrankungen des zentralen Nervensystems. Berlin: Springer, 1958:1907–2502.

22. Chisholm IA, Pettigrew AR. Biochemical observations in toxic optic neuropathy. Trans Ophthalmol Soc UK 1970;90:827–838.

23. Cagianut B, Rhyner K, Furrier W, Schnebli HP. Thiosulphate-sulphur transferase (rhodanese) deficiency in Leber's hereditary optic atrophy. Lancet 1981;2:981–982.

24. Shiraki H. Neuropathy due to intoxication with antituberculosis drugs from a neuropathological viewpoint. Adv Neurol Sci 1973;17:120–125.

25. Schmidt IG, Schmidt LH. Studies of the neurotoxicity of ethambutol and its racemate for the rhesus monkey. J Neuropathol Exp Neurol 1966;25:40–67.

26. Pau H. Augenschadigungen durch Myambutol (Ethambutol). Klin Monatsbl Augenheilkd 1974;165:121–126.

27. Place VA, Peets EA, Buyske DA, Little RR. Metabolic and special studies of ethambutol in normal volunteers and tuberculosis patients. Ann NY Acad Sci 1966;135:775–795.

28. Delacoux E, Moreau Y, Godefroy A, Evstigneeff T. Prevention de la toxicite oculaire de l'ethambutol: interet de la zincemie et de l'analyse du sens chromatique. J Fr Ophtalmol 1978;1:191–196.

29. Martin-Bouyer G, Lebreton R, Toga M, Stolley PD, Lockhert J. Outbreak of accidental hexachlorophene poisoning in France. Lancet 1982;1:91–95.

30. Martinez AJ, Boehm R, Hadfield MG. Acute hexachlorophene encephalopathy: clinico-neuropathological correlation. Acta Neuropathol 1974;28:93–103.

31. Lockhart JD. How toxic is hexachlorophene? Pediatrics 1972;50:229–235.

32. Towfighi J. Hexachlorophene. In: Spencer PS, Schaumburg HH, eds. Experimental and clinical neurotoxicology. Baltimore: Williams & Wilkins, 1980:440–455.

33. Pleasure D, Towfighi J, Silberberg D, Parris J. The pathogenesis of hexachlorophene neuropathy: in vivo and in vitro studies. Neurology 1974;24:1068–1075.

34. Dixon GJ, Roberts GBS, Tyrrell WF. The relationship of neuropathy to the treatment of tuberculosis with isoniazid. Scott Med J 1956;1:350–354.

35. Sutton PH, Beattie PH. Optic atrophy after administration of isoniazid with PAS. Lancet 1955;1:650–651.

36. Noel PRB, Worden AN, Palmer AC. Neuropathologic effects and comparative toxicity for dogs of isonicotinic acid hydrazide and its methanosulfonate derivative. Toxicol Appl Pharmacol 1967;10:183–198.

37. Takayama K, Schnoes HK, Armstrong EL, Boyle RW. Site of inhibitory action of isoniazid in the synthesis of mycolic acids in *Mycobacterium tuberculosis*. J Lipid Res 1975;16:308–317.

38. Uhthoff W, Metzger E. Die Sehgifte und die Pharmakologie des Sehens. In: Bethe A, Bergmann G, Embden G, Ellinger A, eds. Handbuch der normalen und pathogischen Physiologie. Berlin: Springer, 1931:12(2):812–833.

39. Imre G. Glial proliferation on the papillary surface in workers exposed to lead intoxication. Szemeszet 1967;104:133–135.

40. Tennekoon G, Aitchison CS, Frangia J, Price DL, Goldberg AM. Chronic lead intoxication: effects on the developing optic nerve. Ann Neurol 1979;5:558–564.

41. Ritchie JM. The aliphatic alcohols. In: Gilman AG, Goodman LS, Rall TW, Murad F, eds. Goodman and Gilman's The pharmacological basis of therapeutics. 7th ed. New York: Macmillan Publishing, 1985:372–386.

42. Tephly TR, Makar AB, McMartin KE, Hayreh SS. Methanol; its metabolism and toxicity. In: Majchrowicz E, Noble EP, eds. Biochemistry and pharmacology of ethanol. New York: Plenum Press, 1979;1:145–264.

43. Benton CD Jr, Calhoun FP Jr. The ocular effects of methyl alcohol poisoning: report of a catastrophe involving three hundred and twenty persons. Trans Am Acad Ophthalmol Otolaryngol 1952;56:875–885.

44. Rossazza C, Delplace MP, Boulanger JF, Leboucq F. Recuperation visuelle importante mais-

transitoire apres une intoxication par le methanol. Bull Soc Ophtalmol Fr 1983;83:545–548.

45. Muller H. Histologische Untersuchung eines Auges bei akuter todlicher Methylalkoholvergiftung. Klin Monatsbl Augenheilkd 1950; 116:135–145.

46. Sharpe JA, Hostovsky M, Bilbao JM, Rewcastle NB. Methanol optic neuropathy: a histopathological study. Neurology 1982;32:1093–1100.

47. Pick L, Bielschowsky M. Uber histologische Befunde im Auge und im zentral Nervensystem des Menschen bei akuter todlicher Vergiftung mit Methylalkohol. Berl Klin Wochenschr 1912;1:888–893.

48. McLean DR, Jacobs H, Mielke BW. Methanol poisoning: a clinical and pathological study. Ann Neurol 1980;8:161–167.

49. DeReuck J. The human periventricular arterial blood supply and the anatomy of cerebral infarctions. Eur Neurol 1971;5:321–334.

50. Nicholls P. Formate as an inhibitor of cytochrome *c* oxidase. Biochem Biophys Res Commun 1975;67:610–616.

51. Askalonowa T. Die Einwirkung normaler und toxischer Plasmoziddosen auf die Netzhaut (nach klinischen und experimentellen Ergebnissen). Vestn Oftalmol 1937;10:91–94.

52. Krassnow M, Lewkojewa E, Dosorzewa P. The effect of plasmocid on the organ of vision in the light of clinical experimental and pathologic anatomic findings. Vestn Oftalmol 1937;10:73–83.

53. Sipe JC, Vick NA, Schulman S, Fernandez C. Plasmocid encephalopathy in the rhesus monkey: a study of selective vulnerability. J Neuropathol Exp Neurol 1973;32:446–457.

54. Alajouanine T, Derobert L, Thieffry S. Etude clinique d'ensemble de 210 cas d'intoxication par le sels organiques d'etain. Rev Neurol 1958;98:85–96.

55. Pesme P. Complications oculaires observees chez quatre enfants intoxiques par le "Stalinon". Arch Fr Pediatr 1955;12:327–328.

56. Barnes JM, Stoner HB. The toxicology of tin compounds. Pharmacol Rev 1959;11:211–231.

57. Scheinberg LC, Taylor JM, Hertzog I, Mandell S. Optic and peripheral nerve response to triethyl-tin intoxication in the rabbit: biochemical and ultrastructural studies. J Neuropathol Exp Neurol 1966;25:202–213.

58. Hedges TR, Zaren HA. Experimental papilledema: a study of cats and monkeys intoxicated with triethyl tin acetate. Neurology 1969;19:359–366.

59. Torack RM. The relationship between adenosine triphosphatase activity and triethyl-tin toxicity in the production of cerebral edema in the rat. Am J Pathol 1965;46:245–262.

60. Barnes JM, Stoner HB. Toxic properties of some dialkyl and trialkyl tin salts. Br J Industr Med 1958;15:15–22.

61. Gorgone G, Inserra A, Barlotta F, Malfitano D. Indagini elettroretinografiche nella intossicazione sperimentale da acetato di amile. Ann Ottalmol Clin Oculist 1970;96:313–319.

62. Agnello F. Amaurosi tossica da felce maschio. Rass Ital Ottalmol 1939;8:210–221.

63. Georges A, Gerin Y, Denef J. Study of the toxic effects of purified fern extracts. In: Baker SB de C, Tripod J, eds. Sensitization to drugs; proceedings of the European Society for the Study of Drug Toxicity. Vol X. Amsterdam: Excerpta Medica, 1969:218–226.

64. Freedman A, Sevel D. The cerebro-ocular effects of carbon dioxide poisoning. Arch Ophthalmol 1966;76:59–65.

65. Freedman BJ. Papilloedema, optic atrophy, and blindness due to emphysema and chronic bronchitis. Br J Ophthalmol 1963;47:290–294.

66. Newton DAG, Bone I. Papilloedema and optic atrophy in chronic hypercapnia. Br J Dis Chest 1979;73:399–404.

67. Caffi M, Bettaglio M, Pasotti C. Contributo alla conoscenza del solfocarbonismo sperimentale. Rass Ital Ottalmol 1962;31:49–60.

68. Seto Y. Influence of carbon disulfide on the ERG in rabbits. Acta Soc Ophthalmol Jpn 1958;62:951–961.

69. Merigan WH, Wood RW, Zehl D, Eskin TA. Carbon disulfide effects on the visual system. 1. Visual thresholds and ophthalmoscopy. Invest Ophthalmol Vis Sci 1988;29:512–518.

70. Saida K, Mendell JR, Weiss HS. Peripheral nerve changes induced by methyl n-butyl ketone and potentiated by methyl ethyl ketone. J Neuropathol Exp Neurol 1976;35:113.

71. Ide T. Ocular changes in mice caused by carbon disulfide poisoning. Acta Soc Ophthalmol Jpn 1958;62:85–108.

72. Kittel V, Cornelius C. Sehnervenschadigung durch chloramphenicol. Klin Monatsbl Augenheilkd 1969;155:83–87.

73. Cogan DG, Truman JT, Smith TR. Optic neuropathy, chloramphenicol, and infantile genetic agranulocytosis. Invest Ophthalmol 1973;12:534–537.

74. Werner R, Kollak A, Nierhaus D, Schreiner G, Nierhaus K. Experiments on the binding sites and the action of some antibiotics which inhibit ribosomal functions. In: Drews J, Hahn FE, eds. Drug receptor interactions in antimicrobial chemotherapy. New York: Springer-Verlag, 1975:217–234.

75. Miller NR. Walsh and Hoyt's Clinical neuro-ophthalmology. 4th ed. Baltimore: Williams & Wilkins, 1982; Vol 1:289–307.

76. Kravitz D. Neuroretinitis associated with symptoms of ergot poisoning; report of a case. Arch Ophthalmol 1935;13:201–206.

77. Gundlach AL, Krstich M, Beart PM. Guanine nucleotides reveal differential actions of ergot derivatives at D-2 receptors labelled by [^{3}H]-spiperone in striatal homogenates. Brain Res 1983;278:155–163.

78. Birch-Hirschfeld A. Zum Kapitel der Intoxikations-Amblyopien (Methylalkohol, Opto-

chin, Granugenol). Zentralbl Augenheilkd 1916;35:1–12.

79. Sattler CH. Augenveranderungen bei Intoxikationen. In: Schieck F, Bruckner A, eds. Kurzes Handbuch der Ophthalmologie. Berlin: Springer, 1932;7:229–290.

80. Rall TW, Schleifer LS. Oxytocin, prostaglandins, ergot alkaloids, and other drugs; tocolytic agents. In: Gilman AG, Goodman LS, Rall TW, Murad F, eds. Goodman and Gilman's The pharmacological basis of therapeutics. 7th ed. New York: Macmillan, 1985:926–945.

81. Kramer SG, Potts AM, Mangnall Y. Dopamine: a retinal neurotransmitter. II. Autoradiographic localization of H³-dopamine in the retina. Invest Ophthalmol 1971;10:617–624.

82. Ehinger B, Floren I. Quantification of the uptake of indoleamines and dopamine in the rabbit retina. Exp Eye Res 1978;26:1–11.

83. Osborne NN. Noradrenalin, a transmitter candidate in the retina. J Neurochem 1981;36:17–27.

84. Jess A. Die Gefahren der Chemotherapie fur das Auge, insbesondere uber eine das Sehorgan schwer schadigende Komponente des chinins und seiner Derivate. Albrecht von Graefes Arch Ophthalmol 1921;104:48–74.

85. Singer TP, Von Korff RW, Murphy D, eds. Monoamine oxidase: structure, function, and altered functions. New York: Academic Press, 1979:210–238.

86. Jones OW III. Toxic amblyopia caused by pheniprazine hydrochloride (JB-516, Catron). Arch Ophthalmol 1961;66:29–36.

87. Mizuno K. Etiology and treatment of retinitis pigmentosa. Acta Ophthalmol Jpn 1960;64:2186–2195.

88. Bacon P, Spalton DJ, Smith SE. Blindness from quinine toxicity. Br J Ophthalmol 1988;72:219–224.

89. Zahn JR, Brinton GF, Norton E. Ocular quinine toxicity followed by electroretinogram, electrooculogram, and pattern visually evoked potential. Am J Optom Physiol Opt 1981;58:492–498.

90. Holden WA. The pathology of experimental quinine blindness. Trans Am Ophthalmol Soc 1898, Publ 1899;8:405–411.

91. Casini F. Il metabolismo respiratorio della retina nell' intossicazione sperimentale da chinino. Arch Ottalmol 1939;46:263–279.

92. Manschot WA. Ophthalmic pathological findings in a case of thallium poisoning. In: Francois J, ed. Occupational and medicative hazards in ophthalmology. Basel: Karger, 1969:348–349 (Ophthalmologica Suppl to v. 158).

93. Walsh FB, Hoyt WF. Clinical neuro-ophthalmology. 3rd ed. Baltimore: Williams & Wilkins, 1969:81–97.

94. Andre T, Ullberg S, Winqvist G. The accumulation and retention of thallium in tissues of the mouse. Acta Pharmacol Toxicol 1960;16:229–234.

95. Inturrisi CE. Thallium-induced dephosphorylation of a phosphorylated intermediate of the (sodium plus thallium-activated) ATPase. Biochim Biophys Acta 1969;178:630–633.

96. Cavanagh JB, Fuller NH, Johnson HR, Rudge P. The effects of thallium salts, with particular reference to the nervous system changes. Q J Med 1974;43:293–319.

97. Hurst EW. The lesions produced in the central nervous system by certain organic arsenical compounds. J Pathol Bacteriol 1959;77:523–534.

98. Lazar NK. Effect of tryparsamide on the eye; an experimental and clinical study and report of a case. Arch Ophthalmol 1934;11:240–253.

99. Sanderson PA, Kuwabara T, Cogan DG. Optic neuropathy presumably caused by vincristine therapy. Am J Ophthalmol 1976;81:146–150.

100. Green WR. Retinal and optic nerve atrophy induced by intravitreous vincristine in the primate. Trans Am Ophthalmol Soc 1975;73:389–416.

101. Shelanski ML, Wisniewski H. Neurofibrillary degeneration induced by vincristine therapy. Arch Neurol 1969;20:199–206.

102. Oehninger C, Rodriquez Barrios R, Gomez Haedo CA. Optic neuritis caused by arsenicals; treatment with B.A.L. Br J Ophthalmol 1955;39:422–428.

103. Strandvik B, Zetterstrom R. Amaurosis after broxyquinoline. Lancet 1968;1:922–923.

104. Teleky L. Gewerbliche Vergiftungen. Berlin: Springer, 1955:109–137.

105. Recknagel RO, Glende EA Jr. Carbon tetrachloride hepatotoxicity: an example of lethal cleavage. CRC Crit Rev Toxicol 1973;2:263–297.

106. Smith AR. Optic atrophy following inhalation of carbon tetrachloride. Arch Industr Hyg 1950;1:348–351.

107. Osuntokun BO. An ataxic neuropathy in Nigeria. A clinical, biochemical and electrophysiological study. Brain 1968;91:215–248.

108. Homeida M, Babikr A, Daneshmend TK. Dapsone-induced optic atrophy and motor neuropathy. Br Med J 1980;281:1180.

109. DeGowin RL. A review of therapeutic and hemolytic effects of dapsone. Arch Intern Med 1967;120:242–248.

110. Hubner AH. Ueber Dinitrobenzolvergiftungen. Munch Med Wochenschr 1918;65:1285–1287.

111. Nieden A. Ueber Amblyopie durch Nitrobenzol- (Roburit-) Vergiftung. Centralbl Prakt Augenheilkd 1888;12:193–200.

112. Lindemann K. Bericht uber einen Fall von Erblindurg durch Einatmen von Nachschwaden von Dynamitsprengung im Grubenbetrieb. Zentralbl Augenheilkd 1927;61:72–79.

113. Ahmed MM. Ocular effects of antifreeze poisoning. Br J Ophthalmol 1971;55:854–855.

114. Vainshtein BI. Ophthalmological diagnosis of acute poisoning due to antifreeze. Vestn Oftalmol 1967;80:62–63.

115. Friedman EA, Greenberg JB, Merrill JP, Dammin GJ. Consequences of ethylene glycol poisoning: report of four cases and review of the literature. Am J Med 1962;32:891–902.

116. Hepp P. Ueber Quecksilberathylverbindungen und uber das Verhaltniss des Quecksilberathyl - zur Quecksilbervergiftung. Naunyn-Schmiedebergs Arch Exp Pathol Pharmakol 1887;23:91–128.

117. Fink WH. The ocular pathology of methyl-alcohol poisoning. Am J Ophthalmol 1943;26:694–709, 802–815.

118. Hansson O, Herxheimer A. Neuropathy and optic atrophy associated with halquinol. Lancet 1981;1:450.

119. Behrens MM. Optic atrophy in children after diiodohydroxyquin therapy. JAMA 1974;228:693–694.

120. Fleisher DI, Hepler RS, Landau JW. Blindness during diiodohydroxyquin (Diodoquin) therapy: a case report. Pediatrics 1974;54:106–108.

121. Pittman FE, Westphal MC. Optic atrophy following treatment with diiodohydroxyquin. Pediatrics 1974;54:81–83.

122. Webster LT Jr. Drugs used in the chemotherapy of protozoal infections. In: Gilman AG, Goodman LS, Rall TW, Murad F, eds. Goodman and Gilman's The pharmacological basis of therapeutics. 7th ed. New York: Macmillan, 1985:1052.

123. Lund A. Case of toxic amblyopia after inhalation of methyl acetate. Ugeskr Laeg 1944;106:308–311.

124. Klaassen CD. Nonmetallic environmental toxicants: air pollutants, solvents and vapors, and pesticides. In: Gilman AG, Goodman LS, Rall TW, Murad F, eds. Goodman and Gilman's pharmacological basis of therapeutics. 7th ed. New York: Macmillan, 1985:1628–1650.

125. Eross S, Szobor A. Ophthalmological and neurological signs of chronic methyl bromide poisoning. Orv Hetil 1953;94:944–946.

126. Chavez CT, Hepler RS, Straatsma BR. Methyl bromide optic atrophy. Am J Ophthalmol 1985;99:715–719.

127. von Oettingen WF. The toxicity and potential dangers of methyl bromide with special reference to its use in the chemical industry, in fire extinguishers, and in fumigation. Washington, DC: Government Printing Office, 1946; National Institutes of Health Bull 185.

128. Spencer PS, Schaumburg HH. Experimental neuropathy produced by 2,5-hexanedione—a major metabolite of the neurotoxic industrial solvent methyl n-butyl ketone. J Neurol Neurosurg Psychiatry 1975;38:771–775.

129. Spencer PS, Couri D, Schaumburg HH. n-hexane and methyl n-butyl ketone. In: Spencer PS, Schaumburg HH, eds. Experimental and clinical nerve toxicology. Baltimore: Williams & Wilkins, 1980:456–475.

130. Clarke E. Optic atrophy following the use of arylarsonates in the treatment of syphilis. Trans Ophthalmol Soc UK 1910;30:240–251.

131. Anderson J, Fuglsang H, de C Marshall TF. Effects of suramin on ocular onchocerciasis. Tropenmed Parisitol 1976;27:279–296.

132. Heuner W, Petzold E. Severe poisonings from an oxygen breathing apparatus (from trichloroethylene?) Zentralbl Arbeitsmed Arbeitsschutz 1952;2:4–11.

133. Meyer H. Untersuchungen uber die Giftwirkung des Trichlorathylens, besonders auf das Auges. Klin Monatsbl Augenheilkd 1929;82:309–317.

134. Savic S, Baaske H, Hockwin O. Biochemische Veranderungen am Kaninchenauge bei Vergiftung mit Trichlorathylen. Albrecht von Graefes Arch Ophthalmol 1968;175:1–6.

135. Harley RD, DiGeorge AM, Mabry CC, Apt L. Idiopathic hypercalcemia of infancy: optic atrophy and other ocular changes. Trans Am Acad Ophthalmol Otolaryngol 1965;69:977–992.

136. Kassem A, Hussein HA, Abaza H, Sabry H. Optic atrophy following repeated courses of tartar emetic for the treatment of bilharziasis. Bull Ophthalmol Soc Egypt 1976;69:459–463.

137. Rokos L. Eye complications in poisoning by 'kosso' (Hagenia abyssinica). Ethiop Med J 1969;7:11–16.

138. Sattler CH. Bromural- und Adalinvergiftung des Auges. Klin Monatsbl Augenheilkd 1923;70:149–152.

139. Manthey KF. Augenveranderungen nach chronischen Abusus bromhaltiger Schlafmittel. Klin Monatsbl Augenheilkd 1978;172:400.

140. Belousova RV, Rafalovich SN. Optic atrophy after intoxication caused by seeds of the castor plant. Vestn Oftalmol 1949;28(3):40–41.

141. Olsnes S, Refsnes K, Pihl A. Mechanism of action of the toxic lectins abrin and ricin. Nature 1974;249:627–631.

142. Roper JP. The presumed neurotoxic effects of Catha edulis—an exotic plant now available in the United Kingdom. Br J Ophthalmol 1986;70:779–781.

143. Biesin A. Vergiftungsgefahr und Idiosynkrasie bei Darreichung von Oleum chenopodii. Munch Med Wochenschr 1929;76:661–664.

144. Tate GW Jr, Martin RG. Clindamycin in the treatment of human ocular toxoplasmosis. Can J Ophthalmol 1977;12:188–195.

145. Tally FP, Snydman DR, Gorbach SL, Malamy MH. Plasmid-mediated, transferable resistance to clindamycin and erythromycin in Bacteroides fragilis. J Infect Dis 1979;139:83–88.

146. Hamilton AS, Nixon CE. Optic atrophy and multiple peripheral neuritis developed in the manufacture of explosives (binitrotoluene). JAMA 1918;70:2004–2006.

147. Simon G. Optikusatrophie nach Glibenclamid. Dtsch Gesundh Wes 1975;30:898–901.

148. Lebrun P, Malaisse WJ, Herchuelz A. Modalities of gliclazide-induced Ca^{2+} influx into the pancreatic B-cell. Diabetes 1982;31:1010–1015.

149. Hsu CY, Brooker G, Peach MJ, Westfall TC. Inhibition of catecholamine release by tolbutamide and other sulfonylureas. Science 1975;187:1086–1087.

150. Bruce GM. Permanent bilateral blindness following the use of hexamethonium chloride. Arch Ophthalmol 1955;54:422–424.

151. Goldsmith AJB, Hewer AJH. Unilateral amaurosis with partial recovery after using hexamethonium iodide. Br Med J 1952;2:759–760.

152. Danopoulos E, Melissinos K, Katsas G. Serious poisoning by hexachlorocyclohexane; clinical and laboratory observations on five cases. Arch Industr Hyg Occup Med 1953;8:582–587.

153. Gombos GM. Bilateral optic neuritis following minoxidil administration. Ann Ophthalmol 1983;15:259–261.

154. Ardouin M, Urvoy M, Raoul T, Herve MC. Etude electroretinographique d'un cas d'intoxication par les I.M.A.O. Bull Soc Ophtalmol Fr 1967;67:920–924.

155. Bumke O, Krapf E. Vergiftungen durch anorganische und organische sowie durch pflanzliche, tierische und bakterielle Gift. In: Bumke O, Foerster O, eds. Handbuch der Neurologie. Bd 13(2): Infektionen und Intoxikationen. Berlin: Springer, 1936:694–827.

156. Sedan J. Papillite aigue hemorrhagique au cours d'un intoxication suraigue par l'aspirine. Bull Soc Ophtalmol Fr 1958;58:333–336.

157. Sykowski P. Streptomycin in miliary choroidal tuberculosis. Am J Ophthalmol 1952;35:414–415.

158. Gardiner PA, Michaelson IC, Rees RJW, Robson JM. Intravitreous streptomycin: its toxicity and diffusion. Br J Ophthalmol 1948; 32:449–456.

159. Mitsuhashi S, ed. Drug action and drug resistance in bacteria. Vol. 2. Aminogycoside antibiotics. Baltimore: University Park Press, 1975:197–209.

160. Bryan LE, Kwan S. Mechanisms of aminoglycoside ototoxicity in animal models. In: Weston A, Neu HC, eds. The aminoglycosides: microbiology, clinical use and toxicity. New York: Marcel Dekker, 1982:419–451.

161. Appelbaum A. An ophthalmoscopic study of patients under treatment with thioridazine. Arch Ophthalmol 1963;69:578–580.

162. Bonaccorsi MT. Atrophie optique et atteinte systemique: deux cas de reactions secondaires aux phenothiazines chez des enfants. Laval Med 1967;38:84–88.

163. Meier-Ruge W, Kalberer F, Cerletti A. Mikrohistoautoradiographische Untersuchungen uber die Verteilung von tritiummarkierten Phenothiazinen im Auge. Experientia 1966;22:153–155.

164. Baldessarini RJ. Drugs and the treatment of psychiatric disorders. In: Gilman AG, Goodman LS, Rall TW, Murad F, eds. Goodman and Gilman's The pharmacological basis of therapeutics. 7th ed. New York: Macmillan, 1985:387–445.

165. DiSaia PJ. Pregnancy and delivery of a patient with a Starr-Edwards mitral valve prosthesis. Obstet Gynecol 1966;28:469–472.

166. Whitlon DS, Sadowski JA, Suttie JW. Mechanism of coumarin action: significance of vitamin K epoxide reductase inhibition. Biochemistry 1978;17:1371–1377.

167. Prineas J. Peripheral nerve changes in thiamin-deficient rats; an electron microscope study. Arch Neurol 1970;23:541–548.

168. Swank RL, Adams RD. Pyridoxine and pantothenic acid deficiency in swine. J Neuropathol Exp Neurol 1948;7:274–286.

169. Chisholm IA, Bronte-Stewart J, Foulds WS. Hydroxycobalamin versus cyanocobalamin in the treatment of tobacco amblyopia. Lancet 1967;2:450–457.

CHAPTER 9

Intraocular Metastatic Tumors

Jerry A. Shields, Devron H. Char, Wallace S. Foulds, Evangelos S. Gragoudas, Thomas A. Weingeist, and Eric P. Shakin

INTRODUCTION

Because many more cancer patients survive for longer periods of time than ever before, metastatic tumors to various sites, including the eye, are being recognized more frequently. Consequently, it is important for the ophthalmologist to be aware of the epidemiology, clinical features, diagnostic techniques, management, and prognosis of patients with intraocular metastases.

Epidemiology

Metastatic cancers are now believed to be the most common form of intraocular malignant tumor (1, 2). Although they are more common than either uveal melanoma or retinoblastoma, many intraocular metastases are never diagnosed because they occur in terminally ill patients who do not seek ophthalmic consultation.

Metastases to intraocular tissues occur almost exclusively in adults. They develop more commonly in women because breast cancer accounts for most cases of intraocular metastasis (3–7). Intraocular metastases in children are extremely rare.

Primary Tumors that Metastasize to Intraocular Structures

The vast majority of tumors that metastasize to the eye are carcinomas. Occasionally, malignant melanoma may account for ocular metastasis. Sarcomas metastatic to the eye are exceedingly rare.

The primary tumors that account for most intraocular metastases are breast cancer in women and lung cancer in men (1, 5). Less often, cancers of the gastrointestinal tract, kidney, and thyroid gland may metastasize to the eye. Cutaneous melanomas usually metastasize to the eye as part of disseminated melanomatosis. Carcinoid tumors that metastasize to intraocular tissue are usually of bronchial origin, although they occasionally originate in occult primary sites such as the ileum or thymus gland. Genitourinary tumors such as uterine, prostate, and bladder carcinomas rarely metastasize to the intraocular structures. Almost one-third of patients with intraocular metastasis have no history of a primary cancer when they present to the ophthalmologist (2, 4, 5). In about 10% of cases of intraocular metastasis, the primary site is never found, even after extensive clinical evaluation (4, 5).

Sites of Intraocular Metastasis

The great majority of metastatic tumors to the eye affect the posterior uveal tract, most often the macular area (1–5). Metastases to the retina, optic disc, or vitreous are relatively rare.

CHOROIDAL METASTASIS

Most choroidal metastases occur in the posterior pole, and they can produce painless blurred vision due to macular involvement.

Clinical Features

Ophthalmoscopic examination characteristically reveals one or more homogeneous, creamy yellow lesions deep to the retina (Fig. 9.1). With the exception of metastatic melanoma, choroidal metastases lack intrinsic pigmentation, although overlying alterations in the retinal pigment epithelium (RPE) are common. Most larger symptomatic lesions produce a nonrhegmatogenous retinal detachment (Fig. 9.2). The tumor configuration can range from placoid to dome-shaped, but it almost never assumes a mushroom shape. If an amelanotic tumor is mushroom-shaped, it is much more likely to be an amelanotic melanoma rather than a metastatic tumor (2). In contrast to uveal melanomas, metastatic tumors can be bilateral and multifocal (Fig. 9.3).

Metastatic choroidal tumors produce chronic degeneration of the overlying RPE, leading to characteristic geographical, golden brown deposits on the tumor surface. These deposits are more pronounced after treatment with radiotherapy or chemotherapy (Fig. 9.4). They have been shown to be composed primarily of macrophages containing lipofuscin pigment liberated from damaged RPE cells (8). Larger choroidal metastases can produce a total retinal detachment that may preclude a clear view of the underlying tumor.

Melanomas metastatic to the choroid do not conform to the typical features described above (9, 10). They are more likely to be gray, brown, or black in color, as opposed to the amelanotic appearance of other metastatic tumors.

Diagnostic Approaches

The clinical diagnosis of metastatic choroidal tumor can usually be made by rec-

Figure 9.1. Fundus photograph of carcinoma metastatic to choroid.

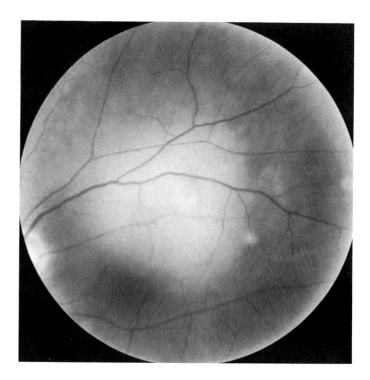

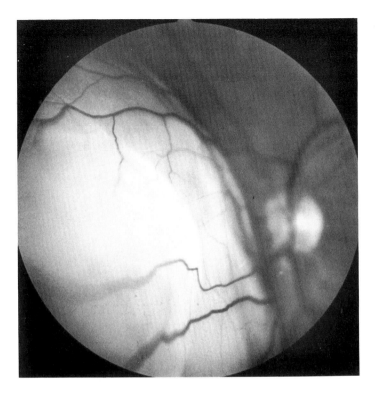

Figure 9.2. Fundus photography of large choroidal metastasis with overlying bullous retinal detachment.

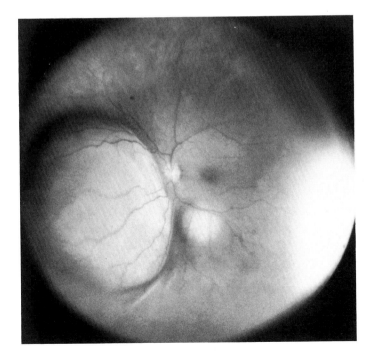

Figure 9.3. Equator-plus fundus photograph showing large choroidal metastatic tumor nasal to the optic disc and a smaller one inferotemporal to optic disc.

Figure 9.4. Typical, golden brown pigment deposits over a choroidal metastasis in the macular area. These are generally more pronounced after the tumor has been treated.

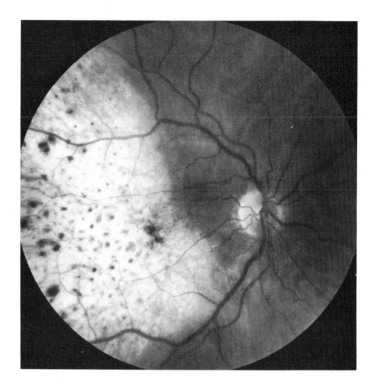

ognizing the typical ophthalmoscopic features. However, many cases are atypical and difficult to differentiate from amelanotic choroidal melanoma, choroidal hemangioma, and other lesions. In general, metastatic tumors show a slightly more rapid growth pattern, whereas melanomas tend to grow more slowly. Certain ancillary studies facilitate the diagnosis.

Fluorescein Angiography

Although there are numerous exceptions, fluorescein angiography of a choroidal metastasis characteristically shows relative hypofluorescence of the lesion in the arterial filling and early venous phases and progressive mottled hyperfluorescence in the late venous phase (Fig. 9.5). This picture contrasts with that of amelanotic choroidal melanomas and hemangiomas, which usually show mottled hyperfluorescence at a slightly earlier stage (2).

Ultrasonography

Ultrasonography can also facilitate the diagnosis of choroidal metastasis. With A-scan, the tumor typically shows a high initial spike and medium to high internal reflectivity within the lesion, with a high scleral spike at the posterior aspect of the tumor (Fig. 9.6). With B-scan, the lesion shows a placoid or dome-shaped configuration with acoustic solidity, no choroidal excavation, and no mushroom shape. These findings contrast with those of a choroidal melanoma, which generally shows acoustic hollowness and choroidal excavation (2).

Computed Tomography

Computed tomography (CT) can often demonstrate metastatic tumors to the uvea. However, since many choroidal metastases are placoid or flat, this technique has

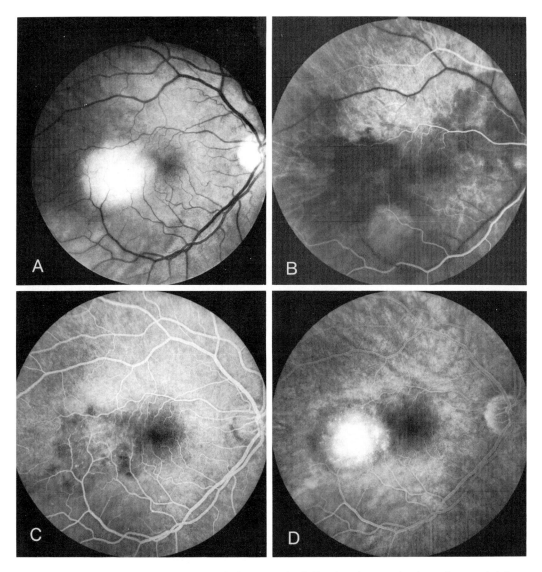

Figure 9.5. Fluorescein angiogram of choroidal metastasis. **A**. Fundus photograph prior to fluorescein injection. **B**. Arterial phase. **C**. Venous phase. **D**. Late phase.

limitations with regard to specific diagnosis.

Magnetic Resonance Imaging

Magnetic resonance imaging (MRI), because of its ability to detect melanin, may ultimately prove helpful in the diagnosis of intraocular metastasis and its differential diagnosis. However, at present, the value of this technique for intraocular tumor diagnosis has not been clearly defined.

Radioactive Phosphorus Uptake (^{32}P) Test

The radioactive phosphorus uptake (^{32}P) test can usually differentiate benign from malignant intraocular tumors and thus may be helpful in the diagnosis of metastatic carcinoma to the choroid (11). Although

Figure 9.6. A-scan ultrasonogram of choroidal metastasis. Note the medium-high internal reflectivity of the tumor (*between arrows*).

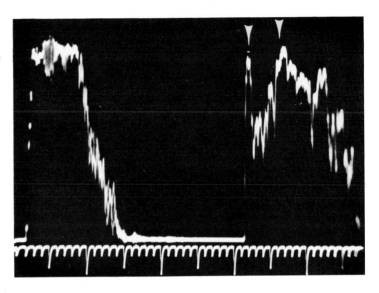

the ^{32}P test cannot differentiate melanoma from metastatic tumor, it can differentiate metastatic tumor from benign conditions such as posterior scleritis. With the advent of fine needle aspiration biopsy for the diagnosis of selected intraocular tumors, the test is employed less frequently today.

Intraocular Biopsy

Biopsy of intraocular tumors is controversial (14). In recent years, fine needle aspiration biopsy (FNAB) has gained popularity in the diagnosis of selected intraocular tumors. This technique is particularly useful in differentiating amelanotic choroidal melanoma from metastatic carcinoma when the diagnosis is equivocal or when a systemic primary malignancy is not detectable (2, 12, 13).

Systemic Evaluation

Any patient with a suspected intraocular metastasis should have a thorough systemic evaluation. This evaluation should include breast examination, mammography, chest x-ray, abdominal CT, and other appropriate studies directed toward detecting other tumors in predisposed organs. Plasma carcinoembryonic antigen

(CEA) levels may be helpful in suggesting occult gastrointestinal neoplasms.

Management

There seems to be a misconception among some physicians that the diagnosis of uveal metastasis is an automatic indication for external beam radiotherapy. However, there are several treatment options for uveal metastasis in addition to radiotherapy. In some cases, a clinically inactive choroidal metastasis will be discovered in an asymptomatic eye of a patient who has received prior chemotherapy for the primary cancer. In such instances, we often withhold active treatment and recommend only periodic observation of the lesion to detect future signs of growth or reactivation.

If a patient with a symptomatic choroidal metastasis has an untreated primary tumor, chemotherapy may control the intraocular metastasis without radiotherapy. If the metastatic tumor is larger and more active and has produced visual loss due to a serous detachment of the retina, radiotherapy may be appropriate (4, 5). In general, 3500 to 4000 GCA (rad) are delivered to the whole eye in fractionated doses over a 3- to 4-week period (2, 4, 5). Most metastatic tumors respond rather dramatically to such treatment (Fig. 9.7).

Prognosis

The visual prognosis for patients with metastatic carcinoma to the choroid varies with the location and extent of the tumor (2), and it is often quite good. The systemic prognosis, however, is generally more guarded. Patients with uveal metastases from breast carcinoma have a somewhat longer survival time than do patients with uveal metastases from carcinoma of the lung, gastrointestinal tract, or kidney or from metastatic melanoma.

CILIARY BODY METASTASIS

Ciliary body metastasis can be contiguous with metastases to the iris or choroid. Because of their more cryptic location, tumors that affect primarily the ciliary body can attain a larger size than do metastases to the choroid or iris (15). Furthermore, ciliary body metastases have an uncanny propensity to produce a clinical picture of chronic iridocyclitis that is generally unresponsive to corticosteroids. Some ciliary body metastases have a large sentinel vessel on the overlying sclera, similar to that seen with some ciliary body melanomas (Fig. 9.8). The diagnostic approaches, management, and prognosis are essentially identical to those of choroidal metastasis.

IRIS METASTASIS

Metastatic tumors to the iris are generally detected when they are relatively small. In the early stages, one or more yellow iris lesions may be present (Fig. 9.9). In contrast to choroidal metastasis, metastasis to the iris can be extremely friable and can shed tumor cells into the aqueous, sometimes producing a deposit of cells in the inferior portion of the anterior chamber, resembling a hypopyon. Hence, these lesions can simulate an intraocular inflammatory reaction that can lead to the erroneous diagnosis of endophthalmitis.

Ultrasonography has little or no diagnostic value in the diagnosis of metastasis to the iris because of the small size and anterior location of the tumor. Fluorescein angiography may show a very vascular lesion, but there is no convincing evidence of its diagnostic usefulness. Fine needle aspiration biopsy is a convenient and relatively safe method of establishing the diagnosis in selected cases.

The management of metastasis to the iris is similar to that of choroidal or ciliary body metastasis. Because these anterior uveal tumors tend to produce secondary glaucoma, it may be necessary to resort to the earlier use of radiotherapy.

RETINAL METASTASIS

In contrast to uveal metastases, retinal metastases are extremely rare (2, 16). True retinal metastasis results from tumor emboli in the retinal blood vessels. The emboli cause retinal vascular obstruction accompanied by diffuse growth of tumor cells into the adjacent retinal tissues, which results in a patchy, yellow lesion, sometimes with surrounding hemorrhage or exudation. Metastatic melanoma to the retina may have a brown or gray color.

Little is known about the results of ancillary diagnostic studies for retinal metastasis. Fluorescein angiography is expected to show early relative hypofluorescence and late patchy hyperfluorescence.

OPTIC DISC METASTASIS

Metastatic tumors exclusively confined to the optic disc are also quite rare. Most metastases that involve the optic disc result from direct extension from a juxtapapillary choroidal metastasis or, rarely, from an orbital metastasis that affects the retrolaminar portion of the optic nerve. Clinically, one sees a swollen optic nerve head with yellow-white material, which represents the tumor (Fig. 9.10) (17). Secondary obstruction of the central retinal vein may occur, leading to dilated retinal veins accompanied by hemorrhages and

Figure 9.7. Response of choroidal metastasis to radiotherapy. **A**. Pretreatment photograph. **B**. Appearance of lesion about 6 weeks after treatment.

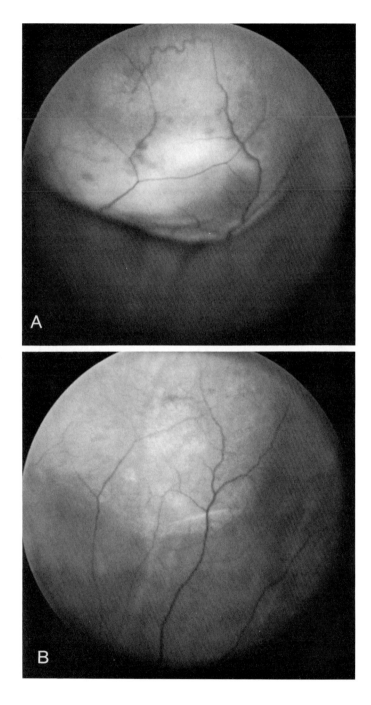

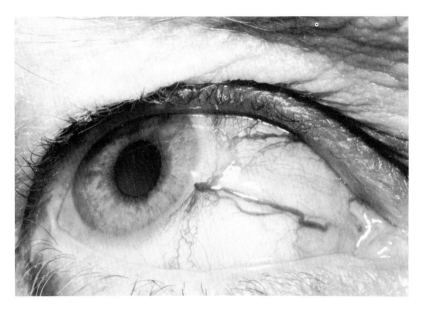

Figure 9.8. Dilated episcleral vessel over ciliary body metastasis from bronchogenic carcinoma.

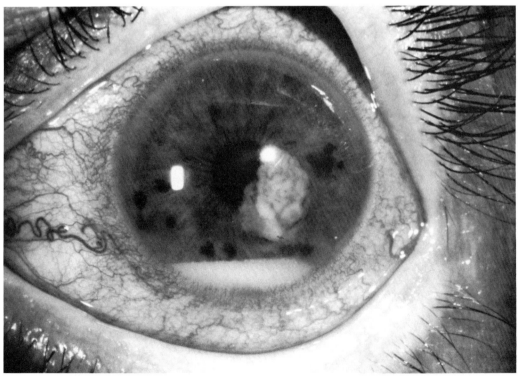

Figure 9.9. Metastatic carcinoma to the iris. Note the layer of tumor cells inferiorly, producing a pseudohypopyon.

Figure 9.10. Optic disc metastasis from a breast carcinoma.

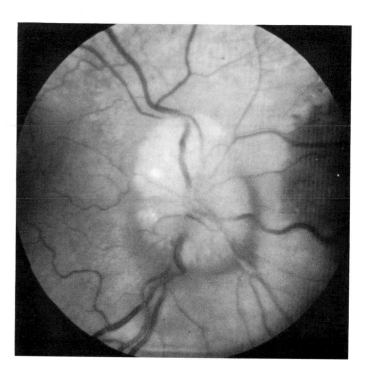

macular edema. Fluorescein angiography typically shows early hypofluorescence of the tumor with late hyperfluorescence, in contrast to papilledema and optic neuritis, which would be more likely to show earlier hyperfluorescence.

VITREAL METASTASIS

Metastatic tumors affecting the vitreous are also extremely rare. Most cases of vitreal metastases result from extension into the vitreous from a metastasis in the retina or ciliary body. It is noteworthy that metastatic cutaneous melanoma has a peculiar propensity to affect the retina and the vitreous simultaneously (2, 18). Another malignancy with a propensity for retinovitreal involvement is large cell lymphoma (reticulum cell sarcoma) (19), which is possibly not a true metastatic lesion but rather a primary lesion with concurrent involvement of the central nervous system. The vitreous cells can lead to the erroneous diagnosis of intraocular inflammation.

SUMMARY AND CONCLUSIONS

Metastatic tumors to the intraocular structures represent the most common form of intraocular malignancy. Most intraocular metastases originate from carcinomas of the breast or lung and spread to the uveal tract, usually the posterior choroid, where they produce painless visual loss. Metastases to the ciliary body and iris may simulate uveitis. Metastatic tumors to the retina, optic disc, and vitreous are exceedingly rare. In almost one-third of cases, there is no history of a primary tumor when the patient presents with uveal metastasis; in about 10%, no primary tumor is ever found. Most intraocular metastatic lesions have rather typical clinical features and usually can be diagnosed with the aid of indirect ophthalmoscopy or slitlamp biomicroscopy. Fluorescein angiography, ultrasonography, and other ancillary studies may facilitate the diagnosis. In many cases, the intraocular tumors can be controlled with chemotherapy as part of the systemic treatment. If chemotherapy fails to control the intraocular tumor, then radiotherapy may be necessary. The systemic prognosis is generally quite poor, but most patients retain useful vision for the remainder of their lives.

References

1. Bloch RS, Gartner S. The incidence of ocular metastatic carcinoma. Arch Ophthalmol 1971;85:673–675.
2. Shields JA. Diagnosis and management of intraocular tumors. St. Louis: CV Mosby, 1983:278–321.
3. Ferry AP, Font RL. Carcinoma metastatic to the eye and orbit. I. A clinicopathologic study of 227 cases. Arch Ophthalmol 1974;92:276–286.
4. Stephens RF, Shields JA. Diagnosis and management of cancer metastatic to the uvea: a study of 70 cases. Ophthalmology 1979;86:1336–1349.
5. Shakin EP, Shields JA. Metastatic cancer to the uvea. A survey of 270 cases. In preparation.
6. Freedman MI, Folk JC. Metastatic tumors to the eye and orbit; patient survival and clinical characteristics. Arch Ophthalmol 1987;105:1215–1219.
7. Mewis L, Young SE. Breast carcinoma metastatic to the choroid; analysis of 67 patients. Ophthalmology 1982;89:147–151.
8. Shields JA, Rodrigues MM, Sarin LK, et al. Lipofuscin pigment over benign and malignant choroidal tumors. Trans Am Acad Ophthalmol Otolaryngol 1976;81:OP871–881.
9. Font RL, Naumann G, Zimmerman LE. Primary malignant melanoma of the skin metastatic to the eye and orbit; report of ten cases and review of the literature. Am J Ophthalmol 1967;63:738–754.
10. de Bustros S, Augsburger JJ, Shields JA, et al. Intraocular metastases from cutaneous malignant melanoma. Arch Ophthalmol 1985;103:937–940.
11. Shields JA. Accuracy and limitations of the ^{32}P test in the diagnosis of ocular tumors: an analysis of 500 cases. Ophthalmology 1978;85:950–966.
12. Augsburger JJ, Shields JA. Fine needle aspiration biopsy of solid intraocular tumors: indications, instrumentation, and techniques. Ophthalmic Surg 1984;15:34–40.
13. Augsburger JJ, Sheilds JA, Folberg R, et al. Fine needle aspiration biopsy in the diagnosis of intraocular cancer; cytologic-histologic correlations. Ophthalmology 1985;92:39–49.
14. Foulds WS, Lee WR, Roxburgh STD, Damato BE. Can chorio-retinal biopsy be justified? Trans Ophthalmol Soc UK 1985;104:864–868.
15. Shields JA, Shakin EP, Shields CL. Metastatic malignant tumors. In: Gold DH, Weingeist TA, eds. The eye in systemic disease. Philadelphia: Lippincott, 1990;299–303.
16. Young SE, Cruciger M, Lukeman J. Metastatic carcinoma to the retina; case report. Ophthalmology 1979;86:1350–1354.
17. Brown GC, Shields JA. Tumors of the optic nerve head. Surv Ophthalmol 1985;29:239–264.
18. Robertson DM, Wilkinson CP, Murray JL, Gordy DD. Metastatic tumor to the retina and vitreous cavity from primary melanoma of the skin; treatment with systemic and subconjunctival chemotherapy. Ophthalmology 1981;88:1296–1301.
19. Char DH, Ljung BM, Miller T, Phillips T. Primary intraocular lymphoma (ocular reticulum cell sarcoma); diagnosis and management. Ophthalmology 1988;95:625–630.

CHAPTER 10

Retinal and Choroidal Changes in Pregnancy

Janet S. Sunness, J. Donald M. Gass, Lawrence J. Singerman,
Richard R. Ober, Gisele Soubrane, and Lloyd M. Aiello

Most women go through pregnancy without any obvious change in their vision, and, in fact, the retina and retinal vascular bed generally appear unchanged (1). When a pregnant woman develops a retinal disorder, or undergoes a change in a preexisting retinal disorder, one is inclined to consider pregnancy as a possible precipitating factor in the change. In certain cases, such as those involving toxemia of pregnancy, the relationship to pregnancy is clear. More often, however, there are not enough natural history data to determine whether a certain disorder is more common during pregnancy or whether the course of a disorder is truly modified by the pregnancy. Potential fetal risks also may preclude a full, but not essential, evaluation of a given condition. For these reasons, our knowledge of the effects of pregnancy on the retina and choroid is limited. The general principle for any retinal disorder is to treat the condition as one would in a nonpregnant woman, so long as no risk to the fetus is involved. It would be valuable, however, to obtain more information about retinal disorders in pregnancy. This information would contribute to the optimal treatment of the pregnant woman, as well as to our knowledge of other related phenomena, such as the effects of hormones on various disorders, which may apply to both pregnant and nonpregnant patients.

SYSTEMIC CHANGES IN PREGNANCY

During pregnancy, there are many hormonal changes due to both modifications in hormonal secretion by the mother and abundant production of hormones by the placenta (2, pp 119–137, 201–205; 3). Among these changes are increases in the production of cortisol, aldosterone, renin, angiotensin substrate, and angiotensin II. Human placental lactogen, along with increased corticosteroid production, may account for the diabetogenic effects of pregnancy. The placenta produces increased levels of melanocyte-stimulating hormone. Although a direct connection between these changes and the development of retinal and choroidal disorders has not been proven, such changes as the possible exacerbation of diabetic retinopathy and ocular melanoma have been attributed to these hormonal alterations.

Hematological and cardiovascular changes are also prominent in pregnancy. There is an increase in blood volume, both in circulating erythrocytes and in plasma volume. There is typically an increase in the level of clotting factors. There is an increase in cardiac output, along with a decrease in arterial blood pressure, a decrease in vascular resistance, and an increase in resting pulse rate (2, pp 191–197). Some of these factors are thought to be related to the development of central serous chorioretinopathy and to the effect of pregnancy on retinal vascular disorders.

The pregnant woman can be considered as being in a state of relative immune suppression. Decreases in both cell-mediated immunity and humoral immunity have been found (4–6). These immunological modifications may be related to the response of the eye in certain inflammatory conditions.

RETINAL AND CHOROIDAL DISORDERS ARISING DURING NORMAL PREGNANCY

Central Serous Chorioretinopathy

There are a number of case reports of central serous chorioretinopathy (CSC) de-

veloping at varying times during pregnancy (7–10). Because CSC is generally more common in men than in women by a factor of 10:1 (11, p 46), the clinical impression is that it may be more common during pregnancy, but there has not been an adequate evaluation of this. Hormonal changes (8) or changes in blood volume along with hypercoagulability (10) have been postulated as being causal factors related to CSC in pregnancy. In all case reports, the CSC has followed a typical course that results in resolution with only minor, residual pigmentary changes. In some patients, CSC has recurred in the same eye in one (9) or more (8) subsequent pregnancies, but it has not recurred outside of pregnancy.

Figure 10.1 shows the evolution of a case

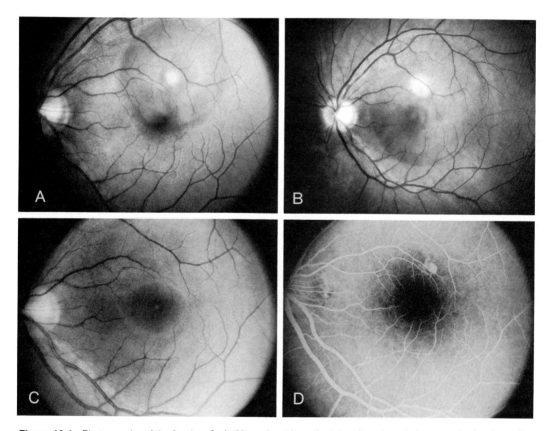

Figure 10.1. Photographs of the fundus. **A.** At 29 weeks, this patient developed central serous chorioretinopathy, with a pigment epithelial detachment and deposition of fibrinous material. **B.** Two weeks later, the area of subretinal fluid enlarged to involve the fovea. Three weeks postpartum, the red-free photograph (**C**) and fluorescein angiogram (**D**) showed resolution of the detachment.

of central serous chorioretinopathy during pregnancy. At 29 weeks of gestation, this patient presented with central serous choroidopathy along with a pigment epithelial detachment and fibrinous material within the area of detachment (Fig. 10.1A). Visual acuity at the time was 20/40. Over the next 2 weeks, the area of subretinal fluid enlarged, with involvement of the fovea and a decrease in vision to the 20/200 level (Fig. 10.1B). By 3 weeks after delivery, the detachment had resolved, with return of visual acuity to 20/30 (Figs. 10.1C and D). The right eye remained normal throughout, with 20/20 acuity.

Choroidal Melanoma

There is an increase in melanocyte-stimulating hormone during pregnancy. This may be the cause for the trend of a greater than expected incidence of ocular melanomas presenting during pregnancy (12). There are reports in the literature of both the development of choroidal melanomas and the exacerbation of preexisting melanomas during pregnancy (12–17). There is no evidence that termination of pregnancy is beneficial. Although cutaneous melanoma has metastasized to the placenta and the fetus (15), there is no report of similar metastasis of a uveal melanoma.

Figure 10.2A shows the left eye of a 33-year-old woman when she presented in her third month of pregnancy with a 6-month history of decreased vision and metamorphopsia. At that time, visual acuity was 20/50; by ultrasound, the lesion was 2.2 mm elevated; and there was a sensory retinal detachment overlying the lesion. At the patient's next visit 6 months later (Fig. 10.2B), visual acuity had decreased to 1/200, and there was a retinal detachment behind the lens. The lesion was 2.7 mm elevated. Two months later, there was a total retinal detachment, and ultrasound examination showed a collar-button lesion (Fig. 10.2C). The eye was enucleated, and the pathological diagnosis was malignant melanoma.

Other Retinal Vascular Conditions

A study of retinal arterial occlusions included two young, pregnant women, both of whom had a past history of a migraine disorder (18). There is a case report of a woman with retinal phlebitis, with no known etiology, early in pregnancy (19).

RETINAL DISORDERS ASSOCIATED WITH A SYSTEMIC COMPLICATION OF PREGNANCY

Hypertensive Disorders of Pregnancy (Preeclampsia, Eclampsia (Toxemia))

Preeclampsia is the occurrence, generally in the latter half of pregnancy, of hypertension, edema, and proteinuria. It is seen in about 5% of first pregnancies in healthy women. Risk factors for preeclampsia include old or very young age, multifetal pregnancies, and hemolytic disease of the newborn. Preeclampsia is more common in women with preexisting diabetes, chronic hypertension, or renal disease. It is associated with an increase in perinatal mortality (2, pp 525–560). Eclampsia is the development of seizures late in pregnancy or in the immediate postpartum period in a preeclamptic woman. The term "toxemia" includes preeclampsia and eclampsia. In the past, lacking the diagnostic capabilities of today, the retinal status of patients with preeclampsia was used as a measure of overall systemic disease. Today, other modalities are used for this purpose, but visual disturbances are quite common in toxemia and may be a significant complaint of a toxemic woman. Because of this, the ophthalmologist is required to have a knowledge of the possible situations that may develop.

Visual complaints such as scotoma, diplopia, photopsia, and dimness of vision have been reported in 30% to 50% of women with eclampsia and in 20% to 25% of women with preeclampsia (20, 21). In the postpartum period, visual disturbances may be a sign of an impending seizure in a preeclamptic patient (22). Though

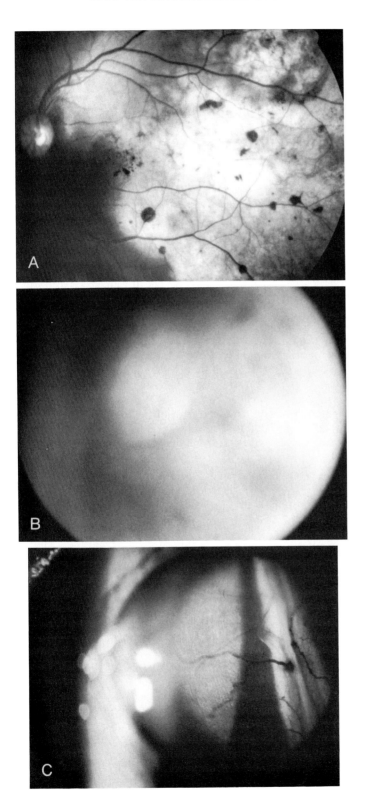

Figure 10.2. A 33-year-old woman presented in the third month of pregnancy with a 6-month history of decreased vision and metamorphopsia. **A.** Examination of the fundus disclosed an elevated, solid lesion with overlying detachment. **B.** Six months later, there was an increase in the size of the lesion and detachment. **C.** The eye was enucleated 2 months later, when a total retinal detachment was present and ultrasonography disclosed a collar-button lesion.

photic stimuli (such as the bright light of an ophthalmoscope) may predispose a susceptible patient to a seizure, the risk is small compared with the benefit of a thorough examination when indicated (23).

Retinopathy in Toxemia

The earliest and most common retinal change in toxemia is the development of reversible focal arteriolar spasm (Fig. 10.3), which has been reported in 40% to 100% of patients with preeclampsia (24–26). Reversible, generalized arteriolar narrowing may also be seen (Fig. 10.4) (27, 28). Other signs of retinal hypertensive change, including hemorrhages, exudates, diffuse retinal edema, and papilledema, are uncommon in patients without other systemic disease (21). When arterial width changes are present, there is a disruption in the blood-aqueous and blood-retinal barriers as shown by ocular fluorophotometry (29). Widespread capillary nonperfusion may also occur (30).

Many investigators have found a correlation between the degree of retinopathy and both the severity of preeclampsia (26, 31–34) and fetal mortality (20, 26, 33, 34). Retinal vascular changes are thought to reflect placental vascular insufficiency. Before better techniques for assessing fetal status were available, the presence of severe or rapidly progressive retinopathy was used as an indication for early delivery, because the premature infant was thought to have a better chance of survival independent of a severely compromised placenta (25, 35). On the other hand, the absence of retinopathy or improvement in retinal status in a preeclamptic patient was considered as a recommendation to allow the pregnancy to continue to term (25).

Retinal Detachment in Toxemia

Serous exudative retinal detachments have been reported in 10% of patients with eclampsia and in 1% to 2% of patients with severe preeclampsia (35, 36). The detachments are most commonly bilateral and bullous, but cases of cyst-like detachments

have been reported (37, 38). There does not appear to be a direct relationship between the retinal vascular changes of toxemia and the detachments. Exudative detachments have been reported in the absence of retinal arterial change (37, 39, 40), and even, rarely, in nontoxemic patients (41). Retinal detachment does not seem to correlate with fetal mortality (26). The detachments are thought to be on a choroidal, rather than on a retinal, vascular basis. Evidence for this includes fluorescein angiograms showing areas of choroidal nonperfusion or delayed filling (Fig. 10.5) (42, 43) and multiple foci of subretinal leakage (Fig. 10.6) (11, pp 164–165; 23, 40, 42, 44, 45). Also, some patients have Elschnig's spots (choroidal infarcts) after the detachment has resolved (23, 37, 46).

Most patients with detachments have full, spontaneous resolution in the weeks following delivery. Most eyes regain normal visual function, though occasionally a woman may have residual retinal pigment epithelial change centrally with decreased acuity (47, 48). Some patients develop permanent pigment epithelial changes that, years later, may mimic a heredomacular dystrophy (Fig. 10.7) or tapetoretinal disorder (Fig. 10.8) (27). Optic atrophy following detachment has also been reported (36).

Other Changes Associated with Toxemia

Cases of ischemic papillophlebitis (30) and peripheral neovascularization (49) associated with toxemia have been reported.

Cortical blindness and other causes of severe visual loss may also be seen in pregnant women with and without toxemia (3, 50, 51).

COAGULATION DISORDERS IN PREGNANCY

Retinal changes in pregnancy may be manifestations of systemic coagulation disorders, such as disseminated intravascular coagulopathy, thrombotic thrombocytopenic purpura, and amniotic fluid embolism.

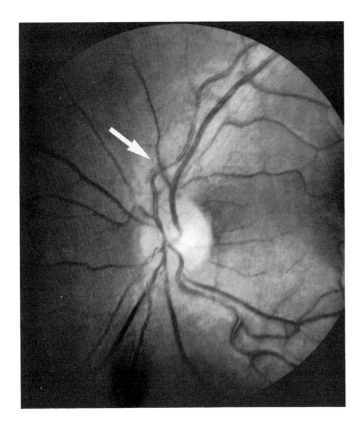

Figure 10.3. Focal arteriolar constriction (*arrow*) in a patient with mild preeclampsia. (Reprinted, with permission, from; Ryan S. Retina. St. Louis: CV Mosby, 1989.)

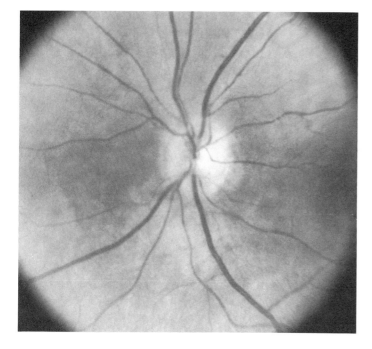

Figure 10.4. Generalized arteriolar narrowing in a patient with severe preeclampsia. (Reprinted, with permission, from; Ryan S. Retina. St. Louis: CV Mosby, 1989.)

Figure 10.5. Arteriovenous phase of a fluorescein angiogram in a preeclamptic patient 14 days postpartum. Delayed filling of the choriocapillaris is seen. (Reprinted, with permission, from; Ryan S. Retina. St. Louis: CV Mosby, 1989.)

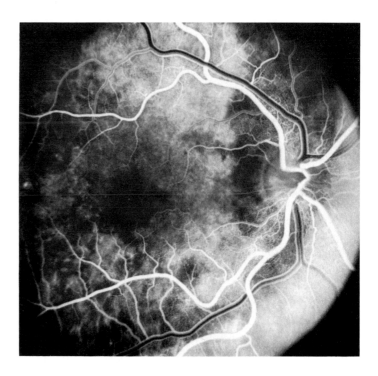

In disseminated intravascular coagulopathy (DIC), which may occur with abruptio placenta, retained dead fetus, and severe preeclampsia (52, 53), there is widespread thrombus formation in small vessels. The choroid is most often involved, generally in the macular and peripapillary regions. There is thrombotic occlusion of the choriocapillaris as well as the choroidal arterioles and venules. Retinal pigment epithelial changes and serious retinal detachments may occur. If the patient survives, vision generally returns to normal with only mild residual pigmentary change (54).

Thrombotic thrombocytopenic purpura (TTP) is a rare disease that includes abnormal platelet consumption and thrombus deposition, leading to thrombocytopenia, microangiopathic hemolytic anemia, and neurological and renal changes. Visual symptoms are reported in 10% of cases. Retinal signs include sensory retinal detachment, arteriolar constriction, optic disc edema, hemorrhages, and exudates (55).

Amniotic fluid embolism occurs during labor, delivery, or the early postpartum period. It is a catastrophic event with high mortality. Almost all survivors develop DIC (56), with signs as described above. There is a report of a patient with bilateral retinal arteriolar occlusions, thought to be due to entrapment of particulate matter in the vessels (57). One patient developed severe retinal and choroidal ischemia that left one eye with no light perception, presumably secondary to massive blood loss from an amniotic fluid embolism (58).

OTHER DISORDERS DEVELOPING DURING LABOR, DELIVERY, AND THE EARLY POSTPARTUM PERIOD

Purtscher's-like Retinopathy

A picture of retinal arteriolar embolization after a precipitous delivery in a normotensive woman has been reported (Fig. 10.9) (11, pp 346–347). This picture was associated with a generalized seizure, suggesting the presence of cerebral involvement as well.

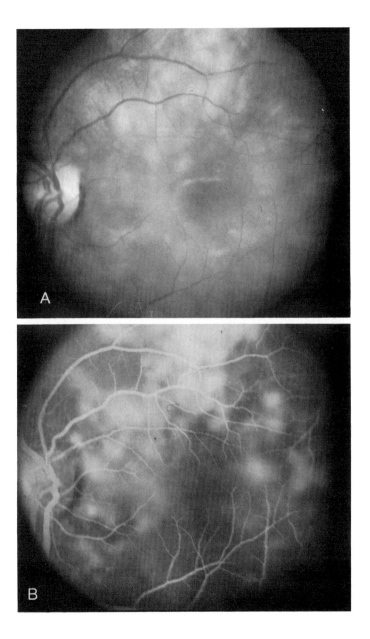

Figure 10.6. A 42-year-old woman with eclampsia developed loss of vision 3 days after cesarean section. She had bilateral bullous retinal detachments. **A.** Patchy white areas of ischemic infarction of the retinal pigment epithelium were present beneath the detachment. **B.** Fluorescein angiogram showed multiple areas of leakage at the level of the RPE. (Reprinted, with permission, from; Gass JDM. Stereoscopic atlas of macular disease. St. Louis: CV Mosby, 1987.)

Acute Macular Neuroretinopathy

This developed in a healthy, 28-year-old woman who had hypertensive agents administered following uterine bleeding after an elective cesarean section (Fig. 10.10) (11, pp 512–513).

Valsalva Maculopathy

The rapid rise of intravenous pressure during delivery may cause a Valsalva maculopathy, with sudden decrease of vision from preretinal, subretinal, or vitreous hemorrhage (Fig. 10.11) (11, pp 564–565).

Figure 10.7. An asymptomatic 63-year-old woman with 20/20 acuity was seen because of suspected macular dystrophy. Multiple Elschnig's spots were present, along with a branched pattern of yellow changes in both eyes. These resulted from severe toxemia with transient bilateral visual loss many years previously, just before the birth of her second child. (Reprinted, with permission, from; Gass JDM. Stereoscopic atlas of macular disease. St. Louis: CV Mosby, 1987.)

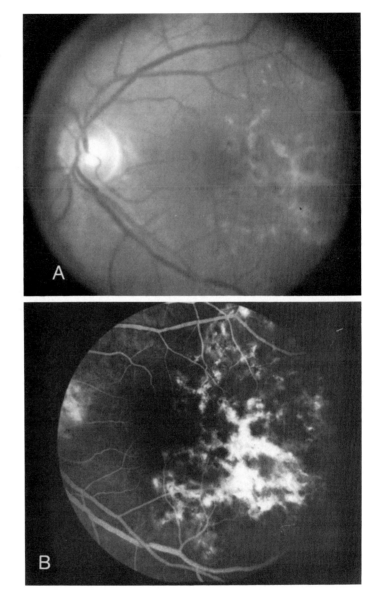

EFFECTS OF PREGNANCY ON PREEXISTING RETINAL CONDITIONS

Diabetic Retinopathy

General Considerations

There are two general guidelines to follow in advising and managing diabetic women planning to conceive. The first is that diabetic women should plan to have their children as early as possible (59), because duration of diabetes is the prime risk factor for the presence (60), severity (61), and progression (62) of retinopathy, as it is for the nonpregnant diabetic woman. The risk of fetal morbidity and mortality in women with advanced diabetic retinopathy is much lower than in the past (59, 60, 63, 64), and, with modern management,

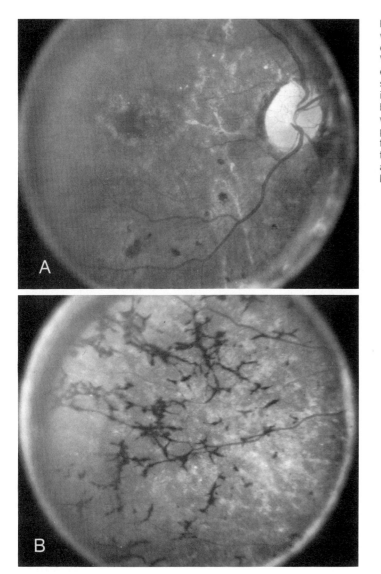

Figure 10.8. At age 18, this woman had eclampsia with bilateral blindness following delivery. Vision returned to 20/400 in each eye. Twenty years later, Elschnig's spots (**A**), narrowed retinal arterioles, and peripheral bone spicule pigmentation (**B**) were present, presenting a pseudo-retinitis pigmentosa picture. (Reprinted, with permission, from; Gass JDM. Stereoscopic atlas of macular disease. St. Louis: CV Mosby, 1987.)

the fetal prognosis in the presence of maternal retinopathy is much improved (60, 65–67). However, there remains evidence that the severity of diabetic retinopathy is a risk factor for an adverse outcome of pregnancy (miscarriage, perinatal death, or severe congenital anomaly) (54).

The second guideline is that blood glucose control is probably very important for fetal well-being (68, 69). In particular, good control of serum glucose should be instituted prior to conception and continued throughout pregnancy. Studies have shown that well-controlled blood glucose and hemoglobin A_{1c} prior to conception and through pregnancy reduce the risk of spontaneous abortion (70), congenital anomalies, and fetal morbidity (71). One study suggests that good glucose control might counteract the adverse effects of proliferative retinopathy or nephropathy on the fetus (68). Good glucose control remains an important guideline

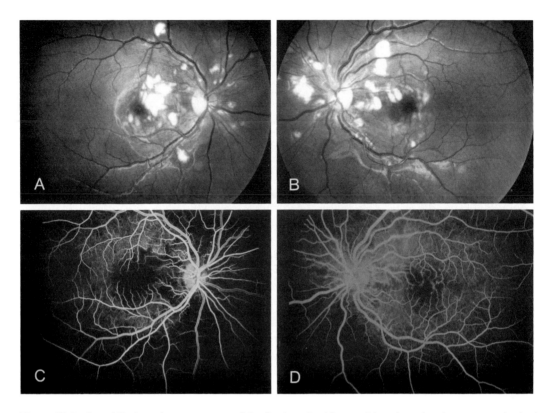

Figure 10.9. **A** and **B** show the appearance of the fundus of a 16-year-old nonhypertensive woman who had precipitous delivery of a live infant following oxytocin administration. She had a generalized seizure 6 hours later. The following morning, she noted blurred vision in both eyes; acuity was hand movements in the right eye and 20/20 in the left. **C** and **D.** Fluorescein angiography showed multifocal retinal arteriolar occlusions in both eyes. Over the next 2 months, the retinal lesions cleared, with acuity returning to 20/40 in the right eye and remaining at 20/20 in the left eye. (Reprinted, with permission, from; Gass JDM. Stereoscopic atlas of macular disease. St. Louis: CV Mosby, 1987.)

despite evidence that tightening of control can transiently aggravate diabetic retinopathy (72).

All pregnant diabetic women should have a baseline ophthalmological examination, ideally prior to pregnancy, but certainly in the first trimester. Follow-up examinations are determined by the retinopathy status at the initial examination. A diabetic woman with background retinopathy should probably be examined once per trimester, and a woman with proliferative disease should be examined monthly.

Recent studies of diabetic retinopathy in pregnancy have found a higher rate of development and progression of retinopathy than did studies performed more than 10 years ago. This is primarily due to refine-

ments in the grading of retinopathy, so that a study now might consider additional microaneurysms on a photograph of the fundus as evidence of increased background retinopathy, or an increase in the amount of neovascularization as evidence of increased proliferative disease. Older studies often documented progression by more dramatic steps, such as the appearance of significantly more background and preproliferative change or the occurrence of vitreous hemorrhage with vision loss. Also, patients in more recent studies are more likely to have had tight glucose control than did patients in older studies, and the tighter control may also have an effect on changes in retinopathy (73).

To determine whether there is truly a

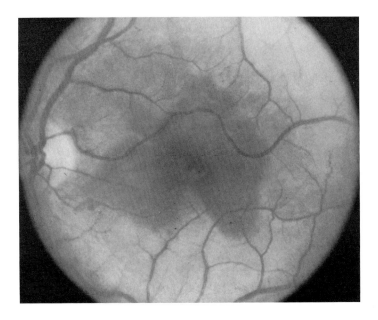

Figure 10.10. A woman had uterine bleeding following an elective cesarean section. She received oxytocin and epinephrine and experienced elevated blood pressure, along with severe headache and extrasystoles. These were treated with intravenous lidocaine and sodium pentothal. On awakening, acuity was 20/200, and the patient noted central scotomata. Her vision improved over the next few days. At 6 weeks postpartum, acuity was 20/20. There were paracentral scotomata and the typical appearance of acute macular neuroretinopathy as shown. The lesions were slightly hyperfluorescent on angiogram. The lesions cleared over the next 6 weeks. (Reprinted, with permission, from; Gass JDM. Stereoscopic atlas of macular disease. St. Louis: CV Mosby, 1987.)

difference in the progression of diabetic retinopathy during pregnancy versus during a 9-month period in an age-matched, nonpregnant diabetic group, one ideally would define matched groups to be followed prospectively. The Retinopathy in Pregnancy Study is following matched groups of insulin-dependent diabetic women, one group of pregnant women and one group of nonpregnant women. The groups are matched with respect to duration of diabetes, degree of retinopathy at

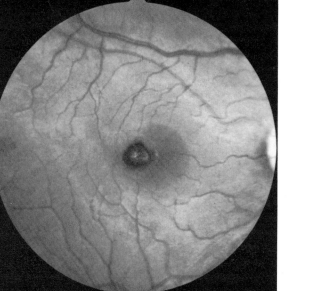

Figure 10.11. Valsalva maculopathy due to straining during delivery.

baseline, and age. A preliminary analysis of 70 women in each group showed that 25 of the 70 pregnant women had more severe retinopathy at their postpartum visit than at their initial visit early in pregnancy, whereas 7 out of the 70 pregnant women had an improvement in retinopathy at their postpartum visit. During the same time period, 15 of 70 nonpregnant, diabetic women experienced worsening of their retinopathy, whereas 21 out of 70 had improvement. The difference between these groups was apparent even after accounting for duration of diabetes, blood pressure, and glycosylated hemoglobin. This difference suggests that there may be a greater tendency for retinopathy to progress during pregnancy, but firm conclusions cannot be drawn yet due to the small size of the preliminary sample (74). One study has shown that the number of past pregnancies does not increase the risk of diabetic retinopathy when duration of diabetes is taken into account (75).

Effects of Pregnancy as a Function of Baseline Retinopathy Status

No Retinopathy at Onset of Pregnancy. A review of nine studies (60, 62, 66, 73, 76–80) reported from 1978 to 1988 included 484 pregnant diabetic women (3). Eighty-eight percent of these women did not develop retinopathy during pregnancy, whereas 7% developed mild or minimal background retinopathy and an additional 5% developed more significant background change. In 23 of these cases, postpartum results were reported, and 57% of the patients developing background change had regression of their retinopathy. One patient (0.2%) developed proliferative retinopathy during pregnancy. She was treated with laser photocoagulation, with partial regression during pregnancy and total regression in the postpartum period.

Gestational diabetics (women who develop diabetes only during pregnancy) do not appear to be at risk for retinopathy (69). A recent study found that women with gestational diabetes had increased tortuosity of their retinal vessels that persisted for at least five months postpartum and was inversely correlated with the hemoglobin A_{1c} level (81).

Minimal Retinopathy at Onset of Pregnancy. Women with minimal retinopathy, that is, fewer than 10 microaneurysms and dot hemorrhages per eye without exudates, were the subject of studies in 1978 (76) and 1980 (82). Together, the studies included 24 women, 2 of whom (8%) developed more microaneurysms during pregnancy. Another 2 had a decrease in microaneurysms during pregnancy. None developed proliferative disease.

Background Retinopathy at Onset of Pregnancy. Background diabetic retinopathy (BDR) often waxes and wanes during pregnancy (60, 66). The changes may be related in part to the institution of tighter blood glucose control (73). Some studies have reported worsening in the second trimester (78, 79, 83, 84) with improvement toward the end of pregnancy and during the postpartum period. A recent fluorescein angiographic study showed an increase in microaneurysms late in the third trimester, with some regression by 6 months postpartum (85). Macular edema can be prominent during pregnancy (86), but it often resolves spontaneously near term and postpartum. One study found that those patients who developed cystoid macular edema tended to have proteinuria of greater than 1 g/day (87).

Figure 10.12 shows the fundus of a 23-year-old woman with a 21-year duration of insulin-dependent diabetes mellitus. Two months prior to her second pregnancy, microaneurysms were visible surrounding the foveal avascular zone. There were small areas of disruption of the perifoveal capillary net (A). At the 35th week of pregnancy, there was no change in the number of microaneurysms (B).

Figure 10.13 shows the right eye of a 28-year-old woman with a 9-year duration of diabetes. There was no increase in the number of microaneurysms from the 28th week of pregnancy (A) to the 35th week (B), but there were late focal areas of leakage around the central avascular zone at

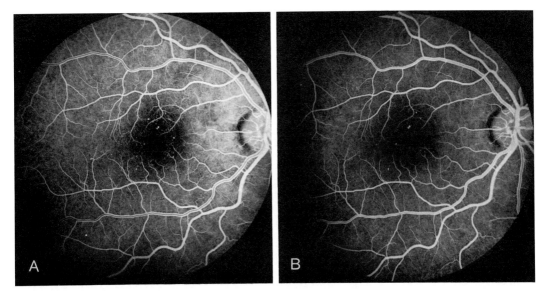

Figure 10.12. Fluorescein angiogram of the macula of an insulin-dependent diabetic woman shows no change in the number of microaneurysms from 2 months prior to pregnancy (**A**) to the 35th week of pregnancy (**B**).

the later time (C). Fifteen months later, there was no increased retinopathy (D) and late frames showed regression of leakage.

A review summarizing studies from 1948 to 1978 (88) of pregnant women with BDR showed a rate of worsening in background change of 10%, which was thought to be no different from the course in a group of nonpregnant diabetic women. A review of 10 studies performed since 1978 (60, 62, 66, 68, 73, 76–80) included 258 women (3). Forty-seven percent of these experienced worsening in background change during pregnancy, most with improvement postpartum. Five percent developed proliferative changes during pregnancy. Follow-up was provided for 8 of these newly proliferative patients; 7 were treated with laser photocoagulation, with postpartum regression of proliferation in 4. One patient was not treated and had spontaneous regression of proliferation in the postpartum period.

The Development of Preproliferative Change. Three studies (60, 78, 79) assessed the new development of soft exudates in women with BDR. Of the 90 diabetic women included in these studies, 43% developed soft exudates during preg-

nancy, and 8% of these women with new soft exudates (3 women) developed proliferative retinopathy (3). Another study of 20 women under tight glucose control found an increase in the number of soft exudates in 35% (73). Soft exudates and large blot hemorrhages often resolve postpartum (60, 79).

Figure 10.14 shows the progression from rare microaneurysms in the periphery to areas of ischemia and intraretinal microvascular abnormalities (IRMA) over the course of the second pregnancy in a 24-year-old woman with an 18-year duration of diabetes. Figure 10.15 shows an increase in preproliferative disease during pregnancy.

Proliferative Retinopathy at Onset of Pregnancy. A review of the literature from 1950 to 1978 (88) found that, in 25% of the 127 reported pregnancies in women with proliferative diabetic retinopathy (PDR), there was progression of PDR during pregnancy. A review of 12 studies (60, 62, 66, 68, 73, 76–80, 88, 89) since 1978 found that 46% of the 122 reported cases of PDR progressed in proliferation during pregnancy. Of the 122 women, 81 had not been treated prior to pregnancy. Of this

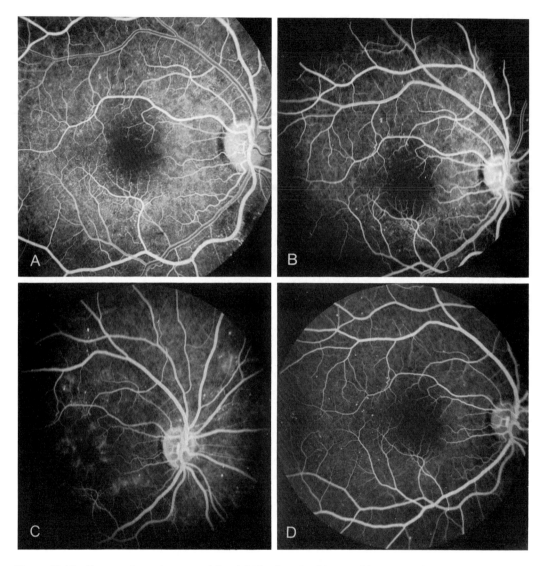

Figure 10.13. Fluorescein angiograms of the right fundus of a 28-year-old woman, with a 9-year duration of diabetes, during and after her third pregnancy. (**A**) shows the appearance at 28 weeks, with numerous micro-aneurysms associated with small areas of ischemia. In the 35th week, there is no increase of microaneurysms on the early frames of the angiogram (**B**). Late frames show discrete perifoveal areas of leakage (**C**). By 15 months postpartum, there is no increase in retinopathy (**D**), and there is regression of leakage in late frames.

untreated group, 58% had progression of PDR during pregnancy. Thirty-five women received some scatter photocoagulation prior to pregnancy, and 26% of these had progression of PDR during pregnancy. Six women had spontaneous involution of neovascularization prior to pregnancy, and none of these progressed in PDR during pregnancy. Finally, 30 of 35 (86%) of women who underwent laser photocoagulation during pregnancy had some regression of their proliferative disease.

No patient with documented complete regression of proliferative disease prior to pregnancy, either spontaneous or laser-induced, has been reported to have progres-

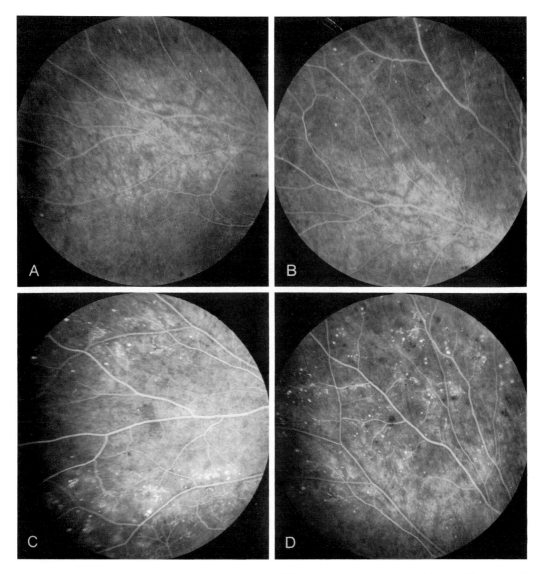

Figure 10.14. Fluorescein angiograms over the course of the second pregnancy of a 24-year-old woman with an 18-year duration of diabetes. (**A**) and (**B**) show the appearance of the periphery in the first month of pregnancy. Only rare microaneurysms were visible. (**C**) and (**D**) show the peripheral areas 2 weeks before delivery. There was a marked increase in microaneurysms, as well as areas of IRMA and ischemia.

sion of PDR during pregnancy (28, 61, 65, 78, 88–91). Therefore, the ideal management of a patient with PDR who wishes to conceive is to treat her PDR prior to conception. The response to panretinal photocoagulation appears to be no different in a pregnant woman than in a nonpregnant diabetic woman (92), nor does prior preg-

nancy affect the response to photocoagulation (91). Given the availability of laser photocoagulation and vitrectomy, termination of pregnancy as a method of treatment of progressive proliferative diabetic retinopathy is no longer a consideration, except perhaps in the most severe, refractory case (28).

Figure 10.15. When first seen prior to pregnancy, this patient had one cotton-wool spot with primarily background changes (**A**). She developed an increased number of cotton-wool spots during pregnancy (**B**). (Courtesy Daniel Finkelstein, MD.)

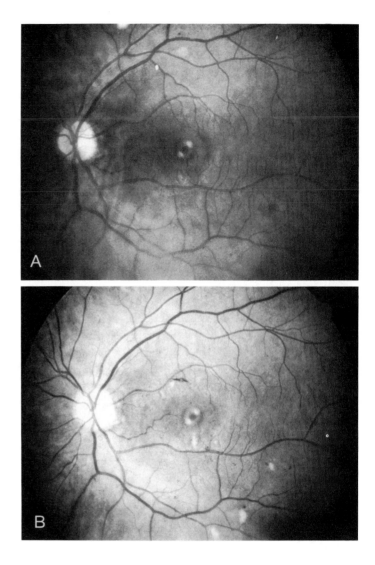

Proliferative retinopathy may spontaneously regress (without treatment) at the end of the third trimester or during the postpartum period (93, 94). For this reason, one study recommends waiting 8 to 12 months postpartum, with careful observation, to see if proliferative disease that develops during pregnancy regresses spontaneously, before any photocoagulation is performed (95). This recommendation is not the consensus, however. Most experts recommend early, aggressive panretinal photocoagulation when three high-risk characteristics (96) are present (62) and perhaps treatment of one or both eyes even

when three high-risk characteristics are not present (62). The possible risk of vitreous hemorrhage associated with the Valsalva action during spontaneous delivery has led one author to suggest that either panretinal photocoagulation should be performed in all patients with active neovascularization with time allowed for regression, or cesarean section should be considered (97). However, there is not adequate documentation in the literature of increased risk of vitreous hemorrhage during delivery to warrant advising a cesarean section on this basis alone, particularly in the modern era when vitrectomy is an available option.

Figure 10.16 shows the fundi of a diabetic woman whose proliferative disease began during pregnancy (**A** and **B**). The proliferative disease regressed spontaneously after delivery. Five years later, the left eye remained stable without therapy, and the right eye was stable following xenon photocoagulation (**C** and **D**).

Figure 10.17 summarizes graphically the changes seen during pregnancy for each type of baseline retinopathy, based on studies since 1978 (5).

High Myopia

One study addressed the concern that perhaps the pressure alteration induced by the Valsalva maneuver during a spontaneous vaginal delivery might put women with pathologically high myopia at risk of a retinal tear or detachment. This study followed 50 pregnant women with myopia of 4.5 or more diopters. When examined during their pregnancies, 8 women had normal fundi; 17 had lattice degeneration; 32 had other peripheral degenerative changes such as snail tracks, cobblestone degeneration, and white-without-pressure; and 11 had peripheral retinal breaks. (Some women had several of these.) The women were reexamined within 2 weeks after delivery, and no changes in eyegrounds were found (98). Thus, at present, there does not appear to be a contraindi-

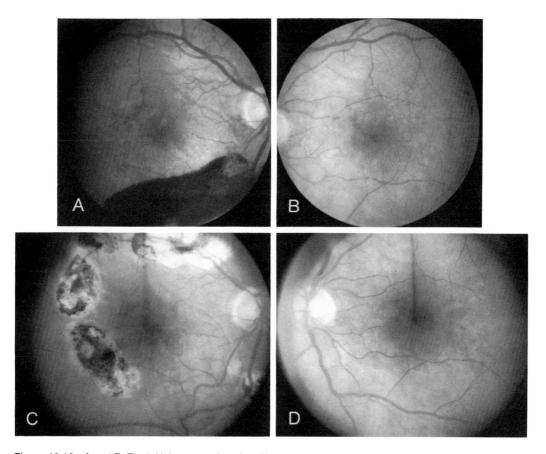

Figure 10.16. A and **B.** The initial presentation of proliferative disease occurred during pregnancy in this patient. Postpartum, there was spontaneous regression of proliferation. **C** and **D.** Five years later, the left eye was stable without treatment, and the right eye was stable following a course of xenon arc photocoagulation.

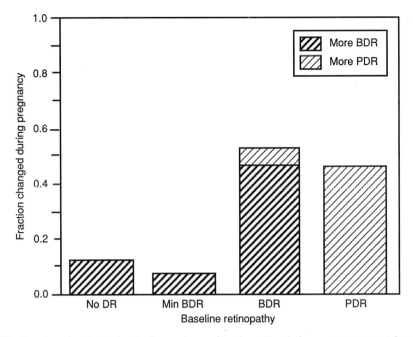

Figure 10.17. Fraction of patients developing a change in retinopathy during pregnancy as a function of type of retinopathy at onset of pregnancy. DR—diabetic retinopathy, BDR—background diabetic retinopathy, PDR—proliferative diabetic retinopathy, min—minimal. (Based on data in Sunness JS, Surv Ophthalmol 1988;32:219–238.)

cation to a spontaneous delivery in a high myope.

Retinitis Pigmentosa

Though there is one case report in the literature of reversible visual field deterioration during pregnancy in a woman with retinitis pigmentosa (RP) (99), in most cases there is only subjective reporting by the patient, years after the fact, as to whether pregnancy modified the course of the disorder. The Retinitis Pigmentosa Study at the Wilmer Institute includes 147 women who have been pregnant. Eight of these patients (5%) reported that their disease progressed more rapidly during pregnancy, and that they did not return to their prepregnancy visual status following delivery. One hundred fourteen (78%) reported no change in their RP during pregnancy. No patient reported improvement. The remaining patients were uncertain whether change had occurred (Palmer, Massof, personal communication). In the

UCLA RP study, 10% of the 107 women with RP who had been pregnant reported visual changes during pregnancy (100). Thus, most RP patients do not notice a significant change during pregnancy.

Sarcoidosis

Perhaps due to the relative immunological suppression that occurs during pregnancy, sarcoidosis may remit somewhat during pregnancy and be exacerbated in the postpartum period (101). Sarcoid retinopathy has initially presented in the postpartum period (102).

Toxoplasmic Retinochoroiditis

Active retinochoroiditis and toxoplasmosis scars in the mother's eye are regarded as evidence of congenital infection of the mother. Since toxoplasmosis appears to be transmitted to the fetus only when the mother acquires toxoplasmosis during the pregnancy itself (82), the presence of retinal evidence of congenital toxoplasmosis in the mother might then preclude transmission of the disease to the fetus. A study of 18 pregnancies in 10 women with toxoplasmic retinochoroiditis confirmed this lack of transmission (103). One woman had only scars; 6 had active involvement before, but not during, the pregnancy; and 3 had recurrent active ocular toxoplasmosis during pregnancy. No infant developed congenital toxoplasmosis. A high, stable toxoplasma hemagglutination titer did not appear to affect the pregnancy. However, no patient in this study had an increasing toxoplasmosis titer during pregnancy, so there are no data on whether this affects the fetus.

Vogt-Koyanagi-Harada Syndrome (VKH)

The limited reports on this condition during pregnancy are conflicting. There is a report of 2 cases first presenting in the second half of normal pregnancies and remitting after delivery without recurrence (104). There is a report of 3 cases of women with preexisting VKH that remitted during pregnancy and worsened postpartum (105).

Pseudoxanthoma Elasticum

Whereas cardiac and gastrointestinal changes have been reported in pregnant women with pseudoxanthoma elasticum, no change in angioid streaks with pregnancy has been reported (106, 107).

Choroidal Hemangioma

A hemangioma of the choroid may grow more rapidly during pregnancy. This growth may occur on a hormonal basis (108). There is a report of a choroidal hemangioma presenting in the fifth month of pregnancy and undergoing spontaneous regression following pregnancy (109).

Choroidal Osteoma

During the last trimester of pregnancy, a woman with a juxtapapillary choroidal osteoma developed a lipid-laden, subretinal exudate and visual loss due to an overlying choroidal neovascular membrane. The exudate disappeared within several months of delivery, and her vision returned. Three years later, despite growth in size of the osteoma, the patient remained asymptomatic (11, pp 178–179).

Choroidal New Vessel Membranes

Though there have been case reports of development or worsening of choroidal neovascular membranes related to drusen (Fig. 10.18), presumed ocular histoplasmosis (J. Donald M. Gass, personal communication), and choroidal osteoma (11, pp 178–179), there has been no study determining whether the occurrence or course of choroidal neovascularization is modified by pregnancy.

USE OF PHARMACOLOGICAL OPHTHALMIC AGENTS IN PREGNANCY

Although no major teratogenicity has been associated with the diagnostic agents commonly used to evaluate retinal and choroidal disease, caution should be exercised in employing any pharmacological agent in pregnancy, and clear benefit to the mother (along with evaluation of potential fetal risk) should be a prerequisite for using any agent.

Fluorescein

In a woman who was 33 weeks pregnant and who underwent fluorescein angiography, fluorescein-stained amniotic fluid was found by amniocentesis (110). This finding shows that fluorescein crosses the placenta and enters the fetus. Fluorescein has also been shown to enter the fetus in pregnant rats (111). However, no teratogenic or embryocidal effects have been observed in rats (111), mice (112), or rabbits (113), and no cases of teratogenic effects from fluorescein angiography have been reported to the National Registry of Drug-Induced Ocular Side Effects (M. Meyer, personal communication). In fact, specific studies have been performed using fluo-

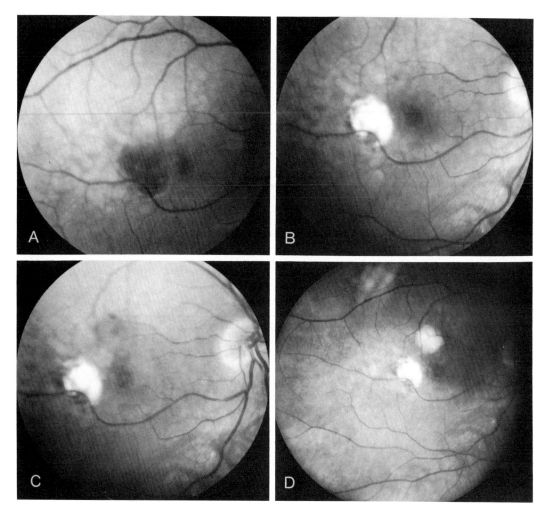

Figure 10.18. This 28-year-old woman with multiple drusen developed a subretinal new vessel membrane, evidenced by subretinal blood, when she was 8 months pregnant (**A**). The area was well-defined and far from the fovea, and she was treated with krypton red laser photocoagulation without a fluorescein angiogram (**B**). A second area (**C**) was treated two days later (**D**). The patient has remained asymptomatic, with 20/20 visual acuity, after 6.5 years of follow-up.

rescein angiography during pregnancy. For example, 1 study quantified the microaneurysms present in diabetic retinopathy during pregnancy (85). In this study, 22 pregnant women had fluorescein angiography without adverse effects on the fetus. Nonetheless, the general recommendation, given the known passage of fluorescein into the fetus, is to use it only when absolutely indicated, such as in the evaluation of a choroidal new vessel membrane being considered for treatment. Even

in this situation, if the membrane is well-defined and far enough from the fovea, some retinal specialists will perform laser photocoagulation without obtaining a fluorescein angiogram (Fig. 10.18).

A recent study (114) showed prolonged secretion of fluorescein in breast milk. A nursing 29-year-old woman required a fluorescein angiogram. Breast milk samples were expressed manually and analyzed for fluorescein concentration. It was found that fluorescein was detectable in breast milk samples up to 76 hours after fluorescein injection. This finding, along with possibly decreased renal clearance of fluorescein by newborns, suggests that caution be exercised in administering fluorescein to lactating women. This would be particularly important for lactating women whose neonates are undergoing phototherapy for hyperbilirubinemia, since a fluorescein-induced phototoxic reaction may occur.

Topical Anesthetics

No cases have been reported to the National Registry of Drug-Induced Ocular Side Effects of teratogenic effects related to these agents (M. Meyer, personal communication).

Dilating Drops

A recent review of ophthalmic medications in pregnant and nursing women (115) reports that fetal hypoxia may be seen following parenteral administration of phenylephrine in late pregnancy or in labor. Minor fetal malformations, including inguinal hernia and clubfoot, have been described in association with systemic administration of phenylephrine. For this reason, phenylephrine was classified by the authors as relatively contraindicated during pregnancy. The risk of phenylephrine causing hypertension in a nursing infant also led the authors to classify this drug as relatively contraindicated in nursing mothers. No data are available as to whether tropicamide and cyclopentolate are associated with fetal problems, but minor fetal malformations have been reported with the systemic use of atropine, homatropine, and scopolamine, so caution is advised in their use. The possibility of an anticholinergic effect in the nursing newborn suggests that these drops are relatively contraindicated in the nursing mother (115).

This information suggests that, in pregnant women, dilating agents should not be used without indication. The risks appear to be in the category of minor fetal malformations, and the data reported above

are associations, not proven causal effects. The data are based on the results of systemic administration of the agents, and the illnesses leading to their administration may have played a part in the development of the malformations. The National Registry of Drug-Induced Ocular Side Effects has had no reports of teratogenic effects secondary to topical use of these agents (M. Meyer, personal communication). When the benefit clearly outweighs the risk, dilating agents should be used with measures to prevent systemic absorption, such as nasolacrimal punctal occlusion for 3 to 5 minutes after application, and removal of excess tears or medication with cotton or other absorbent material before the release of nasolacrimal pressure (115).

ACKNOWLEDGMENTS

Taken in part from Sunness JS. The pregnant woman's eye. Surv Ophthalmol 1988;32:219–238; and from Sunness JS. Pregnancy and retinal disease. In: Ryan SJ, ed. Retina. Vol 2: Medical Retina. St. Louis: CV Mosby, 1989:433–440.

The authors would like to thank Ms. Linda Chandlee for editorial assistance and Ms. Stephanie Napert and Ms. Kelly Wilson for their help in compiling the bibliography.

References

1. Landesman R. Retinal and conjunctival vascular changes in normal and toxemic pregnancy. Bull NY Acad Med 1955;31:376–390.
2. Pritchard JA, MacDonald PC, Gant NF. Williams Obstetrics. 17th ed. Norwalk: Appleton-Century-Crofts, 1985.
3. Duke-Elder S, ed. System of ophthalmology. Vol. IV. The physiology of the eye and vision. St. Louis: CV Mosby, 1968:279–280.
4. Sridama V, Pacini F, Yang S-L, et al. Decreased levels of helper T cells: a possible cause of immunodeficiency in pregnancy. N Engl J Med 1982;307:352–356.
5. Sunness JS. The pregnant woman's eye. Surv Ophthalmol 1988;32:219–238.
6. Tomoda Y, Fuma M, Miwa T, et al. Cell-mediated immunity in pregnant women. Gynecol Invest 1976;7:280–292.
7. Bedrossian RH. Central serous retinopathy and pregnancy. Am J Ophthalmol 1974;78:152.

8. Chumbley LC, Frank RN. Central serous retinopathy and pregnancy. Am J Ophthalmol 1974;77:158–160.

9. Cruysberg JR M, Deutman AF. Visual disturbances during pregnancy caused by central serous choroidopathy. Br J Ophthalmol 1982; 66:240–241.

10. Fastenberg DM, Ober RR. Central serous choroidopathy in pregnancy. Arch Ophthalmol 1983;101:1055–1058.

11. Gass JDM. Stereoscopic atlas of macular diseases; diagnosis and treatment. 3rd ed. St. Louis: CV Mosby, 1987.

12. Seddon JM, MacLaughlin DT, Albert DM, et al. Uveal melanomas presenting during pregnancy and the investigation of oestrogen receptors in melanomas. Br J Ophthalmol 1982;66:695–704.

13. Borner R, Goder G. Melanoblastom der Uvea und Schwangerschaft. Klin Monatsbl Augenheilkd 1966;149:684–693.

14. Frenkel M, Klein HZ. Malignant melanoma of the choroid in pregnancy. Am J Ophthalmol 1966;62:910–913.

15. Pack GT, Scharnagel IM. The prognosis for malignant melanoma in the pregnant woman. Cancer 1951;4:324–334.

16. Reese AB. Tumors of the eye. 3rd ed. Hagerstown: Harper & Row, 1976:235–236.

17. Siegel R, Ainsley WH. Malignant ocular melanoma during pregnancy. JAMA 1963;185:542–543.

18. Brown GC, Magargal LE, Shields JA, et al. Retinal arterial obstruction in children and young adults. Ophthalmology 1981;88:18–25.

19. Spitzberg DH. Retinal phlebitis associated with pregnancy. Ann Ophthalmol 1982;14:101–102.

20. Dieckmann WJ. The toxemias of pregnancy. 2nd ed. St. Louis: CV Mosby, 1952:240–249.

21. Jaffe G, Schatz H. Ocular manifestations of preeclampsia. Am J Ophthalmol 1987;103:309–315.

22. Wagener HP. Arterioles of the retina in toxemia of pregnancy. JAMA 1933;101:1380–1384.

23. Folk JC, Weingeist TA. Fundus changes in toxemia. Ophthalmology 1981;88:1173–1174.

24. Beck RW, Gamel JW, Willcourt RJ, Berman G. Acute ischemic optic neuropathy in severe preeclampsia. Am J Ophthalmol 1980;90:342–346.

25. Mussey RD, Mundell BJ. Retinal examinations: a guide in the management of the toxic hypertensive syndrome of pregnancy. Am J Obstet Gynecol 1939;37:30–36.

26. Trautmann JC. Comment. Surv Ophthalmol 1986;30:273.

27. Gass JDM, Pautler SE. Toxemia of pregnancy pigment epitheliopathy masquerading as a heredomacular dystrophy. Trans Am Ophthalmol Soc 1985;83:114–130.

28. Singerman LJ, Aiello LM, Rodman HM. Diabetic retinopathy: effects of pregnancy and laser therapy. Diabetes 1980;29(suppl 2):1a. Abstract 3.

29. Chaine G, Attali P, Gaudric A, et al. Ocular fluorophotometric and angiographic findings in toxemia of pregnancy. Arch Ophthalmol 1986;104:1632–1635.

30. Price J, Marouf L, Heine MW, Young R. New angiographic findings in toxemia of pregnancy. Evidence for retinal and choroidal vascular decompensation. Poster. Ophthalmology 1986; 93(suppl):125.

31. Duke-Elder S, Dobree JH: System of ophthalmology. Vol X. Diseases of the retina. St. Louis: CV Mosby, 1967:350–356.

32. Landesman R, Douglas RG, Snyder SS. Retinal changes in the toxemias of pregnancy. I. History, vomiting of pregnancy, mild and severe pre-eclampsia, and eclampsia. Am J Obstet Gynecol 1951;62:1020–1033.

33. Riss B, Riss P, Metka M. Die Prognostische Wertigkeit von Veranderungen am Augenhintergrund bei EPH-Gestose. Z Geburtshife Perinatol 1983;187:276–279.

34. Sadowsky A, Serr DM, Landau J. Retinal changes and fetal prognosis in the toxemias of pregnancy. Obstet Gynecol 1956;8:426–431.

35. Hallum AV. Eye changes in hypertensive toxemia of pregnancy; a study of three hundred cases. JAMA 1936;106:1649–1651.

36. Fry WE. Extensive bilateral retinal detachment in eclampsia, with complete reattachment; report of two cases. Arch Ophthalmol 1929;1:609–614.

37. Gitter KA, Houser BP, Sarin LK, Justice Jr. Toxemia of pregnancy; an angiographic interpretation of fundus changes. Arch Ophthalmol 1968;80:449–454.

38. Saito T, Shimizu S. Fluorescence fundus angiography of cyst-like elevations associated with toxemias of pregnancies. Folia Ophthalmol Jpn 1980;31:152–156.

39. McEvoy M, Runciman J, Edmonds DK, Kerin JF. Bilateral retinal detachment in association with preeclampsia. Aust NZ J Obstet Gynaecol 1981;21:246–247.

40. Oliver M, Uchenik D. Bilateral exudative retinal detachment in eclampsia without hypertensive retinopathy. Am J Ophthalmol 1980;90:792–796.

41. Bosco JAS. Spontaneous nontraumatic retinal detachments in pregnancy. Am J Obstet Gynecol 1961;82:208–212.

42. Mabie WC, Ober RR. Fluorescein angiography in toxaemia of pregnancy. Br J Ophthalmol 1980;64:666–671.

43. Ober RR. Pregnancy-induced hypertension (preeclampsia-eclampsia). In: Ryan SJ, ed. Retina. Vol 2. Medical Retina. St. Louis: CV Mosby, 1989:441–448.

44. Fastenberg DM, Fetkenhour CL, Choromokos E, Shoch DE. Choroidal vascular changes in toxemia of pregnancy. Am J Ophthalmol 1980;89:362–368.

45. Kenny GS, Cerasoli JR. Color fluorescein angiography in toxemia of pregnancy. Arch Ophthalmol 1972;87:383–388.

46. Klien BA. Ischemic infarcts of the choroid (El-

schnig spots); a cause of retinal separation in hypertensive disease with renal insufficiency. Am J Ophthalmol 1968;66:1069–1074.

47. Ballantyne AJ, Michaelson IC. Textbook of the fundus of the eye. 2nd ed. Baltimore: Williams & Wilkins, 1970:182–183.

48. Crowther WL, Hamilton JB. Eclampsia with amaurosis due to detachment of retinae. Med J Aust 1932;2:177–178.

49. Brancato R, Menchini U, Bandello F. Proliferative retinopathy and toxemia of pregnancy. Ann Ophthalmol 1987;19:182–183.

50. Carpenter F, Kava HL, Plotkin D. The development of total blindness as a complication of pregnancy. Am J Obstet Gynecol 1953;66:641–647.

51. Monteiro MLR, Hoyt WF, Imes RK. Puerperal cerebral blindness; transient bilateral occipital involvement from pressure cerebral venous thrombosis. Arch Neurol 1984;41:1300–1301.

52. Cogan DG. Ocular involvement in disseminated intravascular coagulopathy. Arch Ophthalmol 1975;93:1–8.

53. Martin VAF. Disseminated intravascular coagulopathy. Trans Ophthalmol Soc UK 1978; 98:506–507.

54. Klein BEK, Klein R, Meuer SM, Moss SE, Dalton DD. Does the severity of diabetic retinopathy predict pregnancy outcome? J Diabetic Complications 1988;2:179–184.

55. Benson DO, Fitzgibbons JF, Goodnight SH. The visual system in thrombotic thrombocytopenic purpura. Ann Ophthalmol 1980;12:413–417.

56. Sperry K. Amniotic fluid embolism; to understand an enigma. JAMA 1986;255:2183–2186.

57. Chang M, Herbert WNP. Retinal arteriolar occlusions following amniotic fluid embolism. Ophthalmology 1984;91:1634–1637.

58. Fischbein FI. Ischemic retinopathy following amniotic fluid embolization. Am J Ophthalmol 1969;67:351–357.

59. Beetham WP. Diabetic retinopathy in pregnancy. Trans Am Ophthalmol Soc 1950;48:205–219.

60. Moloney JBM, Drury MI. The effect of pregnancy on the natural course of diabetic retinopathy. Am J Ophthalmol 1982;93:745–756.

61. Aiello LM, Rand LI, Briones JC, et al. Nonocular clinical risk factors in the progression of diabetic retinopathy. In: Little HL, Jack RL, Patz A, Forsham PH, eds. Diabetic retinopathy. New York: Thieme-Stratton, 1983:21–32.

62. Dibble CM, Kochenour NK, Wocley RJ, et al. Effect of pregnancy on diabetic retinopathy. Obstet Gynecol 1982;59:699–704.

63. White P. Pregnancy and diabetes, medical aspects. Med Clin North Am 1965;49:1015–1024.

64. White P, Gillespie L, Sexton L. Use of female sex hormone therapy in pregnant diabetic patients. Am J Obstet Gynecol 1956;71:57–69.

65. Cassar J, Hamilton AM, Kohner EM. Diabetic retinopathy in pregnancy. Int Ophthalmol Clin 1978;18(4):178–188.

66. Horvat M, MacLean H, Goldberg L, Crock GW. Diabetic retinopathy in pregnancy; a 12-year prospective survey. Br J Ophthalmol 1980; 64:398–403.

67. Watson DL, Sibai BM, Shaver DC, et al. Late postpartum eclampsia; an update. South Med J 1983;76:1487–1489.

68. Jovanovic R, Jovanovic L. Obstetric management when normoglycemia is maintained in diabetic pregnant women with vascular compromise. Am J Obstet Gynecol 1984; 149:617–623.

69. White P. Diabetes mellitus in pregnancy. Clin Perinatol 1974;1:331–347.

70. Mills JL, Simpson JL, Driscoll SG, et al. Incidence of spontaneous abortion among normal women and insulin-dependent diabetic women whose pregnancies were identified within 21 days of conception. N Engl J Med 1988;319:1617–1623.

71. Miller E, Hare JW, Cloherty JP, et al. Elevated maternal hemoglobin A_{1C} in early pregnancy and major congenital anomalies in infants of diabetic mothers. N Engl J Med 1981;304:1331–1334.

72. The Kroc Collaborative Study Group. Blood glucose control and the evolution of diabetic retinopathy and albuminuria; a preliminary multicenter trial. N Engl J Med 1984;311:365–372.

73. Phelps RL, Sakol P, Metzger BE, et al. Changes in diabetic retinopathy during pregnancy; correlations with the regulation of hyperglycemia. Arch Ophthalmol 1986;104:1806–1810.

74. Klein BEK. Diabetic retinopathy during pregnancy. In: Jovanovic L, ed. Controversies in diabetes and pregnancy. New York: Springer-Verlag, 1988:77–89.

75. Klein BEK, Klein R. Gravidity and diabetic retinopathy. Am J Epidemiol 1984;119:564–569.

76. Cassar J, Kohner EM, Hamilton AM, et al. Diabetic retinopathy and pregnancy. Diabetologia 1978;15:105–111.

77. Jervell J, Moe N, Skjaeraasen J, et al. Diabetes mellitus and pregnancy—management and results at Rikshospitalet, Oslo, 1970–1977. Diabetologia 1979;16:151–155.

78. Laatikainen L, Larinkari J, Teramo K, Raivo KO. Occurrence and prognostic significance of retinopathy in diabetic pregnancy. Metabol Pediatr Ophthalmol 1980;4:191–195.

79. Ohrt V. The influence of pregnancy on diabetic retinopathy with special regard to the reversible changes shown in 100 pregnancies. Acta Ophthalmol 1984;62:603–616.

80. Price JH, Hadden DR, Archer DB, et al. Diabetic retinopathy in pregnancy. Br J Obstet Gynaecol 1984;91:11–17.

81. Boone MI, Farber ME, Jovanovic-Peterson L, Peterson CM. Increased retinal vascular tortuosity in gestational diabetes mellitus. Ophthalmology 1989;96:251–254.

82. Perkins ES. Ocular toxoplasmosis. Br J Ophthalmol 1973;57:1–17.

83. Lawrence RD. Acute retinopathy without hyperpiesis in diabetic pregnancy. Br J Ophthalmol 1948;32:461–465.

84. Ward SC, Woods DR, Gilstrap LC III, Hauth JC. Pregnancy and acute optic disc edema of juvenile-onset diabetes. Obstet Gynecol 1984; 64:816–818.

85. Soubrane G, Canivet J, Coscas G. Influence of pregnancy on the evolution of background retinopathy: preliminary results of a prospective fluorescein angiography study. In: Ryan SJ, Dawson AK, Little HL, eds. Retinal diseases. New York: Grune & Stratton, 1985:15–20.

86. Sinclair SH, Nesler C, Foxman B, et al. Macular edema and pregnancy in insulin-dependent diabetes. Am J Ophthalmol 1984;97:154–167.

87. Chang S, Fuhrmann M, and the Diabetes in Early Pregnancy Study Group. Pregnancy, retinopathy, normoglycemia: a preliminary analysis. Diabetes 1985;34(suppl):3a.

88. Rodman HM, Singerman LJ, Aiello LM, Merkatz IR. Diabetic retinopathy and its relationship to pregnancy. In: Merkatz IR, Adam PAJ, eds. The diabetic pregnancy; a perinatal perspective. New York: Grune & Stratton, 1979:73–91.

89. Johnston GP. Pregnancy and diabetic retinopathy. Am J Ophthalmol 1980;90:519–524.

90. Gerke E, Meyer-Schwickerath G. Proliferative diabetische Retinopathie und Schwangerschaft. Klin Monatsbl Augenheilkd 1982; 181:170–173.

91. Singerman LJ. Diabetic retinopathy in juvenile-onset diabetics. 1. Laser therapy in high-risk proliferatives 2. Effects of pregnancy. In: Fine SL, Owens SL, eds. Management of retinal vascular and macular disorders. Baltimore: Williams & Wilkins, 1983:43–46.

92. Hercules BL, Wozencroft M, Gayed II, Jeacock J. Peripheral retinal ablation in the treatment of proliferative diabetic retinopathy during pregnancy. Br J Ophthalmol 1980;64:87–93.

93. Lynn JR, Snyder WB, Vaiser A. Diabetic retinopathy. New York: Grune & Stratton, 1974:271–274.

94. Okun E, Johnston GP, Boniuk I. Management of diabetic retinopathy; a stereoscopic presentation. St. Louis: CV Mosby, 1971:44–48.

95. Serup L. Influence of pregnancy on diabetic retinopathy. Acta Endocrinol Suppl 1986;277:122–124.

96. The Diabetic Retinopathy Study Research Group. Four risk factors for severe visual loss in diabetic retinopathy; the third report from the Diabetic Retinopathy Study. Arch Ophthalmol 1979; 97:654–655.

97. Kitzmiller JL, Aiello LM, Kaldany A, Younger MD. Diabetic vascular disease complicating pregnancy. Clin Obstet Gynecol 1981;24:107–123.

98. Neri A, Grausbord R, Kremer I, et al. The management of labor in high myopic patients. Eur J Obstet Gynecol Reprod Biol 1985;19:277–279.

99. Wagener HP. Lesions of the optic nerve and retina in pregnancy. JAMA 1934;103:1910–1913.

100. Yoser SL, Heckenlively JR, Friedman L, Oversier J. Evaluation of clinical findings and common symptoms in retinitis pigmentosa. ARVO Abstracts. Invest Ophthalmol Vis Sci 1987; 28(suppl):112.

101. Mayock RL, Sullivan RD, Greening RR, Jones RJ Jr. Sarcoidosis and pregnancy. JAMA 1957;164:158–163.

102. Chumbley LC, Kearns TP. Retinopathy of sarcoidosis. Am J Ophthalmol 1972;73:123–131.

103. Oniki S. Prognosis of pregnancy in patients with toxoplasmic retinochoroiditis. Jpn J Ophthalmol 1983;27:166–174.

104. Friedman Z, Granat M, Neumann E. The syndrome of Vogt-Koyanagi-Harada and pregnancy. Metabol Pediatr Ophthalmol 1980;4:147–149.

105. Snyder DA, Tessler HH. Vogt-Koyanagi-Harada Syndrome. Am J Ophthalmol 1980;90:69–75.

106. Berde C, Willis DC, Sandberg EC. Pregnancy in women with pseudoxanthoma elasticum. Obstet Gynecol Surv 1983;38:339–344.

107. Lao TT, Walters BNJ, De Swiet M. Pseudoxanthoma elasticum and pregnancy; two case reports. Br J Obstet Gynaecol 1984;91:1049–1050.

108. Reese AB. Tumors of the eye. 2nd ed. New York: Harper & Row, 1963:366–370.

109. Pitta C, Bergen R, Littwin S. Spontaneous regression of a choroidal hemangioma following pregnancy. Ann Ophthalmol 1979;11:772–774.

110. Shekleton P, Fidler J, Grimwade J. A case of benign intracranial hypertension in pregnancy. Br J Obstet Gynaecol 1980;87:345–347.

111. Salem H, Loux JJ, Smith S, Nichols CW. Evaluation of the toxicologic and teratogenic potentials of sodium fluorescein in the rat. Toxicology 1979;12:143–150.

112. Shirai S, Majima A. Effects of fluorescein-Na injected to mother mice on the embryo. Folia Ophthalmol Jpn 1975;26:132–137.

113. McEnerney JK, Wong WP, Peyman GA. Evaluation of the teratogenicity of fluorescein sodium. Am J Ophthalmol 1977:847–850.

114. Maguire AM, Bennett J. Fluorescein elimination in human breast milk. Arch Ophthalmol 1988;106:718–719.

115. Samples JR, Meyer SM. Use of ophthalmic medications in pregnant and nursing women. Am J Ophthalmol 1988;106:616–623.

INDEX

Page numbers in *italics* denote figures; those followed by "t" denote tables.